Brain Software

The Technology in Patañjali's Yoga Sūtras

Heinz Krug and Gerd Unruh

First Printing	February 2018
German Original Edition	April 2017
Cover Design:	Michael Adamidis
	www.adamidis-art.com
Print:	IngramSpark
Authors' contact email:	heinz@brainsoftware.info
	gerd.unruh@gmx.net
Book Website:	brainsoftware.info

Disclaimer

Information in the Book

Although the authors and the publisher have made every effort to ensure that the information in this book was correct at the time of going to press, the authors and the publisher do not assume and hereby disclaim any liability to any party for any loss, damage, or disruption caused by errors or omissions, whether such errors or omissions result from negligence, accident, or any other cause.

Health

This book is not intended as a substitute for the medical advice of physicians. The readers should regularly consult a physician in matters relating to their health and particularly concerning any symptoms that may require diagnosis or medical attention. Authors and publisher are not liable for any direct or indirect results of any treatments, actions, applications or means for persons, reading this book.

Trademarks and Copyright

ISBN 978-0-9955961-1-5

brainsoftware.info

10 9 8 7 6 5 4 3 2

अहं ब्रह्मास्मि

ahaṁ brahmāsmi

I Am Totality

0

Introduction

Table of Contents

Forewords

Result of a Lifelong Search

This book is the result of a lifelong search for the correct application of the ancient mental techniques known since ancient times as the *siddhis*. This search began for me as a young man, when I had already started to meditate regularly. I discovered the meditation method of Maharishi™[1] Mahesh Yogi and found it to be the most appropriate technique and experienced the deep silence of transcendence right from the beginning of my practice. I even got occasional glimpses into a fantastic mental world that can only be described as heavenly.

I became very successful with the deep silence of meditation. At that time I was still a student in high school. As a result of meditating my grades improved, and everything in my life became easier. When I began my university studies in electronic engineering, I also became much more creative. During my meditations at that time, the most awesome inventions occurred. I actually got some of these ideas patented later on in my life. One of them was the so-called FPGA computer chips, which revolutionized the whole electronics industry.

Three years later I began to practice the *siddhis* regularly. In spite of some initial success with the correct *siddhi* experiences, the practice soon became just a daily grind. We were simply practicing the *siddhis*, hoping that some results would eventually show up. That was not quite satisfactory. I did attend some refresher courses and practiced the *siddhis* exactly the way they had been taught. My thought was to "work to rule!" The result was even more disappointing than before. There were hardly any results at all with

---

[1] Isn't it funny that one always must mention the ™ trademark, even when expressing one's own opinion about Maharishi as a person? Although we are reluctant to do so, due to legal reasons we are urged to mention the trademark owner with each use of the trademark. In this context, see also the disclaimer at the beginning of the book.
Maharishi is a trademark of Maharishi Foundation Ltd. Corporation United Kingdom, P.O. Box 652 St. Helier, Jersey Great Britain JE48Y2.

the *siddhi* practices. It merely became a continuation of meditation, but the results predicted by *Patañjali* were completely missing.

I then spent most of my time on my industrial work Even though I continued to practice the siddhis, but no longer hoped for the predicted results. Admittedly, the deep silence was there. During group practice, there was a certain enthusiasm, especially during the so-called flying technique. On the other hand, nobody could really levitate the body above ground for any length of time more than a few seconds. Yes, there were, very rarely, experiences of somewhat slowed down parabola-like trajectories, but these were not very convincing, and they would not have withstood any real scientific scrutiny.

In those groups, where many people practiced their so-called "program" together, these *siddhas* seemed to get more and more tired over time. They no longer seemed to care about the freshness necessary for the program. They then allowed themselves too little sleep and arrived rather tired for the program. Would one then be surprised that during the relaxation of meditation and the *siddhis* many of them simply fell asleep? Their snoring disturbed me more and more, so I started to do my *siddhi* program alone at home where it was at least quiet. Although I felt fresher with this change, I rarely had many good results. The results seldom came and continued to be unpredictable.

Repair of the Siddhi Machine

Being an engineer, this lack of results did not satisfy me. Why practice a technique for thirty years that ultimately did not function as intended? I decided to approach this situation again, by making the most of my technological, scientific intellect. The thought was, "The machine does not work! The machine needs to be repaired!" But where to start? When repairing something, one always begins with the intended correct functioning or the target state. Where was the correct target state of the *siddhis* to be found? At that point, I remembered the *yoga sūtras* of *Patañjali*. Maharishi™[2] told us that he learned his technique of the *siddhis* from the *yoga sūtras*. It was

---

[2] Maharishi is a trademark of Maharishi Foundation Ltd. Corporation United Kingdom, P.O. Box 652 St. Helier, Jersey Great Britain JE48Y2.

therefore obviously necessary to examine this original work again, but this time more attentively. Maharishi™ had concealed from us that he had fundamentally modified the technique.

My friend Robert was a big help with this new project. Like me, he had a technically trained intellect. We first had to admit that this flying really did not work. One could call it "flying" a thousand times, but saying it, would not make it a reality. Positive thinking alone would not bring the required progress. What remained, was simply hopping, something that one could achieve with just muscular force. Many of our meditating friends had stopped the practice. We had finally arrived at a completely honest analysis of the actual reality of the so-called "flying exercises" at that time.

A marketing professional or teacher or spiritual leader may have wanted to sugarcoat things, but for the engineer who intended to get the machine working again, there was no other way. He first had to assert what the actual state was.

The next step in repairing this situation consisted of finding out why the actual state did not coincide with the target state. Tiredness was one important factor. This only came up after ten or more years of futile effort and is quite understandable. Even before that phase of tiredness during the group program, though, there was never any real flying. Therefore, the tiredness could not have been the actual cause of the failure.

Could it be that flying was impossible in principle? It is certainly not a normal experience for humans to fly without the help of machinery. I had the personal experience of seeing someone actually levitate for several minutes. That happened during the research work I was conducting in the EEG lab at the European University of Maharishi™[3]. At that time, we were measuring and analyzing the brainwaves of the most successful *siddhas*. I knew, therefore, that in principle it was possible for humans actually to fly.

Why could we not fly? The standard answer from *siddhas* that I knew referred to the principle of world consciousness. This stated that as soon as world consciousness reached a higher state of evolution, then the flying

---

[3] Maharishi is a trademark of Maharishi Foundation Ltd. Corporation United Kingdom, P.O. Box 652 St. Helier, Jersey Great Britain JE48Y2.

could manifest. Even though this was a good incentive to motivate larger groups to do their program together, as long as no real flying came about then inevitably one fine day this motivation would no longer suffice.

Therefore I felt this argument that originally came from Maharishi™[4] became ever less relevant. For me, it was rather an act of friendship from him, to be sweet to his students. He just didn't want to say so directly "I am sorry, or it is painful for me, that you are not able to do this." Instead, he found another reason that ultimately we could not change. It was not our fault or our own inability, or us missing some knowledge. It was the bad world consciousness that had been dragged down by stress, wars and the neglect of nature. Through our collective program, though, world consciousness should improve. With this idea, there remained the gleam of a better future, a light at the end of the tunnel.

I now considered that this argument, for other reasons, could also not be fully applied. I had seen a person who was able to levitate, and also there were historical reports of saints from various religions who were able to levitate during a much darker time of humanity, during the middle ages. Mostly these were monks, nuns or others who had devoted their lives to God. Often they had been surprised by their extraordinary abilities, or even wanted to get rid of them. I concluded that it had been quite possible in an even darker time than ours to master and also to demonstrate this flying. Therefore, it had to be possible now as well. It had to be possible to disconnect from the world consciousness enough so that at least some humans would be able to levitate.

Siddhi Technique

The only other cause of error that remained to be researched was the actual *siddhi* technique of flying. Therefore, I marched with my friend Robert into a Vedic library in the town in England where we both lived and fetched the originals of the *yoga sūtras* of *Patañjali*. They were there in *saṁskṛt* and also translated into English. I thought that we should give practicing the *siddhis* a try using the original *saṁskṛt* text. Both Robert and

---

[4] Maharishi is a trademark of Maharishi Foundation Ltd. Corporation United Kingdom, P.O. Box 652 St. Helier, Jersey Great Britain JE48Y2.

I did this, and initially, we thought we had achieved an improvement. The *yoga sūtras* are short formulas which upon application, should immediately bring about the predicted results, as long as the right state of consciousness was there. Within two weeks we gradually noticed that even this new approach did not bring any improvement. Even though there were still some occasional rays of hope, a real breakthrough had not been achieved.

Then I went to the next repair phase. This was another test. I practiced the *siddhis* that I had practiced so far, just the way I had learned it first in the English language, and then in my mother tongue, in German. The result was also not quite convincing, and besides, other friends had already practiced it for years in their mother tongue. I then tried it another way, in my home dialect, in Franconian. That sounded funny, but the results were still missing.

One question that remained was whether the reason would be our lack of consciousness? By then we had meditated regularly morning and evening for thirty years. Was that not yet enough? I know that many of my meditating friends thought like this and are still thinking like this now. Some of them even thought that it would take several lifetimes to master the *siddhis*. What perseverance! I did not have that.

Besides, this could not be the real reason for me, because my beloved master Maharishi™[5] had already confirmed to me twenty years earlier that I had reached the highest state of consciousness, unity consciousness. I never spoke much about it because it would always create some unnecessary envy. For me though, I knew what this meant. Certainly since that time I had not evolved backward in my consciousness. A lack of consciousness could not be the reason. Therefore, there must have been something wrong with the technique.

The most obvious reasons for the lack of success were probably translation mistakes with the *yoga sūtras*. A large part of Vedic knowledge had been lost through translation mistakes. This I had learned from

---

[5] Maharishi is a trademark of Maharishi Foundation Ltd. Corporation United Kingdom, P.O. Box 652 St. Helier, Jersey Great Britain JE48Y2.

Maharishi™[6]. I then began a study of the original *saṁskṛt* of the *yoga sūtras*. There was no way to avoid improving my rather basic skills – at that time – of *saṁskṛt*. I, therefore, began to learn *saṁskṛt* intensively for three years. I acquired five *saṁskṛt* dictionaries and four grammars and began intensive studies. Additionally, there were several online courses and about 50 Vedic books in my library that I had both in *saṁskṛt* as well as in English or in German. I wanted to master the grammar and to have a sufficiently large vocabulary to be able to translate the *yoga sūtras* correctly. It was a lot of work, but the effort paid off. The reading of *devanāgarī* became easier over time; I could decrypt the *sandhis*, read the word connections correctly and also the multifarious declensions. Conjugations became ever more clear, and the whole system gradually opened up to me. What a wonder, with those bad Latin grades that I had previously in school! Somehow *saṁskṛt* was far more systematic and also more likable, and I also had a clear goal in front of me.

Presentation

Now my dear sister Sigrid's contribution came into play. She urged me every weekend to translate a part of the *yoga sūtras*, along with the commentaries of *Vyāsa* and *Śaṁkara*. Initially, we translated from English to German. We used a book whose author, Trevor Leggett, had translated directly from *saṁskṛt* to English: The complete commentary by Śaṅkara on the Yoga Sūtras". Only later I translated all of the *sūtras* and the most important commentaries directly from *saṁskṛt*.

The first translations began in 2007. Sigrid meticulously wrote down everything in her notebook computer. Many of the commentary texts in this book are from that time. I later supplemented them with the direct *saṁskṛt* translations. My criterion always was that I wanted to correctly understand all of the trains of thoughts of the commentators. Then there would be no more logical gaps. Surprisingly, those gaps could all be removed, and that meant hundreds of cases, by finding the correct translation directly from *saṁskṛt*.

[6] Maharishi is a trademark of Maharishi Foundation Ltd. Corporation United Kingdom, P.O. Box 652 St. Helier, Jersey Great Britain JE48Y2.

Our mother Katharina also joined our scholarly club. She had really good experiences with the *siddhis*. Two years later, having read through all of our texts three times and having edited and corrected typing mistakes, we finally had the complete German translation of the English book of Leggett. I never published it. It was all still much too complicated. How would anybody be able to understand it? The language also appeared a bit antiquarian. We then tried, as far as we could, to present in a more simple and modern language those trains of thoughts that had appeared so complicated. Sometimes though, it did not quite work out.

The next phase was that of simplification. Here my friend Gerd Unruh, whom I had known for 30 years came to help. He was interested in creating a complete set of lectures of the *yoga sūtras* with me, in the form of a PowerPoint presentation. We worked mostly via Skype audio conference. He was in Germany while I was in England, though we occasionally met in person for one or two weeks of intensive collaboration.

This set of lectures was really good. It was now time to test it on various audiences. We had made available both a German and an English version. Several of my English and American friends helped us with the English version during three months of intensive collaboration, to get the correct spellings and to bring an elegant style to the text. We needed to remove all the "Germanisms" and of course also to place all commas correctly. Commas, in English, are a real art My mother and sister then traveled to England for a working holiday, to help simplify the German version enough so that it became readable for a general audience.

Gerd tested the German version of courses with German course participants while I did the same in English with my English friends. They all understood and also could apply the new knowledge really well. Many of the course participants were *siddhas* who had striven for decades in vain to experience success from the *siddhi* exercises. Some of them though had never had a single experience with the *siddhi* techniques they had learned before. Behold, now it worked straight away! Over and above those results from the *siddhis,* they also told us that it was the first time in their lives that they had learned so much spiritual knowledge in such a short time.

Some other course participants had never learned any *siddhis* before, and for them, it was almost easier as they had no old habits to forget. On the other hand, they rather lacked the motivation to practice the *siddhis* regularly. At the end of the course, which generally lasted between 7 and 10 days, every course participant had at least some *siddhis* that functioned really well, as if with just the press of a button.

Initial Successes

My repair work now showed the first success. The "*siddhi* machines" were running again, at least partially. For me, in a rather short time, all the *siddhis* I practiced had a really good outcome. Each one worked out within a few seconds, except the very advanced ones like flying. The proof of this *siddhi* still has to be accomplished, so my research is not yet finished. The others at least functioned quite well, and in this book, you can now read the experience reports of these initial course participants.

We already knew about more than enough books containing experience reports of *siddhas*. They were all written rather positively, but what was lacking in most of them were the specific experiences as predicted by *Patañjali*. Experiences like that had come about only casually and seldom with the technique that we had learned 40 years earlier. This was an indication that the correct mastery of the *siddhi* techniques was still lacking.

For us though, it had all changed now. We had gained control over the *siddhis*. It was like a light switch. Switch on – light on; switch off – light off. Now we knew the technique of switching on the light switches of these extraordinary human abilities. We had by now used them successfully thousands of times. It then became easier than ever. The *siddhis* have now become a normal part of our daily life. However, we could not yet fly. Although we knew how we had to switch on the corresponding light switch, we had not yet found the exact place where the light switch was located.

Before our research into the *yoga sūtras,* it was like searching for light switches in a dark room. Now and then one would have a one-hit wonder. But on the next day, it was completely dark again and unclear as to why and how the right result had come about before. Our *siddhi* practices were therefore called research in consciousness. We had been searching for light switches for thirty years, but we had no flashlights in our kit to help us!

Now everything had changed. With the light of the *yoga sūtras,* we were able to see the room correctly. We had gained the knowledge of where most of the places with switches were and how to turn on these switches. By our in-depth research of the *yoga sūtras,* we learned to express the knowledge so simply that we can now reproduce it in this book. By reading this book carefully, you can now gain your own experiences.

I no longer like any big secrecy about the *siddhi* techniques, for what has it actually brought us? It has merely elegantly hidden the fact that the correct knowledge of the *siddhis* had not actually been discovered yet. Why continue this secret system for an unnecessarily long period? Right, true, honest knowledge is required now, more than ever.

Knowledge

Now the question arose of how we could express this newly gained knowledge in such a way that many could understand it. We decided to summarize it in this book, which consists of five chapters: an elaborate introduction followed by four chapters of the *yoga sūtras.* In every chapter, there is theory, practice, as well as tests and experience reports, to demonstrate examples. When we had pretty much finished the book, we taught several courses again to see how this new knowledge would be received. Gerd Unruh, who worked with his professional contacts, noticed that terms like enlightenment, mind, and consciousness simply could not yet be accepted by professionals. These terms were essentially too vague from a scientific viewpoint, or just imprecise or else not defined at all.

Researchers in the field of artificial intelligence can tell you a thing or two about this. Apparently, there are more than four hundred different definitions of the term "knowledge." Here, with the *yoga sūtras,* we have now found a very accurate definition of the term knowledge on several levels. It may be just another definition, but perhaps it is the most original and accurate. Based on our own scientific and technological experiences in researching artificial intelligence, we were very satisfied with this definition of knowledge found in the *yoga sūtras.*

Brain Software

Finally, I had the idea – from the source of pure knowledge – to use the term "brain software." This was the right translation of the term "mind" in this day and age. The mind is something different from pure consciousness. Pure consciousness is the silent observer of the mind, in a way the silent user of the brain software. This concept we have now thoroughly applied at all levels and have been extremely surprised at how well all of the *yoga sūtras* can be explained by it. Some of the more complex contexts we ourselves have correctly understood only with this. Using the expression brain software they now became surprisingly simple and intelligible.

While analyzing the most fundamental natural laws, both from the *yoga sūtras*, as well as modern physics, quite unexpectedly a new perspective, possibly even a paradigm shift towards a unified field theory has originated. This new paradigm is indicated in the commentaries of the *yoga sūtras* 1.23 to 1.29. Probably, I am going to elaborate on this and publish it later in a complete book.

Now you, dear reader, have in front of you this creative, new, yet accurate translation of the *yoga sūtras* of *Patañjali*, along with the elaborate commentaries of *Vyāsa* and *Śaṁkara*. Additionally, we have included our scientific and technological explanations. It is a substantial work based on more than ten years of translating and forty years of the meditation practice of several people. It is also based on our own life experiences in higher states of consciousness. We want to inspire you not merely to consider this work intellectually, but to use it as a practical manual for yourself to explore the *siddhis* and to enrich your life, and with it soon to gain "liberation," the highest state of consciousness.

This procedure is like loading new software into your brain computer. It does not need to take long. Should you happen to come across some of the new places of additional "*siddhi* light switches," we remain eager to hear your feedback. The ability of humans to fly, that is to master the gravitational field, we consider a common project of humanity which should not be reserved for a few in elite circles. In this book "Brain Software" we have described the approximate area where the gravitation light switch should be. If anybody finds out before us where it is exactly, we ask you for an exchange of related thoughts. Should we find it out before you, we will also publish this. Whether or not we would want to do this in book format remains to be seen. For now, just assume that the knowledge will reach you in some adequate form and just possibly even from an orbit around the Earth!

Heinz Krug, February 2018

Research of the SELF As a Goal of Life

The German poet Goethe excellently expressed his search for self-awareness in "Faust" like this:

So that I may perceive whatever holds

The world together in its inmost folds

But Goethe also warned the seeker via Mephisto, the adversary:

Humanities most lofty power,

Reason and knowledge, pray despise!

Let but the spirit of all lies

With works of dazzling magic blind you;

Then, absolutely mine, I'll have and bind you!

Therefore, the approach must be scientific, such that the statements are observable, explainable, predictable and verifiable. Useful findings on this topic I discovered in a Western context in following the books:

(1) Thomas Kuhn: "The Structure of Scientific Revolutions."

(2) Max Planck expressed possible hurdles to research in his "Scientific Self Biography" in this way: "A new scientific truth tends to get established not in such a way, that its opponents become convinced and then declare they have been taught, but rather such that its opponents gradually die out and that the growing generation becomes acquainted with the truth from the beginning."

(3) The mathematician Jaques Hadamard depicts in his book "The Psychology of Invention in the Mathematical Field," the ways how outstanding geniuses of his time, like for example he, Einstein and Brahms arrived at discoveries. The basic method was that they could transform themselves into a state of silent thinking, observing their thought processes as it were. With this they were able, to observe various ideas as in a movie and to select from them according to certain criteria, like the feeling of bliss that came up. Not many humans have this ability.

Yoga – A Research Path of the SELF

In my time as a young student, I came into contact with the meditation technique of Maharishi™[7] Mahesh Yogi. Maharishi™ strived towards giving his system a scientific basis. Due to the meditation techniques that I learned, my studies became easy. During the time of doctoral studies which lasted for a year, I could, due to the meditation techniques, transform myself into a creative state, such that the ideas were springing by themselves – as described in the book by Hadamard.

As a professor of computer science at Furtwangen University (HFU) I intuitively cognized with the help of the meditation techniques future groundbreaking trends in research and teaching. The meditation techniques improve my health, well-being, clarity of thinking and intuitive knowledge.

Support by the Śaṁkarācārya of Southern India

In the year 1999 I had the great luck to become the student of the highly revered and excellent *Advaita-Vedanta* teacher – his *Holiness Śri Śri Bharati Tirtha Mahaswamiji, Śaṁkarācārya* of Southern India. I learned from him *Vedanta* in theory and practice (meditation). His Holiness transformed my mind and my body such that my mental abilities and my health improved enormously. His knowledge helped me in the composition of this book. I am infinitely grateful to him.

Learning of the Yoga Sūtras

I am deeply grateful to my friend Heinz that he included me in his research about *yoga* and the *siddhis*. There I could contribute my findings from India. His hints established the immediate success of my *siddhi* practices. Later on, I taught *siddhis* to professionals. They immediately experienced the results as predicted in the *yoga sūtras*. Understanding of the theory of the *yoga sūtras* is important for success. Therefore, Heinz and I emphasized precise definitions and applications of the *saṁskṛt* terminology.

---

[7] Maharishi is a trademark of Maharishi Foundation Ltd. Corporation United Kingdom, P.O. Box 652 St. Helier, Jersey Great Britain JE48Y2.

EU-India Project

I was involved with computer linguistics, the grammar of *saṁskṛt*, Indian logic (*nyāya*), and ontology (*vaiśeṣika*). As a computer scientist, I was well conversant with the modeling of systems. My Indian wife, Dr. Rashmi Bahadur helped me. She had studied *saṁskṛt* and linguistics in Vārāṇasī, India and therefore could support me with *saṁskṛt*.

In the year 2006, I finished the three-year EU-India project that dealt with syntax and semantics of the language *saṁskṛt* and Indian logic and ontology. The "Sri Shankara Advaita Research Centre" in Sringeri, Karnataka, was a partner in this project under the organizational leadership of V.R. Gowrishankar. His Holiness, the Śaṁkarācārya of Southern India, massively supported the project.

Another partner was a Department of the Ministry of Electronics & Information Technology of the Government of India. We were cooperating with Dr. Om Vikas, the leader of the programme TDIL (Technology Development for Indian Languages). The findings of this project helped me with the translation of the *yoga sūtras*.

Historical Dimension of the Yoga Sūtras

The historical dimension of the technology in the *yoga sūtras* is properly understood, when one's own experiences verify the theory. It goes in steps because the "brain software" (mental abilities) functions together with its "hardware" (physiology), that first needs to be optimized by mental practices, such that in turn an improved brain software can run. It happens with regular practice and serenity.

In the West, the Age of Enlightenment began with the systematic investigation of phenomena: observing, explaining, predicting and verifying. The area of research essentially was confined to matter. The way the human mind - in our terms the "brain software" - functions, so far could not be researched, because there was no possibility, to improve the effectiveness of the mind.

But with the availability of the *yoga* technology and its upgrades of the brain software completely new areas of applications open up as the evidence becomes verifiable. Areas that became stuck also will profit from this rediscovered technology. We see here not only a new paradigm but rather the basis for the successful further development in many fields.

Communication with Natural Laws

Many of you surely have become angry with your computer and scolded it directly like a living being. In nature, you can find many independent systems, that behave intelligently, faultlessly, predictably, and that are more complex than those created by humans. They are called the natural laws. You can view them as software functions. Now go a step further and imagine that you could talk to the natural laws with perfect speech recognition and speech output software; in other words, they would have a communication interface like a computer. You think it is impossible? It is just a matter of getting used to utilizing it! When you first start to communicate with invisible beings, you may be shocked, and think that you are fantasizing. If you apply the communication more often, you get used to it. More than that, if you keep asking natural laws to perform a certain action and it mostly happens like that, you would know that they are to be regarded as real beings. Old legends report it. In the language of our forefathers, they are gods and goddesses, in today's language they are software or natural laws that have a communication interface. One first needs to know them and to establish the interface.

Convince Yourself by Practice and Serenity

You, dear reader, can verify for yourself our descriptions and techniques, simply by practicing. Then you become ever more free and independent of opinions and dogmas. You become healthier, clearer-minded, more intuitive and happier. You are going to improve your mental abilities. In short, you are going to have a fulfilled life and fairly soon. Study the *siddhis*! You have infinite possibilities!

Gerd Unruh, Freiburg, February 2018

Tradition of the Yoga Sūtras

Origin of the Yoga Sūtras

Authors

The *yoga sūtras* (guideline of *yoga*) originate from *Patañjali*. Their most important commentators are *Vyāsa* (around 3000 B.C.) and *Śaṁkara* (around 800 A.D.). The *yoga sūtras* consist of 195 well structured and compressed sentences that were initially orally transmitted and then written down at a later time.

Oral Tradition

The *yoga sūtras* have been orally transmitted for centuries in the *saṁskṛt* language (pronounced: "sanskrit," *a* like in far, *i* like in fit). They have therefore been retained in a compact and well-structured form. The structure of the *yoga sūtras* is hierarchical. The meanings of words are explained in hierarchical levels of generic and specific terms. Hierarchical means in a tree-like structure, with generic terms that are like the stem and specific terms that are like the branches.

Although the *yoga sūtras* are thousands of years old, we were repeatedly surprised by the precision of their formulations. The way they are structured, in a compact and hierarchical form, is the equivalent of state-of-the-art software development.

Structure of the Yoga Sūtras

The Four Chapters of the Yoga Sūtras

Chapter 1:	*samādhi pāda*	Levels of Silence
Chapter 2:	*sādhana pāda*	Removal of Ignorance
Chapter 3:	*vibhūti pāda*	Extraordinary Abilities
Chapter 4:	*kaivalya pāda*	Liberation (*kaivalya*)

Numbering

The *yoga sūtras* were originally written down in *devanāgarī* script so that they could easily be recited. They always end with the number of the *sūtra*. Vedic texts are numbered.

Saṁskṛt Alphabet

The *saṁskṛt* alphabet is structured systematically. It consists of short and long vowels, half vowels, double vowels, consonants, sibilants and a few special sounds. In transliteration, we write the short a as *a*, with *ā* being twice as long. The same applies to *i* and *u*. A specialty is the vowel *ṛ* that is related to the consonant *r* but could be spoken like all other vowels arbitrarily long. However, in practice, it is spoken as long as the *a*. In *saṁskṛt,* the pronunciation corresponds to the script. *Saṁskṛt* has no capital letters. In this book, as a help to the readers, we are adding the English plural –s to untranslated *saṁskṛt* words, to indicate a plural, although in *saṁskṛt* the plural forms are quite different.

Text Structure

In the *yoga sūtras,* there are hardly any verbs. They are mostly just sequences of nouns and adjectives. The *saṁskṛt* language utilizes composite words, the so-called compounds. There is, therefore, a special art for analyzing them correctly. Sometimes an entire sentence consists of only one compound. It is therefore very important to recognize the correct word separations.

Sandhi

As to sorting out these word separations, *saṁskṛt* holds another surprise, in the form of the so-called *sandhis. Sandhis* are adaptions formed between the end of a word and the beginning of the next. They arise from the natural flow of speech. The final sound of a word and the beginning sound of the next word integrate with each other. This occurs according to exact rules. In total, 58 such rules can, in some cases, be applied several times sequentially on the same word gap. The linguistic term for *sandhis* is "euphonic rules." When translating *saṁskṛt,* the *sandhis* are quite a challenge, and more so when several of them have to be solved in reverse order. We took great care in our translation to always solve *sandhis* correctly.

Grammar

saṁskṛt has a very systematic grammar. It is a mathematically precise language. Nouns and adjectives are declined into eight cases (nominative, vocative, accusative, instrumental, dative, ablative, genitive, locative) with a threefold gender (masculine, feminine, neuter) and a threefold number (singular, dual, plural). From this arise 8*3*3 = 72 combinations of word endings. Several of these endings are identical, especially in the dual number. These 72 declensions occur in variations, depending on the ending sound of the word. The most common is the "a" declension. Then, less often, there are the declensions of i, u, ī, ū, and even less ṛ, which is a vowel in *saṁskṛt*. Very rarely there are some irregular declensions on ī, ū, and consonants like t, c, d and with the syllables as, is, us, at, in, an. As icing on the cake, there are 30 more irregular declensions of individual words.

Additionally, there are superlatives, numerals and various pronouns with declensions. If one does not want to learn all this by heart, then one must refer to accurate and appropriate tables.

The conjugation of verbs is far more complex. Fortunately, they do not often appear in the *yoga sūtras* so that we can spare you the exact breakdown of the ten verb classes with their various tenses and modal verb constructions.

We noticed in our research that many other translators of the *yoga sūtras* had little knowledge of these essential rules of grammar. Our approach was quite the opposite. We often found that only by utilizing the complete grammar and *sandhi* rules could we unlock the true meanings of sentences. You should therefore not be astounded when our translations often divert from those of previous translations. Due to the correct and meticulous application of grammar, we are sure that our translations are accurate.

Pronouns

As the *yoga sūtras* had to be transmitted orally and learned by heart, they have necessarily been kept very compact. Therefore, demonstrative pronouns like the words "this" and "that" occur quite often. We have made a point of always establishing the correct grammatical reference to the corresponding word in previous *sūtras*.

Commentaries

The commentaries of the ancient enlightened masters, *Vyāsa* and *Śaṁkara*, were very helpful indeed. We could only understand many of the *sūtras* by referring to them. Many thanks for your help! A large part of our text is derived from these commentators.

Yoga Sūtras These Days

Categories of Knowledge from the Viewpoint of Yoga Technology

(1) **Intuitive knowledge:** Knowledge is cognized directly. In mathematics therefore often it is stated: "by observation, it can be seen that..." Through intuitive knowledge, there can arise conjectures that will be proven years later.

Examples: mathematics, natural sciences, the science of *yoga*.

(2) **Verifiable knowledge:** There are fundamental theories and methods to prove the theories. This leads to well-established knowledge: it can be observed, explained, predicted and validated.

Examples: mathematics, natural sciences, the science of *yoga*.

(3) **Semi-knowledge:** Theories and methods are incomplete. They are validated only partially.

Examples: medicine, psychology, sociology, philosophy, politics.

(4) **Nescience:** It is not possible to validate statements based on blind belief. Therefore suppression or paralysis of society can result.

Examples: religions, ideologies.

Technology of the Yoga Sūtras

A Complete System

Due to the rediscovery of the mental technology in the *yoga sūtras*, it became possible to re-establish the *yoga sūtras* as a complete system demonstrating all the characteristics of a science. The *yoga sūtras*, in this way, have become accessible and verifiable for all.

The Theory

- explains processes in consciousness;
- explains mental processes and predicts them. "Mental" refers to the totality of feeling related, sense oriented and intellectual activities and states of a living being;
- uses clear, unambiguous terms from the *saṁskṛt* language.
- is in itself non-contradictory;
- uses no dogmas and is not a blind belief like "the Earth is flat."

The Practice

- consists of mental exercises;
- leads to success and fulfillment in life;
- improves the capacity of the organism;
- improves brain functioning;
- allows one personally to verify the theory.

Verification by Personal Experience

We have very accurately checked the meanings of words and sentences, and we were also able, in nearly every case, to verify them through personal experiences. We are, admittedly, still working on actualizing some of them, especially the higher *sūtras*, for example, yogic levitation or mastering of the elements. On the other hand, many of these extraordinary *yoga* abilities have indeed become our daily experience.

When we translated certain terms, for example, the word "*citta*" was no longer "mind," but rather "brain software," we delved into some deep thinking about these terms. Both authors are fully trained in computer science backgrounds with training and have lifelong experience developing and teaching computer science and technology. By using the term brain software, we now bring the *yoga sūtras* out of the mystical realm and into the field of modern science and technology.

Yoga is Not a Religion

- All statements of the theory can be verified by anyone in practice by their own experiences.
- At the very beginning of one's involvement, a certain confidence in the effect is required as an inspiration to learn the technique.
- This confidence later will be replaced by knowledge derived from one's own experiences.
- Even a scientist must have confidence in his or her hypotheses before conducting experiments.

Language of Computer Science

Translations

The *yoga sūtras* of *Patañjali* is one of the oldest texts of humanity and has been translated hundreds of times from *saṁskṛt* into various other languages. Many of the translators and commentators had no access to higher states of consciousness and therefore could not cognize the essence of the *yoga sūtras,* nor could they translate them correctly. Many of them were lacking knowledge of the proper precision of grammar, as well.

Even those translators who themselves had experiences of higher states of consciousness and possessed sufficient *saṁskṛt* knowledge of vocabulary and grammar had difficulty in finding an adequate terminology and system of concepts that could properly represent the original *saṁskṛt* texts. Many translators, for example, used the terminology and system of concepts from the field of psychology. The difficulty that arose here is that psychology is simply not familiar with most of the concepts of the *yoga sūtras,* and therefore lacks the proper vocabulary. Similarly, this applies to the field of philosophy, with the additional difficulty that very few readers understand its language and ways of thinking.

Computer Terms

Why then, use terms from computer technology? Computer science, the science of computer technology, describes the construction and functioning of intelligent systems. As the *yoga sūtras* deal with the basics of human intelligence and its evolution, it was self-evident to transfer this thousands of years old system of intelligence into the current system of computer technology. Additionally, the terms of computer technology are simply more accessible to the modern human who deals with them daily.

For example, the term *saṁskāra* in *saṁskṛt* refers to stored impressions that impair processes of thinking and acting. By using the techniques of the *yoga sūtras,* these impressions can be neutralized, such that they have no more effect.

The term "*saṁskāra*" corresponds to a malware program in computer technology. A malware program is an intelligent pattern that activates itself and negatively influences program execution. Examples of malware programs include viruses, worms, trojans, etc. A scanner program can discover these patterns and neutralize them. Thus, the software works correctly again.

In medicine, one would call the "*saṁskāra*" stress or strain in the nervous system.

Software

- Software determines what a data processing hardware does and the way it does it.
- Software comprises, in a structured way, both commands as well as the corresponding data.
- Examples of hardware items are computers, mobile phones, television sets. On the human level, there are networks of neurons, for example, the human brain.
- The hardware executes the commands of the software
- During command execution, the software runs through various states that are reflected correspondingly in the hardware.
- In this way, hardware can work individually.
- Software can be improved through new versions (upgrades).
- Whereas upgrades were previously installed from data storage media (discs, etc.), they are now done via a data line connection.

The Yoga Sūtras Describe Brain Software

- The brain software comprises all mental activities and states.

- The *yoga sūtras* in the language of *saṁskṛt* are short and simple, structured logically and easy to understand.
- Troubles in understanding only came up with the many translations and commentaries. For example, there are vastly different interpretations of the term "enlightenment" that do not at all fulfill any scientific or technological requirements.
- We are translating, for the first time in this book, the *saṁskṛt* terms directly into the language of computer technology, to explain clearly consciousness and the functioning of the brain.
- Thus every modern person can now easily follow and apply the *yoga sūtras.*
- The description of *yoga* in the language of computer technology is not to be understood as an analogy, but rather as a concrete explanation model for brain research.
- Here we would like to distance ourselves from authors who are using certain terms like the word “quantum,” without any scientific precision, but rather as a kind of ambiguous marketing language.
- When we are talking about the quantum computer, we mean the actual physical phenomenon. However, this book was intentionally written in a way that is easy to understand. We have therefore avoided trying to impress readers with mathematical formulas.
- The effects of the brain software in practice can be measured directly on the body.
- In this book, we are developing, for the first time, a scientifically verifiable description of brain software that comprises all aspects of consciousness.
- With this, we are finally bringing *yoga* out of the mystical and into today's real world.

Format of Translations

Sūtra number →

Translation →

Devanāgarī →

Transliteration →

Dictionary with Grammar →

Commentary →

1.1

Now begins the instruction in yoga.

अथ योगानुशासनम्

atha yoga-anuśāsanam

atha (now [comes]) yoga (m. Komp. [defined in 1.2] anuśāsana (n. Nom. Acc. s.: Explanation, Instruction in))

The structure of the *yoga sūtras* is hierarchical, terms are explained in hierarchical levels.

Saṁskṛt words are *italicized*. Most commentaries are from the authors of this book. Commentaries from *Śaṁkara* are *fully italicized*. *Vyāsa's* short commentaries are mostly contained within *Śaṁkara's* commentaries. If you see the term "brain software" in *Śaṁkara's* commentaries, this is just our translation of the word *citta*.

Research of Your Brain Software

We begin with the research of who you are, with the research of the SELF.

I search for my SELF

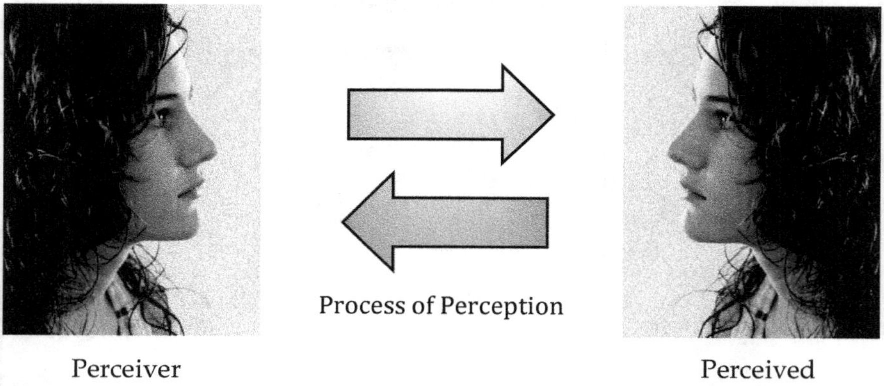

In this search, you are both the perceiver and the perceived. Through this search for your SELF, you are creating a recursion (self-call) in your brain software. Depending on the version of your brain software different results will occur. By examining these results, we can identify the version of the brain software.

Are you ready for the test? Yes – then let us begin.

How do I find my SELF?

I am searching with my mind for the unchanging identity, the "I," the "SELF" in me. I am finding in me: ego, memory, intellect, intuition, sensory perceptions and feelings. Am I not much more? Where is my unchanging identity?

Observation 1

I observe my body like an object.

I am not my body because my body constantly changes and I stay unchanged.

⇨ Therefore I am the observer of my body.

Observation 2

I observe the life energy like an object.

I observe for example that my body gets life energy (*prāṇa*) from breathing. The life energy is an object, which my body takes in, similar to the power supply in a computer.

But I am not the life energy.

⇨ I am the observer of the life energy.

Observation 3

I observe that I am using my sense organs.

I am not my sense organs because they are merely my input devices, whose functioning I can observe. The sensory perception changes with waking, dreaming or sleeping. These three states of consciousness each change the software of the input processors in my brain. In sleep, the sensory perception is switched off, in dreaming it is nonreal and in the waking state it projects my environment.

I can observe these changes in my sensory perception.

⇨ I am the observer of my sense organs.

Observation 4

I observe, how I am using my organs of action.

I am not my organs of action because they are merely my output devices, which perform actions, whose way of functioning I can observe. The actions change with waking, dreaming and sleeping. These three states of consciousness each change the software of the output processors in my brain. During sleep, actions are reduced or unconscious, like the breathing. In the dream state, they are only indicated, for example as muscular jerks. In waking they act upon my environment.

I can observe these changes in my ability to act.

⇨ I am the observer of my organs of action.

The five sense organs and the five organs of action together are called the ten *indrīyas*.

Observation 5

I observe my input-output software.

The input-output software is called the *manas*. It controls the five sense organs and the five organs of action. It controls and processes in conjunction with the intellect the sensory perceptions and steers the organs of action. It registers that something is there. It creates thinking activity and feelings from the sensory perception, which are stored as impressions. The impressions often are connected with sensations of attraction or rejection.

For example, what is the taste of raspberry ice cream?

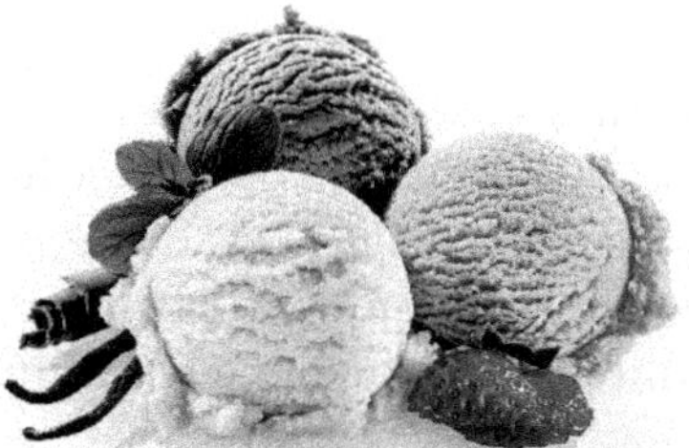

Impressions, in turn, generate a multitude of new thoughts. The impression of one good experience with raspberry ice cream can lead to the expectation, that other kinds of ice cream may also taste good.

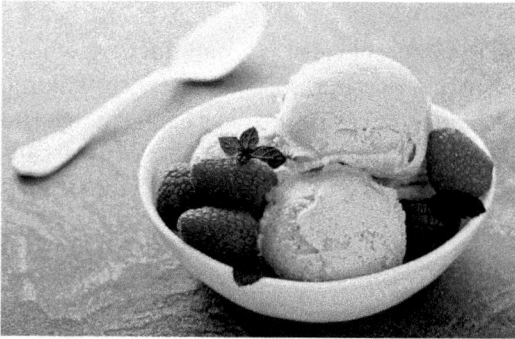

Observation 6

I observe my intellect.

My intellect (the *buddhi*) understands, distinguishes and decides. It includes the intuition. The intellect is the main component of the brain software. It uses and manages all knowledge and information storage in brain, heart, nervous system and other organs.

I observe, that my intellect changes with tiredness, food, medicine, etc.

But I do not change. Therefore I am not my intellect.

⇨ I am the observer of my intellect.

Observation 7

I observe my memory.

My memory (the *smṛti*) stores knowledge, information, and impressions.

I observe how my memory power changes with tiredness.

But I do not change. Therefore I am not my memory.

⇨ I am the observer of my memory.

Observation 8

I observe my brain software.

In *saṁskṛt,* the term *citta* is used for the brain software. The *citta* comprises the intellect (the *buddhi*), the input-output component (the *manas*) and the knowledge and experience storage (the *smṛti*). The brain software changes as its components change in the way we have described it above.

But I do not change. Therefore I am not my brain software.

⇨ I am the observer of my brain software.

Observation 9

I observe my limited "I."

My limited "I," my ego, appears as the identification with body and brain software and is called *asmitā*. It is an incomplete version of the brain software because it lacks the access to the universe-computer. The *asmitā* expresses itself as "I" do this, "I" see, "I" feel, "I" remember, "I" decide, etc. The equivalent to the *asmitā* or the ego is a computer that cannot connect to the global network or global grid.

Here now is a method, to distinguish the ego from the SELF

My "I" knows various thinking activities in the waking and the dreaming state. But in a deep sleep, my "I" only knows the simple thought of non-existence. In deep sleep, there are no other thoughts. Not even the thought, "I am now in a deep sleep," is possible. Thus "I" cannot remember any thoughts during my deep sleep.

But upon awakening, I remember for example: "I have slept well and long." Therefore there must be another level of my consciousness, which has a memory of the deep sleep during the awakening and therefore can do this evaluation. This other level of my consciousness must be a state of ME, which is also conscious during deep sleep. I am the conscious observer of the deep sleep.

Therefore my ego changes, as it is active in waking and dreaming, but not during deep sleep. My SELF does remember the deep sleep.

- ⇨ I, as my unchanging SELF, am the conscious observer of my changing ego.

Summary of observations

My constant point of reference is the I, my SELF that is ever existing. I have, step-by-step, recognized all my abilities as changing, whereas I stay the same as the unchanging observer.

> All mental activities and states run in the brain software. I am not identical with this brain software, but I am the observer and user of this brain software.

Saṁskṛt	**English**	**Computer Science Terms**
ātman	SELF	User of the brain software
citta	Brain software	All components of the brain software
buddhi	Intellect	Main component of the brain software
asmitā	Ego	Ego component of the brain software
smṛti	Memory	Memory
manas	Perception-action processing	Input-output component
indriyas	5 Sensory, 5 organs of action	5 Input, 5 output components
avidyā	Ignorance	Class of malware
śarīra	Body	Hardware

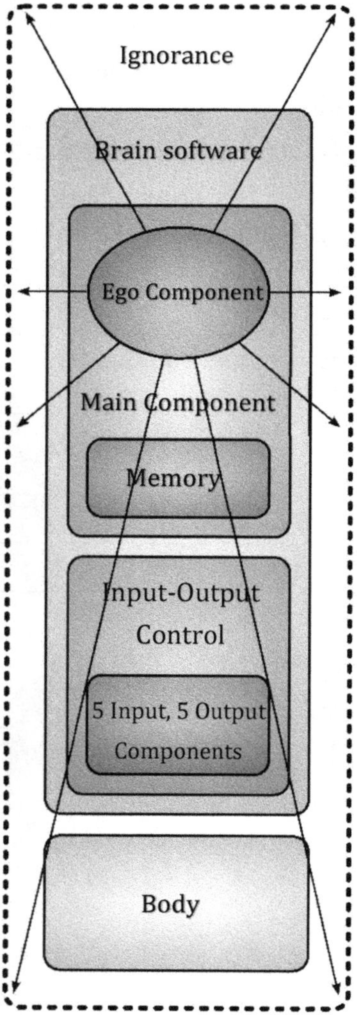

Brain software version 3

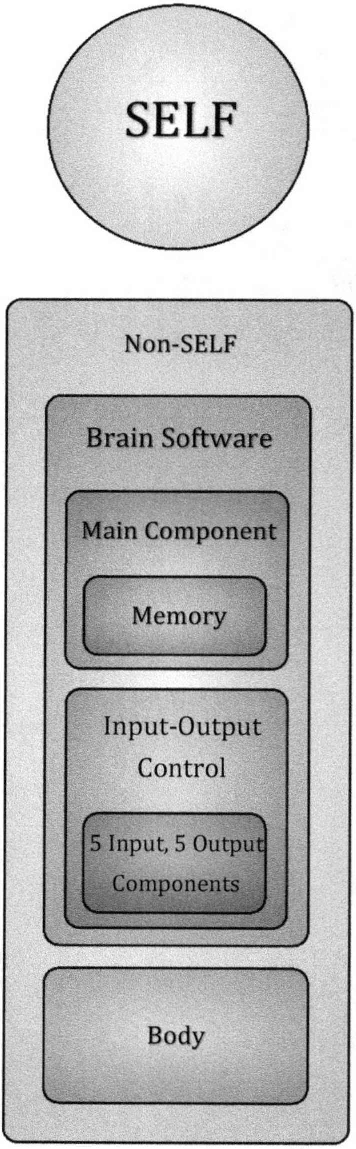

Brain Software Version 5

Test of Your Version of Brain Software

We have now researched the various components of the brain software. The SELF is the uninvolved observer of the brain software.

We describe the SELF as the user of the brain software.

Intellectually all of this is clear. The question remains to what extent this is your daily experience. You can check this from the extent you are experiencing this uninvolved observer status. From this, you can conclude the version of your brain software. There are a series of simple tests.

All these tests only you can do. In principle, there is no method, by which an outsider can evaluate the version of your brain software. It is important that you do this test for yourself because depending on the result of this test you can decide, what would be the next higher version of brain software you require.

The various brain software versions ideally get installed successively. That does not necessarily mean that it takes a long time; only that it is useful to keep the sequence. For example, it can happen that following the experience of brain software version 4 you have temporary experiences of versions 6 or 7. However, these are stabilized only once the version 5 is stable. Therefore, in any case, it is useful, first to stabilize version 5.

Brain Software Versions 1 to 3

Brain software version 1 causes the deep sleep, version 2 the dream state, version 3 the waking state. These three versions are common experiences so that no test is required.

Test for Brain Software Version 4

I can be for some time conscious without any mental activity.

⇨ If yes, version 4 is functioning.

This version also has the name "transcendental consciousness," because it transcends any mental activity. This state is experienced in the transition states between waking, dreaming state, and deep sleep. It is the waiting state or observing state, the idle mode of the brain software, which is experienced as quiet and blissful wakefulness.

Test for Brain Software Version 5.1

For someone who has discovered the SELF, there exists a consciousness during sleep, but no thoughts about the process of sleeping. This consciousness is more silent than thoughts, is infinite and without the perception of time. Others do not notice this consciousness in sleep. During all sleeping phases, including deep sleep, I am the silent observer of my non-activity.

⇨ If yes, version 5.1 is functioning.

Test for Brain Software Version 5.2

During the dream state, I am the silent observer of all my dreams.

⇨ If yes, version 5.2 is functioning.

Test for Brain Software Version 5.3

During the waking state, I am the silent observer of all activity.

⇨ If yes, version 5.3 is functioning.

Complete Test for Brain Software Version 5

I always exist as the observer during the sleep, the dream state, and the waking state.

⇨ That means that version 5 is running in a completely stable way.

This version also has the name "cosmic consciousness." The term "cosmic" originates from the experience that I am unboundedness. With the progress of the development of consciousness usually, versions 5.3, 5.2 and 5.1 stabilize in this sequence. The version 5 runs stable only when in the deepest state of deep sleep a consciousness remains.

This version 5 of the brain software requires that the quantum computer in the brain is activated and running.

Quantum Computer

A quantum computer utilizes the quantum principle of entanglement for data transmission with infinite speed and the quantum principle of superposition to process arbitrarily many processes in parallel. With this a quantum computer, at least theoretically, can process data infinitely fast. However, practically such quantum computers have not been built, and the research is still in an early phase.

Test for Brain Software Version 6

With the brain software version 6, extremely refined sensory perceptions and activities are possible.

It shows up for example in an extremely refined sense of hearing that allows me to perceive in an inner dialogue the answers of higher beings. Also, I can feel, see and talk with heavenly beings. I can also feel, see and neutralize negative and disturbing energies. The refinement of perception is a progressive process that goes along with the switching off of malware programs in the brain software and the corresponding purification of the body.

I can, for example, notice with my refined intuition in version 6 that a friend wants to call me, then the phone rings and I am talking to him in version 5.3. In this way, I confirm, that the perception in version 6 is not merely imagined.

⇨ If yes, version 6 is functioning.

Version 6 can occasionally occur before version 5, but it becomes stable only once version 5 is stable as well. Version 6 also has the name "refined cosmic consciousness." The quantum computer in the brain has access via the universe-computer to a multitude of cosmic resources.

Test for Brain Software Version 7

Everything happens within my SELF. The difference between subject and object no longer exists. Knowledge is correct and immediately appears when required.

⇨ If yes, version 7 is functioning.

Version 7 can occasionally appear before versions 5 or 6 but becomes stable only when version 5 is already stable. Version 7 is also called "unity consciousness" because I and everything else is in unity. There does not exist any difference between ME and the world. All is happening within ME. All is cognized, as an expression of my SELF. My brain uses the cosmic computer. I recognize that all in the subjective and objective universe is identical with consciousness.

Test for Brain Software Version 8

Version 7 has expanded in every respect into infinity.

⇨ If yes, version 8 is functioning.

Version 8 also has the name "*brahman* consciousness," because *brahman* is a term in *saṁskṛt* for the all-encompassing universe-computer. The universe-computer has infinite resources available. Then the cognition of the SELF is complete.

Brain Software	State of Consciousness	Test
Version 1	Deep sleep	Common experience
Version 2	Dream state	Common experience
Version 3	Waking state	Common experience
Version 4	Transcendental consciousness	You can consciously experience a state of total silence without thoughts.
Version 5	Cosmic consciousness (CC)	You are the absolutely silent, non-judging, and wakeful experiencer of all actions and silence.
Version 5.1	Deep sleep in CC	You are the wakeful experiencer of the deep sleep state without any mental activity. If you are not awake in a deep sleep, then you have not yet reached version 5.
Version 5.2	Dream state in CC	You are the wakeful experiencer of all dreaming thoughts.
Version 5.3	Waking state in CC	You are the wakeful and absolutely silent experiencer of all thoughts in your brain software and actions of your body.
Version 6	Refined cosmic consciousness	You have refined sensory perceptions which you can verify as true experiences in version 5.3. For example, you can perceive, that now a friend is going to ring you. Then the telephone rings and you are talking with this same friend.
Version 7	Unity consciousness	Everything happens within your SELF. The difference between subject and objects no longer exists. Knowledge is perfectly correct and appears where ever and whenever it is required. If you do not perceive the world in this way, then you are not yet in unity consciousness. The unity becomes stable as soon as cosmic consciousness is stabilized too. It means, for example, if your consciousness does not stay awake during sleep then your unity is not real but rather an intellectual concept within brain software version 3.
Version 8	*Brahman* consciousness	Unity consciousness is expanded to infinity.

Upgrade Of Brain Software

Brain Software and the SELF

In *yoga,* the SELF is called the *ātman*, the *puruṣa*, or the *brahman*. The SELF is the silent, blissful observer of all mental and physical processes. The goal of the technology of *yoga* is first to enliven this intellectual insight of the SELF and then to implement it into an immediate, practical life reality.

In *yoga,* the SELF comprises everything, not only the individual. The SELF recognizes everything as SELF, both the limited universes as well as the infinite.

⇨ Therefore the SELF is far more than merely the observer. The SELF is the basis of all.

The SELF is the user of the brain software that runs on the quantum computer in the brain and links with the universe-computer. The brain software uses the *manas* (input-output component), the *buddhi* (main component) and the *smṛti* (memory).

The intellect (*buddhi*) acts on behalf of the SELF. However, if the intellect assumes to be the SELF, this is in *yoga* a definition of ignorance (*avidyā*).

Samādhi is a state of total serenity, total balance, where the SELF is recognized as pure consciousness. It is a state "as if empty," that means without mental activity, only observing its existence, fulfilled with silent, blissful wakefulness.

> *Samādhi* is the idle mode of the brain software, where all the resources are available, yet inactive.

Samādhi occurs in several stages if in addition to the empty state there are mental activities as well.

Components of the Brain Software

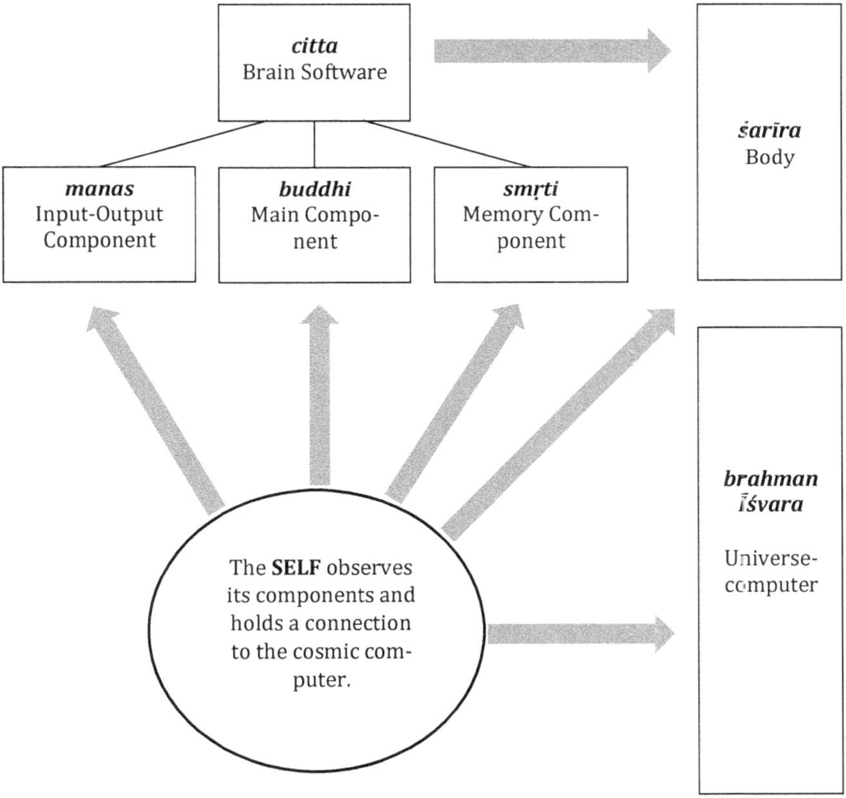

Brain Software Changes the Physiology

In computer technology there is special hardware that allows, changing the hardware via the software such that another processor can replace the current processor. With this new "hardware," another software may run far more efficiently. This technology is called *Field Programmable Gate Array (FPGA)*. It ranges from circuits of low complexity, like for example a simple synchronous counter, up to highly complex circuits like microprocessors. FPGAs are utilized in all areas of digital technology, mostly when fast signal processing and flexible changes to the circuitry are important, for example, implementing late improvements of functionality, without directly changing the physical hardware.

The brain software functions similarly. It can change its basic physiology such that it can run new and more efficient software on the universe-computer.

Heinz Krug, one of the authors of this book, has been significantly involved in the development of FPGA technology.

An Upgrade Is Very Simple

If you have done these tests, by now, you will recognize the version of your current brain software.

Only YOU can recognize that. An outsider can never deduce your current version from your actions. The higher versions contain, in addition to the enormous improvements, all the possibilities and abilities of the previous versions as well. We are going to describe these extensively. Now you have determined the version of your brain software. If you have not, take a few minutes of your time, and do it now. As we have stated previously, the theory can only be understood, if you perform these simple practices as well.

You can upgrade your brain software utilizing fairly simple exercises of the *yoga* technology. For this, you do not need to meditate for a lifetime. Even though you may have practiced advanced *yoga* techniques, like for example the *siddhis*, for decades without any concrete results, you can learn within a few hours how these *siddhis* work, namely like in a "button press operation."

We are going to give you hints for these exercises. The exercises are simultaneously purifying the body. It is a continually evolving process.

> Therefore it is important, to practice, for example once or twice a day, until achieving the corresponding goal of the exercise.

Therefore it is important, to practice, for example once or twice a day, until achieving the corresponding goal of the exercise.

As long as your brain does not yet work with version 8, you cannot even imagine the range of infinite possibilities that are available to you with the higher versions. From the moment when you activate your quantum computer by upgrading your brain software, and you connect with the universe-computer, the extraordinary abilities starting from version 5 are available to you.

Examples are: continuous deep inner bliss and wakefulness; complete control over your feelings; perceiving the thoughts of other persons; understanding the language of animals; perceiving hidden things; perceiving past and future; perceiving and healing the state of all the organs in the body; seeing higher beings and talking to them; perceiving any correct knowledge within the source of all knowledge.

Definition of Terms Related to Brain Software

Short Definitions

We are now defining the terms of the *yoga* theory and *yoga* practice, required for an understanding of brain software.

Vṛtti – Thinking process

In brain software versions 1 to 3 the mental activities are occurring in five kinds of thinking processes (*vṛttis*): Correct knowledge (*pramāṇa*), misunderstanding (*viparyaya*), imagination (*vikalpa*), deep sleep (*nidrā*) and memory (*smṛti*). *Yoga* is a state, where these five are all calmed down.

Kleśa – Illusion

The thinking process, called "misunderstanding" can relate to anything. If it is an essential misunderstanding of life, it is called illusion (*kleśa*). Illusions come in five types (2.3). Ignorance (*avidyā*) about one's nature, the SELF, is the cause of the four other *kleśas*, namely the limited "I"-consciousness or ego, longing, hate, and survival instinct.

The SELF is the silent, uninvolved observer of all. When the SELF, the *puruṣa*, the silent observer is "noticed" permanently, there is no ignorance (*avidyā*).

Saṁskāra – Impression

An impression (*saṁskāra*) consists on the one hand of stored memory and connections to illusions (*kleśas*) and the other of the corresponding thinking patterns (*vāsanās*).

Both parts of a *saṁskāra* get stored in the brain software (*citta*) and the physiology. *Saṁskāra* part 1 shows up as a memory connected to an illusion, *saṁskāra* part 2 shows up as a thinking pattern in the form of virtue (*dharma*) and vice (*adharma*). In this context, see *yama* (2.30) and *niyama* (2.32).

Example: Someone has done something wrong due to hate (*kleśa*), that in turn generates part 2 of a *saṁskāra*, in the form of a vicious thinking pattern, or it further strengthens an existing *saṁskāra*. As long as this person has not removed the original hate, and therefore has not escaped the illusion, this viciousness is going to bring bad luck and suffering in his present or future life. However, once he has removed the hate, utilizing the practice of *yoga*, the vicious thinking pattern will be removed as well. Then only the memory (*saṁskāra* part 1) of the action remains but does no longer cause any suffering (3.18).

Vāsanā – Thinking pattern

A *saṁskāra* has a twofold nature, on the one hand, it consists of memory and the illusions which are causing it, and on the other hand, it has the name *vāsanā* if it causes the ripening (*vipāka*) in the form of virtue (*dharma*) and vice (*adharma*).

Karma – Action

As long as someone uses only brain software versions 1 to 3, the *kleśas* are the cause of *karma*, which means of thinking, speaking, and acting. *Kleśas* cause virtuous (*dharma*) or vicious (*adharma*) actions. When *kleśas* are active, *karma* results in merit (*puṇya*) or guilt (*pāpa*).

> As you sow, so shall you reap.
>
> [Cicero, de oratore 2,65,261; 55 B.C.]

Karmāśaya – Store of karma

The store of *karma* is similar to a field where the seeds sprout and ripen. It is the store of results of actions (fruits) in the form of merit (*puṇya*) and guilt (*pāpa*). It is located in the *citta*. The fruits ripen for some time before they generate special thinking processes, which in turn influence new activities.

The store of *karma* corresponds to an associative memory in the brain, heart, and nervous system.

Removal of the binding effect of karma

Karma is pretty complicated and gets simplified only by upgrading to higher versions of the brain software. With those higher versions, the suffering creating thinking processes, *saṁskāras* and *kleśas* are gradually switched off. Then the binding effect of *karma* no longer applies. The user of the brain software from version 7 is someone who is free or emancipated because he has freed himself from the binding effect of *karma*. He is called "freed in life" (*jīvan mukti*) because he has achieved freedom while living on Earth.

Detailed Definitions

Vṛtti – Thinking process

The five thinking processes are

1. Correct knowledge (*pramāṇa*). Its definition is direct perception through the five sense organs, correct logical inference, and knowledge from reliable authorities (1.7).
2. Misunderstanding (*viparyaya*) is a kind of memory that does not agree with the facts (1.8). The illusions (*kleśas*) explained below are grave kinds of misunderstandings to be switched off in higher versions of the brain software.
3. Imagination (*vikalpa*) is a thinking process following on from words that do not refer to any real entity (1.9).
4. Deep sleep (*nidrā*) is a primitive thinking process where only one thought of nonexistence is repeated (1.10).
5. Memory (*smṛti*) is a thinking process that does not forget previous contents of experience (1.11). The content of experience can be any one of the thinking processes 1 to 5.

saṁskṛt	English	Thinking Process
pramāṇa	Correct knowledge	Perception, logic, authority
viparyaya	Misunderstanding	Contradiction to facts
vikalpa	Imagination	Reference to words, not facts
nidrā	Deep Sleep	Nonexistence
smṛti	Memory	Repetition of previous contents of experience

The five kinds of illusions (kleśas)

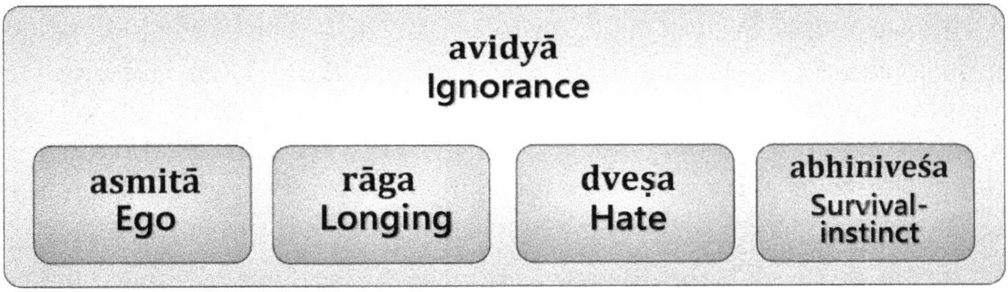

Classification of kleśas

The most influential *kleśa* is the ignorance (*avidyā*) about one's nature. It is the cause of the other four *kleśas*. They are limited "I"- consciousness or ego, longing, hate, and survival instinct.

Avidyā - Ignorance

is to consider the ephemeral as eternal, the impure as pure, unhappiness as happiness, the non-SELF as the SELF (2.5).

Asmitā - Limited „I"-Consciousness

or ego is the identification with the body, intellect, perception organs and organs of action. It shows up as limitedness, pride, stubbornness, egocentricity, infatuation, arrogance, sense of inferiority, self-pity, sadness, and in considering the body and its environment as the SELF. The environment also includes family, friends, possessions, home, work, and lifework.

Rāga – Longing

appears as addiction, wanting to repeat happiness by satisfying the senses, appears in craving, jealousy, amusement, lust, envy, greed, yearning, and passion.

Dveṣa – Hate

shows up as repulsion, aversion, rejection, aggression, anger, rage, and wrath.

Abhiniveśa – Survival Instinct

appears as fear, fear of death, panic and clinging on to earthly existence.

Illusions induce suffering

A firewall is to be activated via the intellect, the main component of the brain software (2.17), to avoid future suffering (2.16). The term firewall in computer technology describes a protection program that shields off unwanted influences. The firewall in the brain software consists of removing the ignorance by separating the connection between the perceiver and the perceived (2.17), (2.25). It is a recognition process and can happen fast.

If someone rejects the intellect in principle, to achieve freedom quickly, this is not constructive. The firewall cannot be established in the higher SELF, where there is only deep silence. The shielding function of the firewall, however, is an activity that can function only in the intellect, which means in the brain software. Our goal is indeed, to remove the fault of the intellect, but we do need the intellect as a tool to achieve that.

Saṁskāra – Impression

The perceived, no matter whether in reality, in television, cinema, or in computer games reaches the store of *citta* in the form of *saṁskāras*. Activated *saṁskāras* influence one's behavior for example, in the form of fear or anger.

Each *saṁskāra* gets stored together with a memory of the situation and the causative illusion at the time of its formation. The *saṁskāra* activates automatically in a suitable environment. Normally the memory is hidden and can only be retrieved by certain *siddhi* techniques (3.18).

The more intensive the attention and intention for a specific activity are, the more shocking the experience, the more intense is the resulting impression. The impression also becomes stronger with repeated attention and intention. In this way, habits are arising. The stronger the habits are, the less they can be controlled, and the more thought power is required to remove them. They are steering the thoughts, the language, and the actions and let the world appear only in a certain, habitual way.

Saṁskāras assume the control of the brain software as soon as they get activated. Then they are called *vāsanās*. They manifest in the form of strong desires, inclinations, or tendencies and they influence thinking and action. Then they become as it were "scripts" or "screenplays" from the personal producer, from the "I."

Saṁskāras manipulate the brain software such that it produces thinking processes (*vṛttis*) as the effects of their underlying illusions (*kleśas*). In this way, further thoughts and actions arise that again lead to new *saṁskāras*, and the cycle continues, until one applies the *yoga* technology, to interrupt it.

Examples of activities caused by *saṁskāras* our: smoking, excessive consumption of sweets, alcohol addiction, wanting to be dressed always in the latest fashion, shyness towards people, fear of flying, rejection of children, wanting to do everything yourself, not being a team player, withholding knowledge, hating foreigners, fan behaviour, style of car driving, excessive preference for anything.

Even though freedom is limited by *saṁskāras*, there still exists a power of veto of the intellect (*buddhi*), to decide freely anyway and to accept guidance from higher principles.

Without any mental techniques, it is nearly impossible to identify or dissolve *saṁskāras*. *Saṁskāras* are carried into future lives if they fit with the timing and the circumstances of a future birth. The unsuitable *saṁskāras* stay hidden and inactive.

Beginning with brain software version 5 the *saṁskāras* more and more lose their influence. The desires become more and more cosmic, in tune with the universe. In practice, one can describe it as: "as it just happens." Then the incentive is the evolutionary force of the universe.

Karma – Action

For the user of brain software version 3 (waking consciousness) the effect of activity is like a line engraved in stone, depending on the degree of wakefulness and previous experiences.

For the user of brain software version 5, the effect is like a line drawn in water. The SELF has been found in the waking state, dream state, and in the deep sleep state, however, the perceiver and the world are different. It also is called duality.

For the user of brain software from version 7 (unity consciousness), the effect of activity is like a line drawn in the air. The perceiver sees the world as the SELF. It only consists of unity. He sees 99.9% as the unbounded SELF and 0.1% as items. The items bring about only minimal, momentary "disturbance" of the unity.

> "What you see, is what you become":
> He/She sees the SELF and remains the SELF.
> The perception process happens within the SELF.

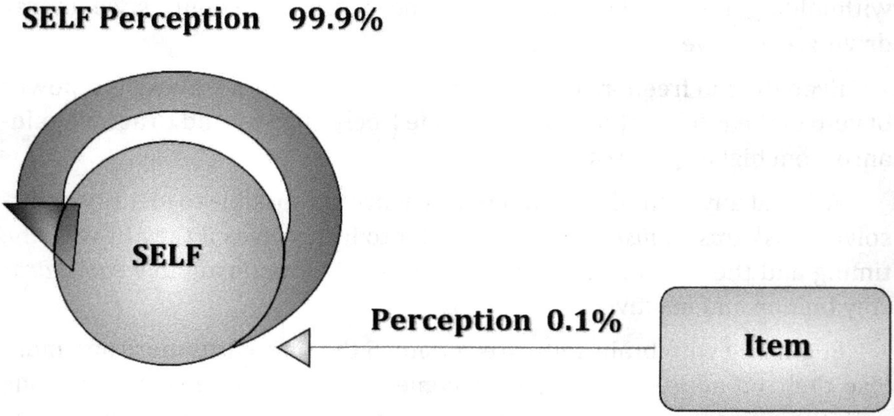

Karmāśaya – Store of karma

The roots of the store of *karma* are the illusions (*kleśas*). Especially in the case of longing (*rāga*) and hate (*dveṣa*) the six-spoked wheel of *saṁsāra* (existence) is kept moving (4.11).

Therefore the aim is, to erase the *kleśas* and thereby to neutralize the effect of the *saṁskāras*. Acting out the *saṁskāras* does not erase them. The fastest method is to destroy the rim that holds together the six spokes of the *karma* wheel (4.11). It happens by removing the ignorance, which means, by cognizing the SELF. The method for it is *viveka khyāti* (2.26).

Merits that follow from virtuous activities can lead to heaven but get used up there, and then the game starts again from the beginning, and this cannot be the final goal. Therefore it is wiser to erase both virtuous as well as vicious *saṁskāras*, to gain freedom from all *karma*.

In the wheel of *saṁsāra* (existence) the world is seen in the network of previous impressions, which can be escaped only with great difficulty. With grey glasses everything is grey. However, the fewer malware programs (*saṁskāras*) that are stored in the brain software, the purer and clearer are perception and insight.

Perception process

The components of any perception are

- *Perceiver:* *ṛṣi*
- *Perception Process:* *devatā*
- *Perceived:* *chandas*

The information from the perceived travels through the perception process to the perceiver. The totality of all three of them has the name *saṁhita*. For the user of brain software version 3, the expression would be: "what you perceive is what you become" (1.4). The perceiver (*ṛṣi*) takes on the qualities of the perceived (*chandas*).

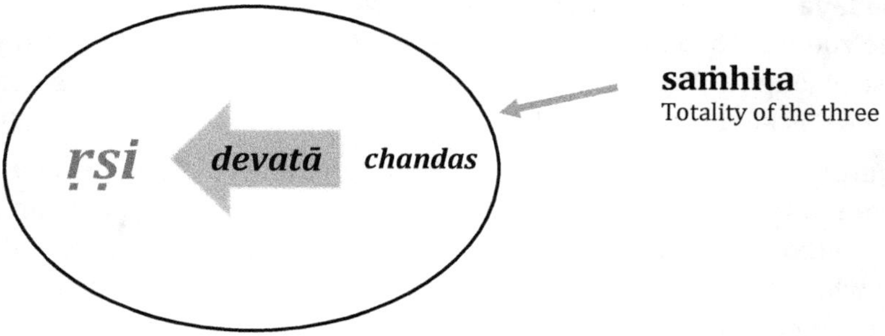

Guṇa – Relative tendency

There are the three relative tendencies that are called the *guṇas*. They correspond to the fundamental components of perception, *ṛṣi, devatā, and chandas*:

- *Sattva* with *ṛṣi* qualities Clarity, Insight
- *Rajas* with *devatā* qualities Movement, Activity
- *Tamas* with *chandas* qualities Solidity, Persistence

The *guṇas* act together in various, changing proportions. Therefore they are called relative.

The effect of the guṇas on the brain software

A *vṛtti* is a thinking process in *citta*, which means in the brain software. *Citta* in its original form is *sattva*. It can, however, be superimposed with *rajas* and *tamas*. The following *guṇa* combinations tend towards special qualities of the brain software.

- *sattva + rajas + tamas*: Preference for power and sensory items.
- *sattva + tamas*: Mischief, ignorance, longing, sleep, laziness, lack of power, weakness, misunderstanding, inability.
- *sattva + rajas*: Merit, limited knowledge (*pramāṇa*), power.
- *sattva*: Pure consciousness, infinite organizing power.

1

Samādhi Pāda

Levels Of Silence

Thinking Processes – Vṛttis

First of all a hint regarding the commentaries

The commentaries of *Vyāsa* and *Śaṁkara* are always written in *italics*. They are sometimes very extensive and cover the smallest details. We are very well aware that this writing style appears unusual to many readers and is not easily understood at least at the first reading. If you like, you can read our shorter summaries (not italics) at the beginning without losing the central theme, and postpone the extensive commentaries to a later time, after having acquired the basic understanding of the *yoga sūtras*.

1.1

Now begins the instruction in yoga.

अथ योगानुशासनम्

atha yoga-anuśāsanam

atha (now[comes]) yoga (m. comp. [defined in 1.2]) anuśāsana (n. nom. acc. s.: instruction)

Yoga is a higher state of consciousness that we are describing, to adapt it to modern times, as a higher version of the brain software.

Here are the commentaries of *Vyāsa* und *Śaṁkara*:

(Vyāsa) The word "now" here means a beginning and the theme that is beginning now is an interpretation of yoga.

(Śaṁkara) In who are neither karma nor its operation, but from whom they come about,

whom the illusions of humanity can never withstand nor touch, whom the eye of time that reckons all, cannot encompass,

that Lord of the world, slayer of the demon Kaiṭabha – to him I bow.

Who is omniscient, all-glorious and all-powerful,

who is without illusion, and who rewards actions with their fruits,

the Lord who is the cause of the rise, end, and maintenance of everything, that teacher of teachers, to him I bow.

No one would follow the exercises and restrictions of yoga unless the goal and the means to this goal were set out. The commentator Vyāsa explains, what these have been for the sūtra author Patañjali so that humans can be led towards the practice.

In medicine, there is a clarifying description. In the classics of medicine the exposition comes under four headings:

- The Disease
- The Cause of the Disease
- The Healthy State
- The Healing

In addition to that, medical science explains these things in terms of prescripts and restrictions. So it is in yoga. See sūtra 2.15: "Change, fear, saṁskāras, suffering, that arise from activity patterns in the conflict of the [three] guṇas (the relative tendencies) to the discriminating (vivekin) are nothing but suffering." It corresponds to the first heading (diagnosis of the disease).

The corresponding fourfold division of this work of yoga is as follows:

- The thing that is to be escaped that is the disease is *saṁsāra*, the world jungle, full of pains.
- Its cause is the connection between the perceiver and the perceived, caused by ignorance (*avidyā*).
- The means of liberation is the unshakeable knowledge that they are different. As soon as the correctly discriminating cognition (*viveka khyāti*) appears, the ignorance disappears.

- When the ignorance disappears, there is a complete end to the connection between the perceiver and the perceived. That is the goal, the liberation that is also called the unity of consciousness (*kaivalya*). This *kaivalya* corresponds to the healthy state.

1.2

Yoga [is] the calming of thought processes (vṛttis) in the brain software (citta).

योगश्चित्तवृत्तिनिरोधः

yogaḥ citta-vṛtti-nirodhaḥ

yogaḥ (m. nom. s.: yoga) citta (n. comp.: brain software) vṛtti (f. comp. : thought process) nirodha (m. nom. s.: stilling, calming, settling, suppression)

This is the definition of *yoga*. This *sūtra* 1.2 is the essence of *yoga*. All the following *sūtras*, including the practices, results, etc., are a more detailed description of this *sūtra*. *Yoga* leads to the calming of certain thinking processes. The *yoga sūtras* describe, how someone can gain this state and what the phenomenal results are, brought with it. A completely new vision arises and a completely new experience of the world in success, simplicity, bliss, unboundedness, access to all knowledge, wisdom, and truth.

The calming of the processes in the brain software is called yoga. What is the nature of the brain software? The brain software always strives towards (1) clarity, (2) movement, or (3) steadiness; these are exactly the qualities of the three guṇas. The guṇas are (1) light that reveals, that brings something out; that is the quality of the sattva guṇa. (2) Activity is movement and effectiveness; that is the quality of the rajas guṇa. (3) Steadiness is steady, limited and with resistance; that is the quality of the tamas guṇa. These are the unchanging tendencies of the guṇas (2.18). As the brain software always strives towards one of them, it is based on the continuous transformation of the three guṇas.

The brain software by nature is radiant. The brain software is sattva, and therefore it is called brain software sattva because its main component is sattva.

- *Mixed with rajas and tamas the brain software is pulled towards power and possessions and this preference is called passion. It means that thoughts arise, that concentrate on the passion for power and possessions.*
- *Permeated by tamas, the brain software comes under the influence of unrighteousness, ignorance, attachment, and helplessness.*
- *When the overshadowing by temptation dwindles away, the brain software, still permeated with a degree of rajas, is equipped with righteousness, knowledge, detachment, power, and generates pure thoughts.*
- *Once the last trace of rajas is removed, the brain software is established in its nature and simply becomes the cognition (2.26), that sattva and puruṣa are different (3.35). The yogi is equipped with the rain cloud of dharma (4.29); yogis call it the highest continuous meditation on intuitive insight (prasaṅkhyāna).*

In this state, which we call brahman consciousness, or brain software version 8, the power of pure consciousness (citi-śakti) is unchanging (4.34): pure consciousness alone is power. Therefore it is called the power of pure consciousness. A power that merely manifests in births, suitable for the owner of this power, is no real power. Pure consciousness, however, is the true power, that does not depend on anything else. Therefore it is eternally steady. The first word citi means pure consciousness, and the second word, power (śakti) indicates, that the individual consciousness, as well, has an unchanging nature. The term "change" means that in an owner of qualities (dharmin) one quality (dharma) gives place to another quality. As this pure consciousness never changes, it is called unchanging. Exactly, for this reason, it does not engage in items, because only such things like the brain software, that are changing, engage in items. Items are shown to the pure consciousness only indirectly through the brain software. Therefore pure consciousness never comes into any direct contact with the items. Therefore it remains pure, and therefore it is infinite in space and eternal in time.

Distinct from citi-śakti (pure consciousness and its power) the correctly-discriminating-cognition (viveka khyāti) is changeable. Its nature is sattva guṇa, and all guṇas are changeable. Sattva guṇa means pure sattva. When saying, that its nature is sattva, it means that its nature essentially is there to radiate. Furthermore, it is called sattva guṇa essentially because the thought of the correctly-discriminating-cognition does not deal with any item in the world.

The correctly-discriminating-cognition is a form of knowledge and knowledge essentially is sattva. This knowledge is therefore different and opposed to the qualities of the power of pure consciousness that have been described. The knowledge changes etc. As it is connected to the quality of change, it is inferior to the highest, silent SELF (puruṣa) that is free from change. As the brain software now sees the faults (doṣas) in its nature, the brain software turns away from it completely and renounces even this highest knowledge.

The essence of the knowledge in the main component of the brain software is the SELF. The brain software now is in a state (version 4), in which the items of perception are missing. What is the nature of the SELF in this state?

1.3

Then the perceiver is grounded in his own nature.

तदा द्रष्टुः स्वरूपेऽवस्थानम्

tadā draṣṭuḥ svarūpe avasthānam

tadā (ind.: then) draṣṭṛ (m. abl. gen. s.: seer, perceiver) svarūpa (n. loc. s., nom. acc. d.: own real nature) avasthāna (n. nom. acc. s.: dwelling, grounded)

The intrinsic nature, the SELF in *yoga* has the names *ātman* or *puruṣa*. It is the eternal existence, the being that never changes, beyond space, time, cause, name, and form. The SELF has the following characteristics:

- Unchangeable, eternal, true (*sat*)
- Pure consciousness, perceiver, knower, pure intelligence (*cit*)
- Pure bliss (*ānanda*)
- Unboundedness (*ananta*)

This is far more than merely the observer! "I" am this, infinite, eternal existence, pure consciousness, and pure bliss. This "I," my unbounded SELF, cannot be comprehended by brain software. Therefore I am not my brain software, but I am rather the user of my brain software. Being the user of my brain software, I stay grounded in my nature, and I am not involved in the thinking processes of my brain software.

Then, in the state of freedom [version 8], the power of pure consciousness (citi-śakti) rests in its nature.

To show that the calming of thinking processes in the brain software does not mean a calming of the user of the brain software (puruṣa) and to hint directly at the knowledge about the user, Vyāsa says:

What is puruṣa, the seer of the brain software, in this state wherein there is no more thing for him? Then the observer, the user rests in his nature. When the thinking processes are calmed down, the power of consciousness rests in its own nature.

What is in this calm state, where no thing exists for him, because the thing, the thinking process of the brain software, no longer exists, then, what is the nature of the user? The user (puruṣa) is the seer of the brain software insofar, as he is conscious of the brain software with its changing thinking processes. The nature of the user simply is, to be the knower of the brain software. To know the brain software is the true nature of the user. There is no one else who is cognizing, and there is no other kind of cognizing.

Then, in the calmed state of the brain software, the observer, the user, rests in his own nature. Once the thinking process is calmed down, then the power of consciousness rests in its nature. "Rests in its own nature," means liberation, freedom (kaivalya). Patañjali, later on, will speak about this true nature, when he is going to say, "That [brain software] does not radiate on its own, [because] it is something observed." (4.19)

However, when the brain software is not calmed, but rather active [versions 1 to 6], why does it then appear as if the power of pure consciousness, that is the power of the user, was subdued by changes? It appears like that because things are shown to him.

1.4

Otherwise [not in the yoga state], [ātman appears to] conform to the thinking process (vṛtti).

वृत्तिसारूप्यमितरत्र

vṛtti-sārūpyam itaratra

vṛtti (f. comp.: thought process) sārūpya (n. nom. acc. s.: similarity of form) itaratra (ind.: otherwise)

"What you see, is what you become." For someone, who is not in the *yoga* state, there is a continuous adaptation to perceived things, to the body, and to the brain software. That means ignorance (*avidyā*). A more accurate definition of ignorance follows in 2.5.

Why does the power of consciousness adapt to the mental process in the brain software? It adapts because things are shown to it. Even though in both cases [both, with the version 7, as well as before] there is no distinction about the resting in its own nature, there is a distinction regarding the power of consciousness, as to whether it adapts to the mental process, or not.

Is there not a fault in the changeability of the power of consciousness? The answer is based on the fact that things are shown to it. This seeming change is not inherent, but rather only projected as through a clear crystal, that takes on the color of something that is put near it (1.41).

There is a sūtra of a previous teacher: "There is only one vision." There is only one vision (darśana) of brain software (buddhi) and user (puruṣa). What does that mean? The vision is only cognition (khyāti). The vision is a process of the brain software. It is cognition insofar as it is known to the user. It also is cognition insofar that through it the qualities of both brain software and user are known. The cognition is a tool because the form of the thing gets comprehended by it, and it is a thing insofar as it gets comprehended through its quality of comprehensibility. Similarly, it is something seen, because it is seen, and also it is a vision because things are seen by it; it is knowledge (jñāna) because it gets known and also because things get known through it. In this way, all this should be understood.

It is the same with computer software that on the one hand is used to process information and knowledge, and is, therefore, a tool for knowledge; on the other hand for a programmer, it is also a thing, which he/she can change. For the normal user it can be replaced by other versions when upgrading it: here again, it is a thing.

As with a king, who is a creator, simply by appearing in front of the council, all the ministers become creators and perform their actions.

And as with the Sun, it does not rely on outside influences, to radiate, and does not perform any actions. It creates no new, previously not existing, radiation, while it comes and goes. It simply is, that radiating is its nature. Therefore it has been said, that simply by its presence it illuminates, and jars, etc. appear as bright forms.

For any human, it is the same. The mental processes in the brain software are permeated by puruṣa, the silent user, who is pure vision, due to his nature as consciousness (cit-ātman).

The previous teacher (Pañcaśikhācārya) assumes that knowledge arises from a connection between the user, the SELF (ātman) and the input-output component of the brain software (manas). However, he also calls the user a knower, who permeates the item of knowledge with knowledge, while not performing any action.

Even if he assumes, that new knowledge arises from the connection between the user and the brain software, this knowledge belongs to the user and not to the brain software, because it has been said, that he knows, and not, that his brain software knows. This shows that knowledge belongs to the user and not to the brain software.

If he assumes, that no user was required but rather, that knowledge in the brain software was to be cognized by another knowledge in the brain software, this would lead to an infinite loop. An infinite loop can only be avoided, if the user, the SELF, cognizes the knowledge.

The brain software creates an effect by being permeated with the user, the SELF and being seen by the SELF. That is a beginning-less relationship, and that is the cause of puruṣa's consciousness of the mental processes. There are many such mental processes in the brain software, and they need to be calmed down.

Test

Perceive an item in front of you. The perception causes a thought to arise in your brain software. Now simply verify, whether this thought is completely overshadowing your SELF. If such an overshadowing is still there, 1.4 applies to you. Do this test occasionally, to find out where you are.

1.5

The thinking processes (vṛttis) are fivefold [and] pain-inducing or non-pain-inducing.

वृत्तयः पञ्चतय्यः क्लिष्टाक्लिष्टाः

vṛttayaḥ pañcatayyaḥ kliṣṭa-akliṣṭāḥ

vṛtti (f. nom. p.: thought process) pañcataya (f. nom. p.: fivefold, a group of 5; in the sūtra –tayyaḥ) kliṣṭa (mf(ā)n. comp.: pain generating, inducing) akliṣṭā (f. nom. acc. p.: not pain-inducing, untroubled, undisturbed)

All five kinds of thinking processes can be further divided into those that ultimately lead to a kind of suffering, and those that do not. To avoid suffering, we have to distinguish between various thinking processes. We must remove the causes of the painful thinking processes. The *yoga sūtras* are now going to examine, step-by-step, the causes and how to remove them.

Vyāsa says in his commentary: "The impressions in the store of karma cause illusions and are the field of the pain-inducing [thinking processes]. In the home of cognition, resisting the influence of the guṇas (1.16), the [thinking processes] are without suffering."

The illusory thinking processes are caused by the five illusions (kleśas) (2.3). Impressions (saṁskāras) also have the name karma seeds, and they are favorable, unfavorable, or mixed. They are deposited in the store of karma (karmāṣaya). They have an inherent impetus, to generate results. From the store of karma seeds, ignorance and the other illusions become the seedbed for pain-inducing thinking processes. When these thinking processes finally appear in the brain software, the corresponding karma seed has nearly ripened.

The others are non-illusory impressions and belong to the cognition store (khyātiviṣaya). They withstand the involvement with guṇas. These pure saṁskāras are the field of knowledge. These saṁskāras withstand the involvement with the guṇas, namely sattva, rajas, and tamas (1.16). Directed towards the field of knowledge, they are pure, because knowledge brings about freedom.

They stay pure, even when they occur together with a stream of impure ones. In the gaps between the impure ones, there are the pure ones. In the gaps between the pure ones, there are the impure ones. Impressions (saṁskāras) are generated only by thinking processes (vṛttis) that correspond to them. Although the illusions (kleśas) generate the impressions (saṁskāras), this happens exclusively by means of the thinking processes. Here the word "exclusively" is strongly emphasized. From the saṁskāras, corresponding thinking processes are generated; thus the wheel of thinking processes (vṛttis) and impressions (saṁskāras) turns continuously. The brain software, therefore, is something that has thinking processes and impressions that mutually cause each other. All these processes happen in the brain software, whereas the user simply stays uninvolved. So it is before installing brain software version 7.

But when the brain software has given up its involvement (from version 7), that means, when the activity caused by ignorance has stopped, and the brain software rests alone in its initial state, then it rests having assimilated the quality similar to its user, the SELF (ātman). Then the brain software for some time adapts to the user (ātman), as far as the rest of those saṁskāras that have been activated already (prārabdha karma), allows it.

Otherwise, when the *saṁskāras* have come to an end, the brain software becomes independent of the human brain and continues to run on the universe-computer, where it has infinite resources available (brain software version 8). This process corresponds to grid computing, where any software can run on hardware resources that are spread globally but interconnected.

But, are there not far too many thinking processes, to be calmed down? Answering this the sūtras says, that they are fivefold. Although there exists an infinite multitude of them, pure and impure, yet, they are only fivefold, there are five groups. The calming down can only succeed with practice and serenity, which override them all at once. The calming does not become obstructed due to their large numbers, however, alternatively there is also no real means, to calm them down one by one.

The evolution of brain software versions (V1 - V8):

V1 to V3	Brain software overshadows the user
V4	Brain software in idle mode
V5	Brain software no longer overshadows the user
V6	Brain software with pure and impure thinking processes
V7	Brain software adapts to the user
V8	Brain software runs on the universe-computer

1.6

[The five kinds of thinking processes (vṛttis) are] pramāṇa (correct knowledge), viparyaya (misunderstanding), vikalpa (imagination), nidrā (deep sleep), smṛti (memory).

प्रमाणविपर्ययविकल्पनिद्रास्मृतयः

pramāṇa-viparyaya-vikalpa-nidrā-smṛtayaḥ

pramāṇa (n. comp.: correct knowledge) viparyaya (m. comp.: misapprehension, incorrect knowledge) vikalpa (m. comp.: imagination) nidrā (f. comp. s.: deep sleep) smṛti (f. nom. p.: memory)

The five thinking processes can generate suffering in brain software versions 1 to 3 because the quantum computer is not yet activated. Those thinking processes, creating suffering, are calmed down in the state of *yoga*. This is *yoga*!

We are now going to examine these five kinds of thinking processes. It is very useful, to deal with this extensively because without this fundamental knowledge, applying the *siddhi* practices in chapter 3, some experiences will occur over and over again, whereby the *yogi* may not be quite sure of the exact differences between correct knowledge, imagination, misunderstanding, and memory. Only correct knowledge can be a meaningful goal of *yoga* practice. In the process, we are going to find, that there is infinite knowledge (1.48), which exceeds the knowledge in 1.7.

1.7

Correct knowledge (pramāṇa) is [defined as] direct perception (pratyakṣa), inference (anumāna) [or] knowledge from an authority (āgama).

प्रत्यक्षानुमानागमाः प्रमाणानि

pratyakṣa-anumāna-āgamāḥ pramāṇāni

pratyakṣa (n. comp.: direct perception) anumāna (n. comp.: inference, deduction) āgama (m. nom. p.: knowledge from an authority) pramāṇa (n. nom. acc. p.: correct knowledge)

Each one of these three and their combinations is correct knowledge (*pramāṇa*) but limited in range. Correct knowledge initially starts with direct perception. From these perceived facts, further inferences can then be drawn, which also count as correct knowledge. If those perceived or inferred facts are passed on, then for the reader or the listener, they are the knowledge of an authority. Here it is important, that the knowledge is passed on by a trustworthy person. These are, amongst others, the seers of the Vedic tradition and correctly transmitted, verified scriptures, for example, the Vedas.

It corresponds to the procedures in modern science, namely starting from measurements (perception), drawing inferences, and then passing knowledge on through scientific publications.

In computer technology, correct knowledge corresponds to a knowledge base that is inherently unambiguous and correctly projects reality.

Direct perception (pratyakṣa)

The component of correct knowledge, called direct perception, is a procedure whereby the brain software through a sensory channel takes up information from a thing and then determines the nature of the thing. The sensory channel refers to one of the five senses of perception, for example, hearing. It does not refer to an organ of action like for example the hands that act, but do not produce knowledge, as a result. The word indriya refers to both sense organs as well as organs of action. But Patañjali here wants to explain those thinking processes that result in knowledge. Therefore he only refers to the senses, which generate knowledge, like for example the hearing.

A sense organ is an input channel, by which the brain software gets activated with a thought in a speech form or another form. Therefore the brain software gets activated by this input channel corresponding to the special peculiarity of an outer thing. As a result of this activation of the brain software, the input information is copied and stored as the memory part of an impression. The impression is that of the thing, which is both general as well as specific, but mainly it is determined by its specificity, and this is called direct perception.

In a silent environment, for example, the gentle ticking of a clock comes through the input channel of the ears. The brain software gets activated by this ticking and tries to find out what this ticking is. Then it determines something general, namely that it is the ticking of a clock. Then it determines the specialty: It is the clock hanging on the wall in the living room.

A sensory channel, like for example sight, can process, together with the brain software, both the general as well as the specialty of a thing. Why should it deal here mainly with determining the specialty? Because the following pattern recognition mainly deals with the specialty. That does not mean that the general would not be perceived, but it is considered as negligible. When saying "blue color" then the main thing is to determine, that it is blue but it is the color (the general) which is blue, and this general, a color, gets negligible importance.

Apart from this, the experience of something general also contains cases of doubt and deception. When someone experiences something general, then he could doubt, whether or not it is that special thing, he is searching.

For example, someone hears a clock ticking and could doubt whether it is his clock in the living room.

Misunderstanding (1.8), however, arises from the memory of another special case of the general, which someone perceives right now. Doubt and misunderstanding, however, cannot remain, if someone has correctly determined the special case and therefore it is said, that direct perception mainly deals with determining the specialty. If someone wishes to determine something general, for example, whether this is a cow or a horse so that one possibility gets refused and the other gets confirmed, still it is most important to determine, what specialty this is, that means what special cow or what special horse it is.

If it is true that there are different specialties, then they must be real. All of practical life would collapse if we could not assume a direct perception together with its distinction of place, time and other circumstances. Otherwise, there would be no memory like "I saw this at this time and that at that time and therefore I can determine, what it is." There can be no memory of things or persons or their qualities, as long as they have not been directly perceived. In reality, no one lives through a fantasy that would be removed from the field of practical life. Therefore it is correct to accept perception in such a way as it is commonly accepted. Perception is a reality. Any attempt to call it a mere imagination would be absurd.

Up to here, up to the pattern recognition of the special patterns, the process of perception is the same for all versions of the brain software. However, there are great differences in the data processing that follows. Next comes the explanation by *Śaṁkara*, of perception processing, starting from brain software version 5:

When it is said that perception is happening in the world by a sensory channel, then this is merely a confirmation of what is happening with a common perception [before version 5] *in the world. On the other hand, the direct perception of a yogi or Īśvara is independent of sense organs. But, once the limitations, caused by the illusions, have been removed, there is a simultaneous perception of all things through the brain software sattva* (quantum computer in the brain), *which reaches all things and fields no matter how fine or remote they are.*

Later it will be said (3.54): "And also in that way knowledge arises, born from the discrimination between all that is intuitively perceived in the starry skies and the totality of all at all times." The definition of direct perception, therefore, may not be limited to that which arrives through the sensory channels.

It means that there is a direct perception via another channel, namely via the universe-computer.

Before reaching brain software version 5, the following applies: The result of a perception process is not only the correct knowledge but additionally the user (*puruṣa*) seems to adapt to the thinking process in the brain software (1.4). Resulting from this perception is a state in the brain software that does not distinguish the brain software from its user (*puruṣa*).

Surely you know this from your computer, when the computer does, what it wants and no longer attends to you. Then a malware is running. In brain software, this means a state of ignorance, which will be explained later (2.5).

What does the term "result" mean? A result is not merely a material, as it is, independent of any action; on the contrary, a result means, taking on of another special state of this material. The result arises from a specific action and appears when the action has reached its end.

Here, the material is the brain software, and the result is another state of the brain software. The non-distinction between the user (puruṣa) and the thinking process in the brain software is the main result of a perception [before brain software version 5]. *Therefore it will be said (3.35) "Experience is a thought that does not distinguish between [buddhi-] sattva and puruṣa, although they are absolutely separate."*

We are going to describe later (3.35) how the user (puruṣa) is the silent observer (pratisaṁvedin); namely the silent observer of the intellect (buddhi), the main component of the brain software.

If the knowledge is immediate, it cannot be the result of a connection between the user and the brain software. Here is an example for that: Even though, for different men the same knowledge of the body of a beautiful woman arises, in one of them the feeling comes up, to want to have her, in another one the feeling, to avoid her and in a third one, none of these feelings. There is no guarantee whether the thought, of wanting to have or the thought of avoiding occurs, even though the knowledge is the same in both cases. For the one, who is indifferent, none of those two feelings arises. The feelings of wanting to have or of avoiding come from longing or hate. According to the rule, "no effect without a cause," there are no feelings of wanting to have or avoiding without longing or hate, even though there is the same knowledge of the body of the beautiful woman. It is called indifference. Due to this indeterminacy, the thoughts of wanting to have or avoiding cannot be the results of correct knowledge. See also sūtra 2.3, which defines the five illusions including longing and hate.

For the indifferent, the brain software only perceives the picture of the beautiful woman. It applies vice versa also for women, who perceive a good-looking man. For the non-indifferent, due to perception, malware gets automatically activated in the brain software which leads to a huge variety of activities. This malware is not a result of the present perception, but rather the result of impressions from previous perceptions.

What is the final result of the perception process? The user (ātman) is all-pervading, and because he's fine and extremely pure, he notices the thinking process in the brain software, because he also permeates the brain software. Thus it is clarified, that the silent user (puruṣa), due to his permeating everything, also permeates the form of this thinking process of correct knowledge in the brain software and that this is his knowledge.

> The recognition that this knowledge belongs to the user is the final result of the perception process.

The recognition that this knowledge belongs to the user is the final result of the perception process.

So it is with a picture that I am recording with a mobile device. Naturally, I am assuming, that this picture belongs to me and not perhaps to the software in the device. It is similar to the brain software and the user of the brain software.

Inference (anumāna)

Inference is the thinking process in the brain software that refers to the inclusion of a similar class of things (those which are inferred) and the exclusion of those that belong to another class. Whereas perception mostly deals with the determination of something special, inference deals mainly with the determination of something general (universal). What is inferred? Anything that someone wants to know more about can be inferred. That, which is similar in qualities and nature, is included, and the rest is excluded.

In essence, this is set theory, the way it has been known for millennia. *Śaṁkara* analyses the mechanisms, as to how to draw an inference. He is going to find, that an inference leads to right knowledge, under the condition of course, that it is applied correctly, and therefore, now we are dealing with the basics of logic.

In a relationship, two things are always related to each other. Now, what is the relationship of including or excluding and which two things does it connect? Is an inference only the relationship between a quality and the thing that has this quality? No, because that would not be sufficient to draw an inference. The relationship with the distinctive feature must be such that it includes or excludes. That is a question of the distinctive feature. It depends on, whether the thing possesses the distinctive feature or not, and this leads to the correct inference.

Often, one cannot determine the movement of heavenly bodies by direct perception, but rather only by inference. For example, someone sees the Moon against the starry skies at one place one day and at another place another day. Because the movement is too slow, to be observed directly with naked eyes, we conclude from the observations at the two different places at two different times that the Moon must have moved.

In the case of cat and mouse (hunter and prey) someone concludes, that, when seeing one of them, the other one cannot be present. That is purely an inference. Not seeing one thing at its usual place, the brain software infers that it must be at a different place. From seeing the cat, the absence of the mouse is inferred. There is another well-known example: "When Caitra, a living man, is not seen at home, then he is absent."

Do not get deluded by the simplicity of logic here; it still is logic.

Now the discussion becomes technical

(Objection) The opponent of the discussion wants to show that, besides the three means, mentioned in the sūtra, there are other means for correct knowledge. One of them is the perception of absence. A classic example that is mentioned several times is this: a man searches for a jar, looks into an empty room and concludes from it, that the jar is not present. However, the opponent calls this a direct perception of the absence of the jar.

(Answer) Śaṁkara calls this an inference from the sight of the empty floor and calls the absence of the jar an inferred thought, and not a direct perception.

Śaṁkara analyses in the following five pages the details of correct logic, something we want to spare you.

> The final result of an inference is the cognition in the brain software that this inferred knowledge belongs to the user.

Knowledge from an authority (āgama)

"Knowledge from an authority" means, that an expert conveys something, which he has perceived or inferred, with the intention, to transfer his knowledge to the other. The thinking process whose topic is the meaning of these words, for the listener is the knowledge from an authority.

"An expert": Someone who, encouraged by benevolence towards the other, and who is without any mistake, and whose intention it is, to say something, which he has perceived or that has been inferred by him and intends to convey his knowledge or his experience to another, namely a specific listener.

"By words": The [words] here are to be understood as a sentence, from which a certain meaning arises, that is conveyed in the sentence. The thinking process in the brain software of the listener, whose topic is the meaning of the sentence, mostly deals with the determination of something general, as in the case of inference, because the listener cannot reproduce this special perception.

"Knowledge from an authority" means for the listener: This kind of knowledge follows on from an original knowledge that the speaker had about something. For him, the speaker, it is not the knowledge from an authority, because in his brain software he has perceived something or inferred something on his own. His knowledge has come about through his sensory perception or his inference.

Knowledge from an authority is not direct perception because it is not in the range of the senses and it is not inference because it does not refer to a relationship with a distinctive feature.

Here again, the final result of this process, is the cognition in the brain software, that this knowledge belongs to the user. The brain software has learned the knowledge.

If a listener says dubious things, which he has neither perceived nor inferred, then this is a wrong testimonial; but if the original speaker has perceived it or inferred it, then the testimonial is without any doubt. What does it mean, to speak something dubious? It is something that is neither perceived nor inferred. That is an incorrect testimonial, and it is only a pretense.

Although he (the commentator Vyāsa) has not said much about the pretense in the cases of direct perception or inference, he has pointed out that the knowledge of an authority in some cases may be pretended, and silently assumes that such a pretense is also possible in the previous cases of direct perception and inference, if their representation contradicts the facts.

"If an original speaker has perceived or inferred it": If it comes from Īśvara (1.26), the first original speaker, then there is no reason to doubt it because his testimony, as a speaker of truth, is not in doubt.

The following discussion now deals with the "analogy" that is valued by some schools as an independent means of gaining knowledge. *Śaṁkara*, however, negates this and follows the *sūtra* that does not mention the analogy. An analogy for *Śaṁkara* is a kind of knowledge from an authority. Analogy requires words and therefore is no additional way to gain correct knowledge because it comes under the term knowledge from an authority.

Practice

We all have learned a lot in our lives. Comb through your knowledge base and consider, from where your knowledge comes. As long as it comes from direct perception, correct inference, or a trustworthy authority, you can be confident that it is correct knowledge.

1.8

Misunderstanding is the illusory knowledge that does not conform to facts.

विपर्ययो मिथ्याज्ञानमतद्रूपप्रतिष्ठम्

viparyayaḥ mithyā-jñānam atat-rūpa-pratiṣṭham

viparyaya (m. nom. s.: misapprehension, incorrect knowledge) mithyā (ind.: illusory, misleading, incorrect) jñāna (n. nom. acc. s.: knowledge) atad (mfn.: this, this here) rūpa (n. comp.: form, feature) pratiṣṭha (n. nom. acc. s.: based on, fundament)

In computer technology, misunderstanding corresponds to a knowledge base, which does not project reality correctly.

Ignorance gets dissolved by correct knowledge, for example by correct perception: If someone sees two Moons due to an eye disease, and then is healed, he sees one Moon again. With this, his misunderstanding gets dissolved by correct knowledge.

Misunderstanding can also be dissolved by inference or by knowledge from an authority. We do not need, nor do we want any misunderstanding, because it generates suffering. We want to be happy!

(Objection) The yoga sūtras deal with bondage and how to escape from it, and its cause, the ignorance (avidyā). Therefore, should not the misunderstanding have been explained before correct knowledge?

(Answer) For sure, ignorance is the first thing that must be stopped. However, human endeavors to stop it, are based on the knowledge, what is right and what is wrong. This knowledge of right and wrong must be correct knowledge. Without correct knowledge the evil of misunderstanding could not be perceived and also one would not know anything about its stopping and about the means towards that. Therefore it was right, first to examine the thinking process of correct knowledge. What is right and what is wrong can only be known through correct knowledge. The misunderstanding is described immediately after that because it is more influential than the other thinking processes.

Misunderstanding is incorrect knowledge. These terms are equivalent; they are based on an untrue form; that is the definition. The form of the thing is its true form. Whatever is not its form, is an untrue form of it, an experience of a pretense of it.

Misunderstanding is the thought that merely has the same general with something else, whose specialty at the moment is not perceived. As such the misunderstanding is supported by the memory of another thing that has been previously perceived. The misunderstanding gets connected with the special form of the other thing, whereby a pretense of certainty arises.

Doubt has this form: "There is a similarity between two things," and it arises in the brain software of someone who sees a similarity and tries to understand, which one of the two, it is. Doubt is merely a memory. The doubt, "Is this a pole or a man?" arises merely from the memory of previously perceived, individual things.

Regarding a misunderstanding, it is different because in this case, only one memory is important. At a place where a pole has been erected, a specific thought arises "That is a man," and it arises from the memory of a man, that previously has been stored with the experience of something with a similar height and width.

Although the misunderstanding is similar to something perceived through the senses, it is not correct knowledge because it is based on the memory of something, previously perceived, that now is no longer there.

Why is misunderstanding not correct knowledge? It is incorrect because it is negated by correct knowledge. The topic of correct knowledge is everything, as it is. The fact that something is not correct knowledge is shown by the possibility that it can be deleted through correct knowledge. For example, seeing a double Moon is deleted by seeing, that in fact there is only one Moon.

Does that not amount to the same as a memory? No, because it appears clearly. The memory is caused by a thing that has been perceived at another place, and now appears in the form "This is as it has been perceived." Misunderstanding is not like that. The thought of misunderstanding arises when the memory is there, and when it has a strong similarity in time, place, etc., to a thing that is perceived now, and that clearly appears as "this thing." Thus the misunderstanding has neither the character of correct knowledge, nor that of memory, and it is another kind of thinking process in the brain software.

Now Śaṁkara gives an example, to show how that, what is not correct knowledge, is refuted through correct knowledge. The example is, how seeing a double Moon, is refuted by the sight that in fact there is only one Moon. An abnormal sight sees things differently, from what they are, for example, sees the Moon double. Then by the perception of the thing, as it is, that means the single Moon, the wrong knowledge is refuted. It gets refuted by the seeing of one Moon and additionally supported by the memory that the seeming second Moon does not exist.

1.9

Imagination (vikalpa) is something following on from verbal knowledge, [but] not based on any existent thing.

शब्दज्ञानानुपाती वस्तुशून्यो विकल्पः

śabda-jñāna-anupātī vastu-śūnyaḥ vikalpaḥ

śabda (m. comp.: verbal) jñāna (n. comp.: knowledge) anupāta (m. nom. s.: following) vastu (n. comp., n. Nom. Akk. s.: real object) śūnya (mf(ā)n., m. nom. s.: empty, absent, Null, emptiness) vikalpa (imagination)

The words taken by themselves do refer to real or abstract objects, but seen in combination, in the context of the sentence, they describe something merely imagined that does not refer to reality. Someone makes sense of some words, but without reference to any real thing. In the brain software, then, a mental image arises, or a picture, by the power of the words only (*śakti vāda*).

Examples of imaginations, not corresponding to "real" things are:

- Fiction, like movies from Hollywood, Bollywood, BBC, etc.
- Fairytales, comics, computer games, advertising.
- Human-made laws are purely word-based agreements in a society. They are necessary, but they are not natural laws.
- The concept of possession comes about through human-made laws.
- Anything that is expressed with the genitive form to indicate possession is merely imagination. For example, the farmer's cow is not interested in, to whom it belongs, only that it gets food, water, and shelter.
- In computer technology, imagination corresponds to models that are detached from reality, as in computer games.

Imagination (vikalpa) is not correct knowledge, but merely verbal knowledge. Something that follows on from verbal knowledge arises from the fixed relationship between words, sentences and their meanings. Verbal knowledge does not refer to any true thing, but merely to the words; that means that it expresses nothing, that really exists. Imagination is a thinking process in the brain software without reference to any real thing.

If imagination follows on from verbal knowledge, should it not be counted as knowledge from an authority? Imagination is not any real knowledge because it does not come under the knowledge of an authority because it does not refer to any real item. Although the knowledge from an authority arises from verbal knowledge, it does, however, refer to real things. Therefore, it has a real item which is described by the words. Imagination, on the other hand, has no real item and therefore is not any correct knowledge.

Furthermore, an imagination is the same for the speaker and the listener. In both of them the thought of the imagination has arisen from the words, unlike the knowledge from an authority that applies only to the listener; in the case of the speaker, it is, what he has perceived or inferred.

Furthermore, for someone in samādhi on a finer level, beyond speech comprehension (nirvitarka samādhi 1.43), any imagination, whatsoever, stops. The knowledge from an authority, however, remains available also in this finer samādhi. Thus the thinking process "imagination" differs from the thinking process "correct knowledge." The words from an authority can confer knowledge, subtler than speech. It is not so for an imagination that always remains connected to the grossest level of thinking, the verbal level.

There is no item present in imagination, should it not, therefore, come under the term misunderstanding? It does not amount to a misunderstanding. Why not? It is because it follows from verbal knowledge. Misunderstanding – even though its item is not present – has no connection to verbal knowledge. The misunderstanding has been defined as wrong knowledge because it relates to an untrue form and not to words. The misunderstanding gets removed because it is incompatible with the known knowledge.

Imagination, therefore, is not a misunderstanding. Although a possible item (thing) is not present, all of worldly life is completely upheld by the validity of verbal knowledge, for example, legal texts, which may, however, be interpreted in various ways.

Thus the terms "not based on any existent thing," and "following on from verbal knowledge" together point to an imagination, which is neither correct knowledge nor misunderstanding, although it carries a trace of both in it. Given that there is a trace of both, the imagination has been explained directly following these two, and the memory follows at a later stage.

Practice

If you are not sure whether, a certain activity of your brain software, originates from your imagination, or whether it is a subtle perception, simply check, whether you have thought or heard a verbal text before. If yes, then it merely is an imagination. If no, then you can attribute it to a subtle perception, which comes under the category "correct knowledge."

Experience

Sometimes, during a spiritual practice, it is not quite clear whether it is a real experience or merely an imagination, a fantasy. For this, I have found a pretty simple distinctive feature. Imaginations always follow on from words. Therefore, as long as I do not think any words, the experience cannot be imagined. Then it must be either memory or direct perception.

1.10

Deep sleep is the mental process based on the thought of nonexistence.

अभावप्रत्ययालम्बना वृत्तिर्निद्रा

abhāva-pratyaya-ālambanā vṛttiḥ nidrā

abhāva (m. comp.: nonexistent) pratyaya (m. comp.: thought) ālambanā (n. nom. s.: depending on, base, support, foundation) vṛtti (f. nom. s.: thought process) nidrā (f. nom. s.: deep sleep)

Deep sleep is a state of consciousness (brain software version 1) that is based on the thought of nonexistence. Although the thought of nonexistence is a primitive one, it still is a thought. Therefore in a deep sleep, there are thoughts, and therefore, it cannot be identical with the thoughtless state of brain software version 4. Whereas in brain software version 4 all resources are available, even though they are not activated, this is different in brain software version 1, in deep sleep; here, the resources, like intellect, memory, sense organs and organs of action are not available.

Deep sleep corresponds to the sleep mode in computer technology, where a simple software function without any actions, runs in an infinite loop until it is interrupted from the outside.

This sūtra describes deep sleep: The thinking process that depends on the thought of nonexistence is deep sleep (nidrā). Correct knowledge, misunderstanding, and imagination that have been explained in the previous sūtras are thinking processes in the waking state [brain software version 3]. *The sleep begins, when they stop, therefore the sleep* [brain software version 1] *is now described, following them.*

Upon awakening, a memory can result in the form of "I have slept well; my brain software is calm, and my understanding has been clarified," or, otherwise "I have slept badly; my brain software is dull and is wandering aimlessly," or, again "In deep sleep I have sunk into a numbness; my limbs appear heavy, and my brain software is slow and weak, as if some force has got it under its control."

There would not be any memory upon awakening if it were not caused by some previous experience. Therefore deep sleep is a special thinking process, and like all the others, it also must be calmed in *samādhi*. Once the sleep is calmed in *samādhi*, we call it brain software version 5.1. It is sleep, wherein the infinite SELF stays awake in *samādhi*, while the limited self additionally, very silently, thinks the thought of nonexistence.

The thought of "nonexistence" means the absence of the waking state, but not absolute nonexistence because there could be no experience of that. An experience of nonexistence, in our context, means, that there is a thought of nonexistence. That, what is based on the thought of nonexistence is deep sleep (nidrā), a dreamless state (suṣupta-avasthā).

Should not the dream state (svapna-avasthā) also be attributed to sleep? No, it does not come under sleep, the way it is defined here because sūtra 1.38 is going to distinguish between them: "Also calming by realizing the knowledge of dreaming (svapna) and deep sleep (nidrā)." There, deep sleep (nidrā) only refers to dreamless sleep. It is only the dreamless sleep that rests upon the thought of nonexistence. Dreaming does not rest on this thought, but rather on the memory of something that has been previously experienced. In dreaming, things from memory become lively (1.11).

What, therefore, is dreamless sleep? It is a thinking process that can be remembered upon awakening. When someone wakes up, he remembers for example "I have slept well." This memory is a reflection of the thinking process during sleep.

1.11

Memory is the not losing of an item of experience.

अनुभूतविषयासंप्रमोषः स्मृतिः

anubhūta-viṣaya-asampramoṣaḥ smṛtiḥ

anubhūta (m. comp.: experienced, perceived) viṣaya (m. comp.: content, sensory object, object of attention) asaṁpramoṣa (m. nom. s.: not forgetting) smṛti (f. nom. s.: memory)

Not losing also means not forgetting, and this seeming cyclical definition of memory corresponds to the feedback loops in computer memories. Not losing means not stopping of impressions that have been caused by previous events; not stopping is like a repetition.

There can be memories of all the five experience processes (*vṛttis*). If, for example, a misunderstanding gets replaced by correct knowledge, there can remain a memory of the misunderstanding.

What is memory? Memory is not letting go of a thought, which has been experienced previously. Not letting go means, that there is no losing or disappearing. Memory is described last because it is the consequence of all the five thinking processes.

The term "item of experience" means both the experience and the item. The item of experience can be any of the five thinking processes, including a previous memory. Although the item of experience is no longer present, it generates a memory, due to its similarity with it, the appearance, as if the item of experience was present.

Is it the thought, that the brain software remembers, or rather the item?

Before reaching brain software version 5, the power (*śakti*) of the SELF gets overshadowed by a thought, which in turn leaves unnecessary side-effects in the form of malware in the brain software. Side-effects no longer occur, beginning with brain software version 5, and additionally, in retrospect, they can be removed again with the methods of *yoga*. However, it is more elegant, to avoid them from the start by installing the higher software versions.

A thought arises, and while it disappears, it leaves a *saṁskāra* in the brain software (*citta*). The *saṁskāra* corresponds to its cause and has two forms. The one part that we call data part is nothing but the innocent memory of the item and the *kleśa*, which has caused it. The other part corresponds to an overshadowing or contamination of the thought process by thinking patterns. These thinking patterns give rise to actions (*karma*) of a similar kind. These patterns act continuously in the background, creating contaminated results both in thinking as well as acting. And that is why we call these contaminations malware.

Memory is twofold; which two?

(1) The word "lively (bhāvita)" means, that a thing exists, because it gets continuously brought into life – like a stream of oil that continuously emerges from another substance, like for example from the oilseed.

The malware corresponds to the oilseed; the contamination corresponds to the oil.

Due to the contaminated stream continuously coming to life, it does not require any more effort or attention, to be maintained. That means, the malware runs autonomously in the background. It is, as if alive, and radiates its harmful influence and can only be stopped by special means. One case, where the remembered items do not require any further effort or attention, is, for example, the memories that come lively in dreams.

(2) However, if someone wants to remember something in the waking state, further efforts or attention are required, to uphold the memory.

It corresponds to the innocent data part of the impression in the brain software that does not autonomously contaminate.

All memories originate from the experience of correct knowledge, misunderstanding, imagination, deep sleep, or previous memories. All these are essentially happiness, suffering, or confusion, arising from the illusions, which will be explained later. Longing is the result of pleasure (2.7), hate is the result of suffering (2.8), while confusion is the result of ignorance (2.5). All these thinking processes must be calmed.

Once they are calmed, the *samādhi* radiates in the brain software. Then the user no longer gets blocked by his brain software.

The Methods Of Yoga

Introductory Commentary by the Authors

In our discussion of the thinking processes, we mentioned several times that a thinking process could go in two directions. On the one side it can go in a direction that generates suffering, and on the other side in a direction, where it does not do that. It was mentioned in *sūtra* 1.5: The thinking processes can be pain-inducing or not pain-inducing. The mechanisms, as to how this suffering comes about and how it is avoided, are going to be described in the later *sūtras* for more details.

When now, starting from 1.12, the talk comes to "good" and "bad" thinking processes, it means inducing suffering or not inducing suffering. It is simply more practical, to use shorter words. No ethical judgment is connected to that, really none at all. That is very important because here, no new fears or aversions should come up. Religious or spiritual organizations strangely have repeatedly managed, even in recent times, to create fears amongst their followers, which ultimately can prevent the state of *yoga*. Even when it is only a fear, to be excluded from the organization, upon any wrong behavior, this can inhibit the liberation of the individual self and the experience of the infinite SELF.

This situation is another reason, why we consciously introduced the terminology of computer technology, to avoid any judgment. The various versions of the brain software are not ethically "good" or "bad," but they merely differ in their range of possibilities. As long as they are permeated by malware, they do not have the same abilities as a clean system. As long as the malware exists, further suffering occurs for the person. No one wants to suffer; that is at least, what we assume. Future suffering is to be avoided (2.16). With the progressive removal of malware the brain software functions better and better. The word "better" is not an ethical judgment, but merely a statement about the power of the brain software. Higher versions of the brain software are just more powerful than lower versions.

1.12

By practice and serenity, the calming of those [vṛttis] is accomplished.

अभ्यासवैराग्याभ्यां तन्निरोधः

abhyāsa-vairāgyābhyām tat-nirodhaḥ

abhyāsa (m. comp.: practice) vairāgya (n. ins. dat. abl. d.: serenity) tad (that) nirodha (m. nom. s.: suppression, restraint, confinement, stopping)

Vairāgya (serenity) means to take everything easy, stay cool, not to strain. It is not mood making, but a true feeling of serenity towards all. Take it easy! Take it as it comes!

Before loading the higher versions of the brain software, the active malware programs in the present version must be ended. That means, all automatically running pain-inducing thinking processes must be calmed down.

Serenity means, not disturbing the calming process and also not allowing any exceptions.

The program flow of the brain software flows in two ways. It flows towards the good (not pain-inducing) and the bad (pain-inducing). When carried towards liberation, into the field of distinction, then this is the program flow towards the good. When being absorbed more and more in the jungle of the world (saṁsāra), into the field of lacking distinction, then this is the bad or the contaminated program flow. By serenity, the malware that means the contaminated program flow towards things gets curtailed. By practicing discriminating cognition (2.26), the good program flow of distinction is chosen. Therefore, the calming of the thinking processes in the brain software rests on both, (1) serenity and (2) discriminating cognition.

The calming happens through practice and serenity, whose details are going to be described in the following sūtras. These two are calming down all the five thinking processes because they are opposed to them. Calming (nirodha) means ending (upaśama) of the malware. Then no longer any inadvertent, disruptive program continues to run. The good thinking processes can still be activated when they are needed.

Humans in the jungle of the world (saṁsāra) are always carried, as in a river, by the program flow of the brain software towards experiential items. They are carried towards saṁsāra and end in saṁsāra like a river ends in the ocean. The ending of this river happens by practice and serenity.

Practices

A series of practices will be introduced following from here on, to enable one to reach the state of *yoga* (1.2). If you are already practicing spiritual exercises, you are probably going to recognize them again. If you do not practice any exercises or do not do them regularly, then it is rather unlikely that you are going to reach the *yoga* state.

Practice 1

Check with all your spiritual practices, meditations, breathing exercises, *yoga āsanas*, etc., whether or not you are doing them with a sufficient amount of serenity. With serenity, they are becoming more powerful. Take it easy!

Practice 2

Do not strain in meditation while striving to achieve the results faster. Otherwise, you may get headaches because you lack serenity.

1.13

In that, staying with those two [practice and serenity], there is practicing with zeal.

तत्र स्थितौ यत्नोऽभ्यासः

tatra sthitau yatnaḥ abhyāsaḥ

tatra (ind.: in that) sthita (m. nom. acc. d.: staying, present) yatna (m. nom. s.: eagerness, zeal) abhyāsa (m. nom. s.: practice)

In serenity, with no strain, the practice is performed intensely. Practices are for example effortless meditations.

Steadiness is the calm flow of the brain software without any thinking processes (brain software version 4). It arises from practice. The striving, strength, and enthusiasm towards this calm flow, helps to perform the training for this purpose (upgrading to brain software version 4).

The steadiness which is the origin of calming of the brain software is the result of the striving, and the striving is the practice. The calm flow is like a stream, free of mud, which means, free of malware activities, changing into a pure form of the brain software without the thinking processes. (They all get stopped in brain software version 4).

The practice means to execute the methods of yoga, like self-control, living rules and the others (2.29).

Practice

It is very important, to do the practice daily. Meditate twice a day for at least twenty minutes.

1.14

If [the *yogi*] practices for a long time without interruption carefully and diligently, [he] becomes firmly grounded.

स तु दीर्घकालनैरन्तर्यसत्कारासेवितो दृढभूमिः

sa tu dīrgha-kāla-nairantarya-satkāra-āsevitaḥ dṛḍha-bhūmiḥ

sa (pron. 3rd. pers. m.,: he) tu (ind.: but) dīrgha (mf(ā)n.: long) kāla (m. comp.: time, duration) nairantarya (n. comp.: without interruption) satkārā (m. comp.: carefully, attentively) āsevita (m. nom. s.: practice with diligence) dṛḍha (mfn.: firm. solid) bhūmi (f. nom. s.: Earth, ground, attitude)

In the brain software, there are far more thinking processes than in a supercomputer. Therefore it requires intensive and long practice. The process of calming should not be prematurely interrupted, to achieve the desired effect.

Practicing for a long time, uninterrupted, with diligence – practicing while striving for liberation, with abstinence (brahmacarya), with knowledge and with trust, it will surely be reached. The idea is that the goal cannot suddenly be superimposed with an outward directed saṁskāra.

How does this calming become stable? Vyāsa says: "Practice for a long time without any interruption." The practice does not become stabilized, when it is not performed for a long time or when it is interrupted; therefore both are mentioned here. It is also specified, that the practice has to be done with care. He explains that "stable" means that it does not get suddenly overwhelmed by an outward directed saṁskāra.

Practice

Practice in such a way, so as not to allow any distraction.

Serenity

1.15

Intentionally not longing for seen or heard things is known as serenity (vairāgya).

दृष्टानुश्रविकविषयवितृष्णस्य वशीकारसंज्णा वैराग्यम्

dṛṣṭa-ānuśravika-viṣaya-vitṛṣṇasya vaśīkāra-saṁjñā vairāgyam

dṛṣṭa (mfn. comp.: seen) anuśravika (mfn. comp.: heard) viṣaya (m. comp.: content, sensory object, object of attention) vitṛṣṇa (mf(ā)n.: not longing, free from desire) vaśīkāra (m. comp.: overcoming, subjugating) saṁjñā (f. nom. s.: known, understanding) vairāgya (n. nom. acc. s.: serenity)

Serenity means, not having any longing for seen or heard things. Seen things mean things, items, objects of this world. Heard things mean promises for a future world, for example, coming to heaven. Promises are merely imaginations, based on words (*vikalpa*).

Serenity means to be unmoved by visible things, like women, men, food, and drink, or power. Serenity also means not having any longing for things in a future world, like reaching heaven, the status of the gods, to merge into nature, [to get rid of the last bit of karma by death, and then to reach the highest state of liberation]. *Someone is serene, if, by the power of his meditation, he is aware of the faults in those things. Serenity means self-mastery that neither has to avoid nor to accept anything.*

"Visible things" means both things as well as the direct perception. What are these? Vyāsa depicts it with the examples of women, men, food, drink, or power. Although there is an infinite number of things, nevertheless the most

important kinds of longings are to possess women, men, food, drinks, or power. In those cases, the longing is strongest, and one needs to resist it with corresponding intensity. Similarly, with things, one has heard about, which means, with the things that are specified in the Scriptures – to gain the comforts of heaven, the joy of merging into nature or the pleasure of the invisible state of the gods.

Does not serenity (vairāgya) mean more than the absence of longing (rāga), but rather include freedom from thirst, because the commentary of sūtra 2.7 says: "Longing is thirst, is greed"?

No, because there are four different stages of serenity:

1. *Yatamāna* – *The effort of interrupting the longing.*
2. *Vyatikrānta* – *The thought of having achieved non-longing for some things, but not yet for others.*
3. *Ekendriya* – *Experiencing the longing no longer with the senses, but merely in the brain software.*
4. *Vaśīkāra* – *Mastery of serenity with the end of the third.*

Vyāsa explains:

"Someone who is internally aware of the faults in them": Seeing the faults brings serenity amidst things; whereas, seeing the good points in them, brings longing.

"By the power of his meditation": By meditating, to see their faults.

"Who is completely serene": Who is completely insensitive to things, even if they are directly in front of him, whether earthly or heavenly. The brain software is in a state, free from longing for them, like a crystal, that does not take on the color of things near it.

"This consciousness of mastery": Certainty that they can be mastered. It is a state, where all the desired things are recognized as controllable, a state, where it is recognized that the senses have been controlled; therefore mastery is achieved.

Mastery of the senses will be explained in 2.54, 2.55, and 3.47 and their phenomenal results in 3.48.

Practices

Practice 1

Take it easy!

Practice 2

Occasionally laugh at yourself.

Practice 3

Take those things or experiences, to which you are strongly connected, or if you cannot easily get rid of a longing, consciously go through the four stages of serenity described above. In this way it will be easier, to get rid of the longing and to achieve serenity.

1.16

Beyond that [serenity], from the cognition of puruṣa [there is] an absence of desires for the guṇas.

तत्परं पुरुषख्यातेः गुणवैतृष्ण्यम्

tat param puruṣa-khyāteḥ guṇa-vaitṛṣṇyam

tat (n. nom. acc. s.: that [simple serenity]) para (n. nom. acc. s.: surpassing) puruṣa (m. comp.: silent SELF) khyāti (f. abl. gen. s.: knowing, knowledge) guṇa (m. comp.: quality, attribute, natural tendency) vaitṛṣṇya (n. nom. acc. s.: without desire)

Puruṣa corresponds to the user of the brain software. The *guṇas* are the three relative tendencies that generate the world of the user of the brain software versions 1 to 6, except 4. With brain software versions 7 and 8 there is no more longing for these tendencies – neither for *tamas* nor *rajas*, not even for *sattva*. The absence of desires amidst the *guṇas* means:

- Perceiving the events of the world at a distance
- A state of happiness free of desire.
- Dancing lightness.
- Carefree state of life.
- Life is a game.

Serenity is twofold. The lower one has been described in the previous sūtra in the form of a non-longing for seen or heard things. Someone who is conscious of the faults in things that he has seen or heard about is serene amidst the things.

However, a higher kind of serenity is the following: Someone who, by practicing the cognition of puruṣa has adapted his brain software to this clarity and now sees clearly, is serene even amidst the guṇas, whose qualities are both visible and invisible. The second, higher serenity is nothing but pure knowledge. When it begins, the yogi, to whom this knowledge dawns, thinks:

> There has been achieved, what needed to be achieved; destroyed are the illusions that had to be destroyed; broken is the continued chain of the circle of existence, by which humans are bound, to die and to be reborn.

Serenity is the highest peak of knowledge; it borders on unity (kaivalya 3.50). It is the higher serenity if from the knowledge of puruṣa not even a thirst for the guṇas arises. "Higher," regarding more evolved, means that it comes at a later time than the lower one. It is the highest because it is closest to liberation.

Someone who is aware of the faults in things, that he sees or about which he has heard, is serene amidst the things.

What is the cause of the higher serenity? Its cause is the knowledge of puruṣa. What is its subject? There is not even a thirst for the guṇas, neither for sattva nor the other two.

"Someone, by practicing the knowledge of puruṣa has converged his brain software towards this clarity and now sees clearly": Here the word "this" refers back to the vision of puruṣa, which is pure because it is free from the impurities of illusions. Or, as well, it could refer to the purity of puruṣa, which clarifies the vision, which rests on him, being the subject of the meditation. Both are correct. The brain software of this yogi becomes clear-sighted.

"Serene even amidst the guṇas": That means that the higher serenity applies amidst the guṇas whereas, the lower is a serenity amidst actual things that are seen or heard. The higher includes the lower one because the guṇas are the cause of all things.

"Whose qualities are visible or invisible": In the state of the "great principle (mahat)," [that corresponds to the natural laws (2.90)], the guṇas show visible (manifest) qualities. In the state of pradhāna (guṇas in their quiet state) their qualities are invisible (unmanifest). The yogi stays serene amidst the guṇas in both states.

This yogi, the knower of puruṣa becomes someone, free from averting or accepting anything, and it will be said later (4.29): "One who does not even expect anything from his meditation, by applying correctly-discriminating cognition [reaches] a samādhi with the name "rain cloud of dharma."

Practices

Practice 1

Consider your life as a game.

Practice 2

Occasionally laugh at your higher SELF.

Beginning Samādhi

1.17

Saṁprajñāta [samādhi] is a state of unboundedness accompanied by [four] sequentially [subtler] levels of thinking: speech comprehension (vitarka), subtle thinking (vicāra), bliss (ānanda), limited "I"-consciousness (asmitā).

वितर्कविचारानन्दास्मितारुपानुगमात् संप्रज्ञातः

vitarka-vicāra-ānanda-asmitā-rūpa-anugamāt samprajñātaḥ

vitarka (m. comp.: gross thinking, consideration, reasoning) vicāra (m. comp.: subtle thinking, idea) ānanda (m. comp.: bliss) asmitā (f. comp. nom. s.: i-consciousness, identity) rūpa (n. comp.: appearance, form) anugama (m. abl. s: followed, accompanied by) saṁprajñāta (mfn.: distinguished, discerned, known accurately)

Now the results of the practices and serenity will be described. The higher versions of the brain software are installed, by practices and serenity. All higher versions have brain software version 4 as its basis. It will be described more accurately in 1.18 as *asaṁprajñāta samādhi*. It is the idle mode of the brain software, when no thinking activity occurs, while simultaneously all resources are available. Now, this idle mode can happen together with thinking activity.

It also has the name *samādhi* but depending, on which level the thinking activity occurs, there are several variations of *samādhi*.

EEG Research

Some of the brain resources support the idle mode, whereas others are busy with thinking processes. Brain resources are not limited to certain regions of the brain, but both the idle mode and the thinking processes are functioning in various information networks that can be spread across the whole brain. EEG studies on *samādhi*, transcendental consciousness, found that the whole brain is included in it. Therefore no specific region of the brain would alone be responsible for *samādhi*. The thinking processes, however, are somewhat more specialized and can be attributed to various brain regions for example during sensory perception. If someone, for example, has a visual perception with the eyes, then information travels via the eyes and the optical nerves from the back into the occipital region of the brain and then, like a wave, towards the front, while simultaneously processing of the visual information happens. In *samādhi*, together with this wave, the *samādhi* network is activated in the whole brain, which is present, like the silence of the deep ocean, together with the wave.

Each level of thinking permeates all levels depicted above it. *Vicāra* "subtle thinking" permeates *vitarka* (logical thinking and verbal associations). *Ānanda* (happiness) permeates *vicāra* and *vitarka*. *Asmitā* (limited "I"-consciousness) permeates *ānanda*, *vicāra,* and *vitarka*.

Each thinking level is permeated by *samādhi* and exists simultaneously with the total silence of *samādhi*.

The first level (with vitarka) is the gross experience of the material thing in the brain software. The second is subtle thinking (vicāra) if the experienced item is subtle. Happiness means delight. I-ness is the feeling, to be an individual separate self.

When the thinking process is calmed down by the two described means, namely by practice and serenity, how then would one describe the samādhi following on from it? It is cognizing because it is accompanied by word meanings, subtle relationships, full of delight and I-ness. The word "accompanied" goes with each one of them. Therefore it means accompanied by the experience of the physical, the experience of the subtle, the experience of delight, and the experience of I-ness.

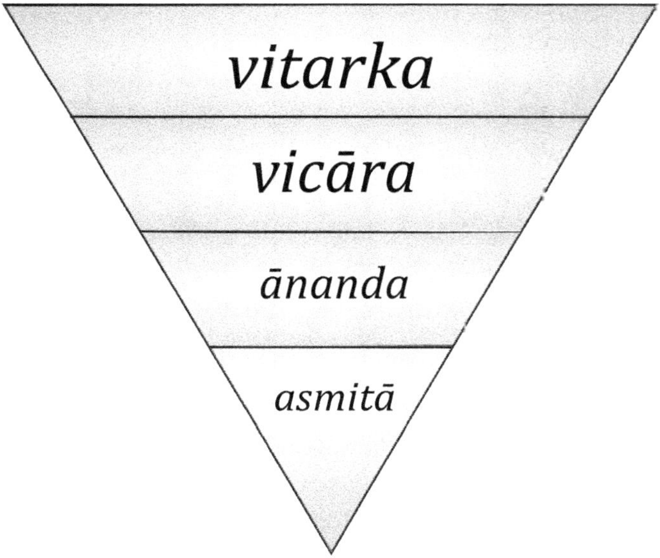

1. *Vitarka samādhi is accompanied by the word meanings. It is the experience of something physical in the brain software. The brain software adapts to the physical item.*
2. *Vicāra samādhi refers to something subtle, for example, energy flows, abstract forms, colors or sounds.*
3. *Ānanda samādhi is far subtler and described as happiness and delight.*
4. *Asmitā samādhi, "I-ness" is the mere thought, that someone has something in common with the universal SELF (ātman). Vyāsa later, in 1.36, is going to give an example: "When someone has discovered the self, that is as fine as an atom, he should be aware only of I-ness."*

Patañjali will add the I-ness (asmitā) to the illusions, when he's going to define asmitā more accurately in 2.6: "Limited 'I'-consciousness is mixing the power of the seer, the unchanging SELF and the power of the process of seeing, the intellectual activity, as if they were only one self (one identity)." How could samādhi be connected with such an illusion, like I-ness?

In other words, how can someone with the brain software versions 5 or 6 continue to have an ego?

It is a valid point, but there is no reason, why samādhi should not also permeate the form of I-ness because that is the appearance of the highest, own cause of individuality when all other things have disappeared.

Although ignorance is the basis of I-ness, it does not lead to ignorance in the thinking of the yogi. That means the yogi, the absolute silent user, no longer allows becoming influenced by his brain software.

For example in the application of the telepathy siddhi (3.19, 3.20), he does not need to take on the ignorance contained in the other's thoughts. Someone who is reading the thoughts of another brain software does not become ignorant, by possible faults of ignorance in the thoughts of the other brain software, when applying the telepathy siddhi. For the yogi, it does not matter whether he observes his own or another brain software. In the brain software of the yogi, rajas and tamas are removed. Therefore he assumes thoughts like "I go" or "I am slim" to be an illusion (kleśa), which is a form of misunderstanding (viparyaya).

Tests

Test 1

Test whether you can spontaneously experience *samādhi*. Sit comfortably and close the eyes. If you can stay like that for a few seconds without any thoughts, you are experiencing *samādhi*. It is version 4 of the brain software. It will be described in detail in 1.18. To be without any thoughts means, without internal language, without pictures, without other sensory experiences, without memories, without going to sleep.

Test 2

If you can experience the silence of thoughts, *samādhi*, at least for some time, check now, whether this silence remains, while additional thoughts are there. Then this is version 5 of the brain software.

Test 3

A *mantra* is a sound that is repeated in meditation in a certain way (1.28). In a *mantra* meditation you can identify several levels of the silence of *samādhi* as follows:

- *Vitarka*: In addition to the silence, the mantra still sounds like a word, or there are verbal thoughts of word meanings with it.
- *Vicāra*: In addition to the silence, there are vibrations, pictures, forms or colors.
- *Ānanda*: In addition to the silence, there is a feeling of happiness.
- *Asmitā*: In addition to the silence, there is a warm glow.

1.18

If one has practiced the thought of stopping before, a residue of saṁskāras remains – that is the other [samādhi].

विरामप्रत्ययाभ्यासपूर्वः संस्कारशेषोऽन्यः

virāma-pratyaya-abhyāsa-pūrvaḥ saṁskāra-śeṣaḥ anyaḥ

virāma (m. comp.: cessation, termination) pratyaya (m. comp.: thought) abhyāsa (m. comp.: practice) pūrva (m. nom. s.: before, former, prior, preceding) saṁskāra (m. comp.: impression) śeṣa (mn. nom. s.: residue) anya (mf(ā)n.: the other)

Asaṁprajñāta samādhi (without any excitations) is the other *samādhi*, where all the thinking processes (*vṛttis*) are calmed down. That means the brain software behaves as if it was switched off. *Asaṁprajñāta samādhi* is the fifth kind of *samādhi* that differs from the previous group of four (*saṁprajñāta samādhi*). *Asaṁprajñāta samādhi* is also called transcendental consciousness. We call it brain software version 4. This version corresponds to the idle mode of the brain software that means it is without thoughts or sensory perceptions, only conscious of itself.

> In this idle mode, the brain software has all its resources available but does not use them. Subjectively it is a state of conscious silence.

Brain software version 4 is wakefulness without any thought activity. The perception of time and space are unbounded and unmanifest. That is different from sleep, where there are still thoughts of nonexistence (1.10).

Stopping means to stop. The composite word thought-of-stopping (virāma-pratyaya) means: Stopping and the thought of it; the form of the thought simply is "stopping," therefore it is called thought-of-stopping. It continues to have the form of thought at a time where the thoughts come to a halt. When the thought comes close to the final stopping and just before it has completely stopped to be any thought at all, it is like a flame. It becomes smaller and smaller while using up its fuel, yet goes on to be a real flame until, in the end, it is merely ashes.

The words "If one has practiced the thought of stopping before" show the relationship to the practice. The words "a residue of saṁskāras remains" explain the state. The result, "the other," follows on from the practice and means the state wherein only saṁskāras remain, whereas the vṛttis are no longer there. It is the samādhi without items that is different from the item-related samādhi which was defined in the previous sūtra.

Asaṁprajñāta samādhi is a state of the brain software in which all the thinking processes have stopped, and only *saṁskāras* remain. The *saṁskāras* in this state are inactive malware programs. This state is empty of any item of experience. It means that nothing but *saṁskāras* remain when the brain software has withdrawn from the thoughts of things. This practice ultimately leads to a state, where the things are as if absent. *Śaṁkara* at this place points to a more advanced state, the *nirbīja samādhi*:

When the brain software without any further support has almost reached pure being, when this happens, it is called nirbīja samādhi which is going to be explained in 1.51.

Nirbīja samādhi is the seedless *samādhi* that means all the seeds for further activities, i.e., the malware programs, are erased. If, however, malware programs are still residing in the brain software, to be activated later, then we refer to it as rest of *saṁskāras*. The nature of *asaṁprajñāta samādhi* is the way it has been described: Although it is silent, it could be interrupted any time by malware.

Levels of Activity of Brain Software Versions 5 and 6

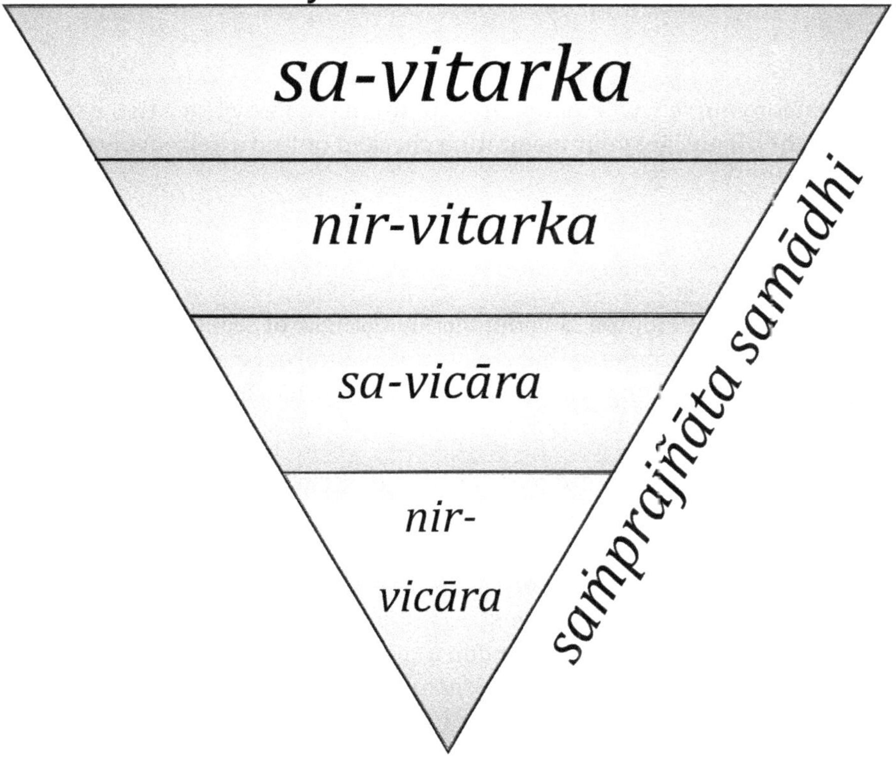

asaṁprajñāta samādhi

EEG of Brain Software Version 4

The brain software version 4 today already can be identified in the brain waves (EEG). It contains very simple brainwave patterns that include the whole brain. The brain communicates intensively in this state, but this cannot be fixed to a pattern in a certain region or partial regions. During thought activities, however, special regions of the brain are activated. If the brain software version 4 runs together with thought activities, we call it version 5. This state with its four varieties has been discussed already in 1.17.

Test

Test for yourself, whether your meditation regularly leads to the silence of thoughts. If not, get your meditation checked or find a better way to meditate.

Practices

Practice 1

In *mantra* meditation, a spontaneous thought of stopping occurs with the letting go of the *mantra* that means not by internal words like "stop" etc. The thought of stopping is an innocent letting go, like forgetting, to think.

Practice 2

The technique of *mantra* meditation is described as follows: Thinking a *mantra*, a word's sound, which increasingly refines and thus increasingly calms down the brain software. Following on from that is the brain software version 4, which corresponds to the *asaṁprajñāta samādhi*. The *saṁskāras*, which we have called malware, stresses, or seeds are calmed at this moment. The right technique for a *mantra* meditation should be learned from a good and experienced teacher. *Mantras* apart from the calming down, do have side effects, so one should not take any arbitrary word as a *mantra* (1.28).

Practice 3

If you cannot yet experience the silence from thoughts regularly, then do the practices 1.21 up to 1.41 because the ability to have silence from thoughts is the basis for all other practices. It is a very important point because all the following practices are based on it.

1.19

[Asaṁprajñāta samādhi] arises from birth in the videhas (the unembodied) and in the prakṛtilayas (nature beings).

भवप्रत्ययो विदेहप्रकृतिलयानाम्

bhava-pratyayaḥ videha-prakṛti-layānām

bhava (m. comp.: from birth) pratyaya (m. nom. s.: caused, cause) videha (m. comp.: without a body) prakṛti (f. comp.: subtle material cause, nature) laya (m. Gen. p.: absorbed)

Videhas are beings without any physical body, who live in heavens due to an excess of *sattva guṇa*, but who are still mixing up the *sattva guṇa* with *puruṣa*. Some religions call them gods, some angels, Arch Angels, etc. The higher beings and those absorbed in *prakṛti* (nature beings, nature spirits, elementals), still have something to accomplish, i.e., to recognize *puruṣa* in the relative, that means to install brain software versions 7 and 8. Although the unembodied carry *saṁskāras* with them, they stay nearly liberated (brain software version 6), because, as soon as their *saṁskāras* ripen, they subordinate under their liberated, heavenly ruler and in this way, escape the influence of the *saṁskāras*.

So far everything sounded fairly scientific; why are we now starting to talk about heavenly beings?

The Quantum Physics of the Phenomenon of Heaven

Astronomy and physics have explored the space of the universe both in the direction of the largest as well as in the direction of the smallest. The largest visible extension of the universe according to today's level of knowledge is 13.8 billion light-years (= 10^{26} m). The smallest divisible length unit of the universe is 10^{-35} m; it is called the Planck length.

10^{-35} m is a mathematical expression for a negative exponent that means 0.000...1 with 34 zeros to the right of the decimal point, which means, it is a very small number. "m" simply stands for meter.

10^{26} m, on the other hand, is a very large number, consisting of a 1 followed by 26 zeros. This is the diameter of the visible universe.

Elementary particles

All the elementary particles discovered so far are divided into two classes, the so-called bosons, and the so-called fermions. The bosons are force particles; the fermions are matter particles. They differ essentially in as to how they behave in groups. Another criterion is their smallest possible size. The bosons can have effects down to a size of 10^{-35} m. In contrast to that, the smallest fermions cannot extend their range to anything smaller than 10^{-19} m. It applies both to electrons as well as quarks. Therefore there exists a limited spatial range between 10^{-35} m and 10^{-19} m, where the forces of the bosons can create effects, but the material fermions have no access to that at all.

The bosons have the quality, to vibrate always at the same energy level. Whenever a new boson joins a group of bosons, they adjust their energy levels until all of them can coherently vibrate together.

The fundamental tendency of fermions is quite different. Fermions always require energy levels differing from all other fermions. Each one must uniquely different from the others, which means it must have its own distinct energy level. When 1000 fermions come together, each one takes its separate place on the energy scale. They also tend towards the formation of hierarchies. Wherever there is a fermion, it does not allow any other fermion to be there. That is a fundamental quality of matter. If a spatial element is already occupied by matter, no other matter particle can come there. If it tries anyway, a fight occurs, and the one matter particle pushes away the other. Here is the fundamental cause of the laws of collision in physics.

Manifest, but not material

This all-permeating range, which follows the internal laws of empty space (*ākāśa*), permeates the whole universe and allows a huge variety of nonmaterial information. It permeates all matter, all energy, as well as the total space of the universe. It ranges across a magnitude of 16 powers of ten in one dimension and 48 powers of ten in three dimensions.

For example, if the smallest of those length units, the Planck length were 1 m long, then the largest of those units that cannot be influenced by matter, would have the diameter of our galaxy, the Milky Way, which contains about 300 billion stars.

In other words: In each of the three dimensions, a magnitude of 16 powers of ten of the smallest length units permeates the nonmaterial space of, for example, an electron. The electron cannot enter into these finer ranges of space because its structure cannot be subdivided below 10^{-19} m; and yet there is a huge variety of nonmaterial space elements in that finer range.

Space as a cosmic network

The nonmaterial space elements, of course, are not only at the position of the electrons but everywhere in the universe. According to the theories of loop quantum gravity, they form a cosmic network. This cosmic network ranges in the space filled up by a single electron lengthwise across 16 powers of ten and volume-wise across 48 powers of ten. Only bosons have access to this range, finer than the size of the electron; fermions have no access.

Vedic description of the phenomenon of heaven

The Vedic literature uses a pictorial language to describe natural laws. Heaven is assumed to be the home of the gods. The gods feel very good there. They only have to fight outside of heaven and, even then, only with the so-called demons. The demons have no access to heaven, but they like to fight, both with the gods and amongst themselves.

Parallels between the Vedic description and quantum physics

Coherence is the fundamental quality that the Vedic literature ascribes to the gods in heaven. They tend towards harmony and coherence.

Heaven would then be the range from 10^{-35} m to 10^{-19} m. There only the bosons can reside and can exchange finest energies amongst each other.

See the graphics on the next page.

The main quality of the demons in Vedic literature is to fight. The main quality of the fermions also is the mutual fight, to dispute their position over and over again.

However, there is a restriction for the fermions, and that is exactly this range of sizes from 10^{-35} m to 10^{-19} m. The fermions cannot get there, simply because they are too large or too gross. Therefore in this range, the gross laws of fermions (demons) do not apply, but rather only the fine, harmony generating laws of the bosons (gods). This area that can be accessed only by the gods, but not by the demons, in Vedic literature is called heaven. Seen physically, it is this finest range of space from 10^{-35} m to 10^{-19} m. In this finest range of space, information exchange can occur without any physical matter but in harmony with the corresponding laws of the bosons. The fermions, however, have no access to this range. They are, so to say, refused at gate 19.

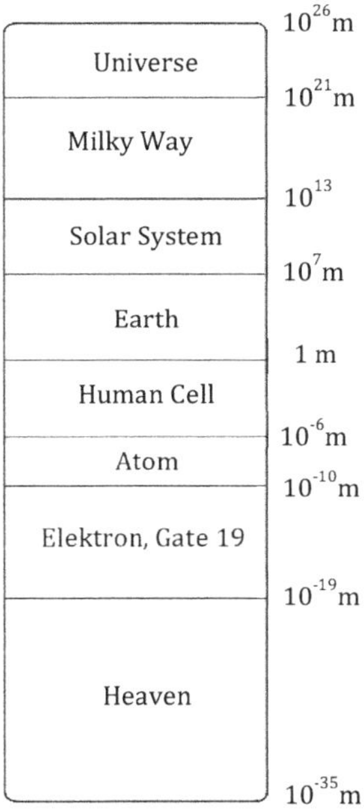

Heaven is Everywhere

With this perspective, the heavens are, therefore, not a special place in the universe, but rather a finer level of the space that permeates the whole universe and in this way is the playground for a huge variety of nonmaterial energy flows and communications.

Let us consider again the smallest volume that can be taken up by a fermion. Expressed in numbers that would be 10^{48} volume units (Planck volumes), that are available for the bosons, for example, available to a light particle, whereas the fermions, for example, electrons in the same range occupy only one spatial element. This huge variety of the finest physical ranges of space is that what we call heaven.

Universe-Computer

The universe-computer has all the information available about these finest, nonmaterial ranges of space. The amount of this nonmaterial information in the form of bosonic energy vibrations, therefore, is 10^{48} times more than what the whole material universe could store. To make that even clearer, it is

1.000.000.000.000.000.000.000.00.000.000.000.000.000.000.000.000

times more information than what the total material universe could contain. This information store is also known as the *ākāśa* Chronicles.

Cosmic software

However, now that communication flows can occur between various space elements, in principle, there can also be software, which gives a pattern to the information flows. Within the 10^{48} space elements per electron volume, there can be very many information flows. These are occurring physically by the so-called vacuum fluctuations. There, in the shortest possible time, up to 10^{44} virtual particles per second are generated and destroyed in each of the smallest space volumes. Overall, this is so well balanced – a quality of the bosons – that it appears as transparent, inconspicuous, empty space. Extended to all the universes, this is the hardware of the universe-computer.

The Power of the Universe-Computer

If the virtual, bosonic waves of the vacuum fluctuations were not balanced, but rather acted like fermions, each cubic centimeter of space would have the mass-energy of 10^{93} grams available. That would be 10^{38} times more than the space energy of our total universe. Thus you get an idea of the power that the universe-computer controls. With the appropriate software, it can completely easily let a new universe pop-up and also dissolve it again, or it could do this for a few thousand or a few billion universes.

The evolution of the gods (videhas)

Now, having described the heavens from a scientific point of view, we return to *Śaṁkara's* commentary.

The gods, free of any material body, experience, to a certain degree, this seeming liberation through the mental, nonmaterial experience of their positive saṁskāras.

There remains a task in their software, which in this case is not a brain software, but similar to distributed computing runs in the space of the whole universe.

The God of the oceans, for example, uses the total water body of all oceans, rivers, lakes, etc. as his hardware. His software then expresses through the information flow within this water hardware. It happens mainly through pressure waves, ions, and water memory. Any sufficiently large, organic, natural system that has, similar to the neurons in our brain, many mutually communicating components, tends towards intelligence. It is the software of these *videhas* (gods), we are discussing here, which expresses the one cosmic intelligence (*Īśvara* 1.24). It is exactly this software that physics calls universally applicable natural laws.

Although the videhas experience a state of seeming liberation, this applies only as long, as their software does not again get whirled up by the power of their task. They transcend this state when the saṁskāras that have caused it stop ripening.

It is similar to the prakṛtilayas (nature spirits), that have united with nature (prakṛti).

Their hardware can consist of partial aspects of nature. For example, there are nature spirits, who are ruling over a river, a mountain, and an air jet or similar natural phenomena. They also are the users of software, which operates in these limited space ranges. They too, like the gods have reached a seeming liberation.

The samādhi is twofold: (1) The result of methods, or (2) the result of birth. The first one is reached by methods and is for the yogis. Although the bodyless gods, in reality, are yogis, this method refers only to those beings that are currently in yoga training, which starts with self-control in 2.29. Their samādhi is reached on the path from trust to strength and memory (1.20).

The bodyless gods use the eight elements of *prakṛti* (nature) instead of bodily hardware. Their software then runs on the information networks of the eight elements, which are earth, water, fire, air, space, cosmic mind (*manas*), cosmic intellect (*buddhi*), and cosmic ego.

Due to the nonmaterial experiences of their saṁskāras, the rest of their saṁskāras, which have come about by inapt practices and serenity, they experience, to a certain degree, a state of seeming liberation. But when, by transcending the sattva guṇa, the saṁskāras that have caused it, stop ripening, then they also throw away these positive saṁskāras.

Regarding the prakṛtilayas who have entered into nature, there is still one task to be accomplished that is to gain the knowledge of the difference between sattva guṇa and puruṣa. Therefore, in this state, their software limits their experiences to a seeming liberation from the saṁskāras, as it is with the gods. This liberation lasts as long as their software does not again start whirling by the power of their task. Their additional task is, to gain knowledge (vidyā) of the difference, as long as they experience this seeming liberation.

Experiences
On this topic see the experience report of *Jaigīṣavya* in 3.18.

1.20

For others before [asaṁprajñāta samādhi] comes trust, strength, memory, [saṁprajñāta] samādhi and intuitive knowledge (prajñā).

श्रद्धावीर्यस्मृतिसमाधिप्रज्ञापूर्वक इतरेषाम्

śraddhā-vīrya-smṛti-samādhi-prajñā-pūrvakaḥ itareṣām

śraddhā (f. comp.: trust) vīrya (n. comp.: strength) smṛti (f. comp.: memory) samādhi (m. comp.: state of restful alertness) prajñā (f. comp.: intuitive clear knowledge) pūrvaka (m. nom. s.: previous, predecessor) itara (mf(ā)n.: for others, residue)

Here the milestones on the way to the un-excited *samādhi* are presented. "Others" means humans or heavenly beings as well, who are in the *yoga* training. Trust regarding the practices protects from doubts. Trust leads to strength and, with this, to an enthusiasm for the training. With strength, the memory in the brain software becomes stable, and *saṁprajñāta samādhi* follows. From this, arises intuitive, clear knowledge of how things really are. From this, in turn, then arises *asaṁprajñāta samādhi.*

Strength concerning brain software corresponds to a stable power supply in a technical computer. The stabilizing of the power supply is an essential requirement for the fault-free functioning of the memory. Only when the memory in a computer works faultlessly, the software can run in a stable way.

For the yogis, whose unexcited samādhi (asaṁprajñāta samādhi) is not there from birth, but rather has to be achieved by a method, it follows on from trust, strength, memory, saṁprajñāta samādhi and intuitive knowledge (prajñā). Trust is clarity of the brain software regarding the attainment of liberation and regarding that, which the yogi has heard about the methods for liberation. It is like the clarity of water after applying the kataka nut, which traditionally purifies dirty water. Like a good mother, trust protects the yogi. It defends him against animosities. If he has this trust and searches for knowledge, that means when his goal is the right vision (saṁyag-darśana), the strength and enthusiasm for the yoga practices increase. When the strength has increased, his memory becomes steady and his recall of things, like the scriptural knowledge (pramāṇa 1.7), becomes very good.

When his memory remains stable, his brain software is undisturbed and stays focused in samādhi. In the brain software in samādhi, extremely clear intuitive knowledge (prajñā) comes about, which has the power to enlighten anything. Vyāsa explains it further: "By which he knows how things really are." The yogi knows how such things, as the SELF (ātman), really are.

"From performing these practices": As mentioned before, from practicing the thought of stopping, comes the vision of the SELF "ātman" and from this the serenity amidst all thinking processes. That is the higher serenity (1.16), and from this comes asaṁprajñāta samādhi.

Here, therefore, the method of 1.18 has been explained in detail.

Test

When you are practicing a *yoga* method, you can use the milestones from this *sūtra*, to check up on your progress. If, for example, you have practiced the *siddhis* of chapter 3 regularly for a month and never achieved *samādhi* and intuitive knowledge, you can be sure that you have not gone beyond the initial stages. Then it is time, to check your method, or to change it. Maybe, you are not taking it easy enough. Serenity is very important to success.

The Methods of Calming

1.21

[For those] with intense striving for [samādhi], [it is] near.

तीव्रसंवेगानामासन्नः

tīvra-saṁvegānām āsannaḥ

tīvra (mf(ā)n. comp.: extreme, intense, excessive) saṁvega (m. Gen. p.: vehemence, intensity, high degree, desire for emancipation) āsanna (m. nom. s.: near, in reach)

Those who have an intense striving to improve their brain software will have a faster download of the upgrades. The milestones of trust, strength, memory, [*saṁprajñāta*] *samādhi*, and intuitive knowledge (*prajñā*) from the previous *sūtra* can be achieved faster with more intensive striving. With intensive practice the result is near, that means imminent. The next *sūtra* is going to explain the differences of intensity of the striving.

Practice

Are you striving intensively, to use the best brain software quickly? If yes, you are correctly exercising this first *yoga* practice. If not, some things may be improved.

1.22

Resulting from a mild, medium, or intensive [striving] there is also a difference [regarding the closeness to asaṁprajñāta samādhi].

मृदुमध्याधिमात्रत्वात्ततोऽपि विशेषः

mṛdu-madhya-adhimātratvāt tataḥ api viśeṣaḥ

mṛdu (mf(u,ī)n.: mild, weak; n. nom. acc. s.: mildness) madhya (mf(ā)n. comp.: medium, middle) adhimātra-tvāt (mfn. abl. s. : excessive, intensive, strong) tataḥ (ind.: due to that) api (ind.: also) viśeṣa (m. nom. s.: difference, degree)

The more intensively someone strives for it, the quicker he attains it. The striving for liberation, in the end, must be let loose, but first of all, it must be there.

To evaluate the progress of your striving for liberation, here are some definitions of terms:

- The six steps of progress for each *yoga* practice are called *sādhana*. They have been enumerated in 1.20 as trust, strength, memory, *saṁprajñāta samādhi*, intuitive knowledge (*prajñā*) and *asaṁprajñāta samādhi*.
- The methods, meaning healing methods, are called *upāya*. They are classified according to their effectiveness as mild, medium or extraordinary. A yogic method always consists of practice and serenity.
- The approach of the *yogi* is called *upakrama*, and it can be done in a lazy, medium, or intensive way.
- The progress of the *yogi* in reaching *samādhi* additionally depends on his *saṁskāras*.

Yogis are of nine kinds according to the methods they follow: mild, medium, or extraordinary; and according to their approach: lazy, medium, or intensive. A soft method can be practiced with lazy, or medium, or intensive striving; the same applies to the medium methods. For those, who practice the extraordinary methods, sūtra 1.21 says: "[For those] with intense striving for [samādhi], [it is] near."

With intensive striving, the methods can be soft, medium or extraordinary and therefore, there is another distinction. For the soft-intensive it is near; for the medium-intensive, it is nearer; for the extraordinary-intensive yogi, who is practicing extraordinary methods, samādhi and the fruit of samādhi are nearest.

Even amongst those intensively striving yogis, there are differences in the speed of their progress, depending on their saṁskāras, which have been generated from previous practices, possibly in previous lives. For the best amongst them, reaching of samādhi is within their grasp.

The purpose of the sūtra is, to strengthen the enthusiasm of the yogis for their methods (practice and serenity). Just as in the world, he who runs the fastest race wins the prize. But then also an enthusiastic mood should arise in all of them, and that is why the commentator Śaṁkara makes clear that all yogis, no matter whether slow or fast, will reach the desired goal. Otherwise, those with slow progress may become fearful or despair due to strenuous efforts or tiredness unless they are told, that the goal can be reached.

Is this the only way in which samādhi can be achieved quickly, or are there also other methods?

Practice

Check the mental techniques for their effectiveness, by getting information about them. Also get an indication of the time, it may take until you achieve results and what exactly these results should be. Do not hesitate to be specific, so you do not waste too much of your precious time. It applies more so when you are going to practice a method regularly for a long time, possibly for years. The milestones for it are described in 1.20. A method has reached its goal if it leads to the absolute silence of *asaṁprajñāta samādhi.*

1.23

Or by attention to Īśvara [samādhi is achieved].

ईश्वरप्रणिधानाद्वा

īśvara-praṇidhānāt vā

īśvara (m. comp.: Supreme Being) praṇidhāna (n. abl. s.: focus on, orientation towards, attention) vā (ind.: or)

By connection of the quantum computer to the universe-computer, the brain software can go into its idle mode. The universe-computer brings the functions of the quantum computer to perfection, helps to erase the remaining malware, and accomplishes all the rest.

Who is *Īśvara*? What does attention to *Īśvara* mean?

The *saṁskṛt* word *Īś* means master, ruler. The word *vara* means the best. "*Īśvara*" therefore means, the best ruler. We have identified *Īśvara* with the universe-computer.

Here now is a scientific explanation. The empty space is also called vacuum. However, it is not completely empty, because it contains the so-called virtual vacuum fluctuations. This finding has ultimately led to the evolution of quantum physics. The zero point energy in a vacuum, first of all, is infinitely large and can be calculated as a finite value only by a so-called renormalization. The vacuum energy emerges from the addition of all vacuum vibrations starting from the smallest space ranges of 10^{-33} cm. The summated energy value is extraordinarily large, namely 10^{107} Joules per cm^3, to be specific. One cm^3 is a volume approximately as large as the front piece of your thumb. The approximate energy converted into mass, amounts to 10^{93} grams per cm^3. Compared to this, the total mass-energy of our universe is only 10^{55} grams. That means that the vacuum energy in 1 cm^3 of space is 10^{38} times more than the weight of the whole universe with its billions of galaxies where each one contains billions of stars, most of them larger than our Sun. Therefore 1 cm^3 of vacuum contains in an unmanifest form

100.000.000.000.000.000.000.000.000.000.000.000.000 times more mass-energy than our universe. Fortunately, we do not notice that at all. The measurable, therefore manifest, part of this energy is merely 10^{-9} to 10^{-11} Joules in a cm^3.

A fantastic force is at work here, restraining those gigantic energies and balancing them to nearly perfect silence. This power we call the power of *Īśvara*. Nothing else can generate as much silence as *Īśvara*. Whereas this power could at any time create an infinite number of universes, here it does not do it, and instead, shows us the perfect silence of the vacuum. This is *Īśvara*. With attention on *Īśvara* we, as human beings, can also enjoy this perfect silence.

This power is undoubtedly present in the universe. Even while the leading physicists today do not quite understand, what vacuum fluctuations are, at least they are admitting that this phenomenon exists and that there is a gigantic difference between the theoretically calculated and the measurable vacuum energy.

We call this phenomenon the universe-computer, and like any computer, it can provide an interface that allows a user to communicate with it. This interface with the universe-computer for the sake of communication with us humans is arranged such, that we can communicate directly with a person with human qualities. That is communication at eye level. While doing this, we establish a communication connection between the quantum computer in our brain and the universe-computer. This communication functions both ways.

Vyāsa and *Śaṁkara* now comment in their old language, how to establish a connection and what results to expect.

Patañjali explains that there is another way: "Or by attention on Īśvara." Here he describes attention. It is due to devotion (bhakti) that Īśvara bends down to him and rewards him. Īśvara comes at eye level with him, and due to his grace, he gives to the yogi, who is completely devoted to him, according to, on what the yogi has meditated. The grace is effortless, due to the mere omnipotence of the Highest. Due to this grace of Īśvara, samādhi and its fruits are quickly attainable and within one's grasp. Who is this Īśvara, who is neither pradhāna nor puruṣa?

Practice

Experience the perfect silence of *Īśvara* by directing your attention to *Īśvara*. Thus you are creating a connection between your brain software and the universe-computer.

Practice 1

In practice you can realize it like this: Consider the universe-computer like an all-knowing and loving person, to whom you can talk. Simply begin a talk as if you would meet for the first time at a festival. Introduce each other, and thus you begin to talk. *Īśvara* can appear to you in any form you would like to see him. That is, as it were, the interface to the universe-computer. He adapts to you. In that way, you can talk, talk in your thoughts then you can listen, as in normal speech, to his answers and then react again from your side with another thought. We also call this the "inner dialogue." We recommend to you, at least in the beginning, to write down those talks, ideally written by hand. Therefore, take an empty paper notebook and dedicate it to the talks with *Īśvara* or the universe-computer. It is quite simple.

What is important in this context, that you really listen in silence and do not keep babbling. While this listening refines more and more, with it, you are directing increasingly finer attention to *Īśvara*. Thus automatically silence emerges, which is the desired result.

It is a form of devotion (*bhakti*). You are giving your brain software completely to the omniscient one so that he – using the speech center in your brain – formulates his answers. You are giving up your complete individuality to perceive the answer. Then, always take the first thought as the answer. The universe-computer works infinitely fast. The human intellect, however, sometimes tries to improve on something. You can confidently forget this, or cross it out. You may recognize the intervention of the intellect, in that it always takes a bit longer than the universe-computer. Therefore filter this out and take the first thought as an answer.

Do a check to see, that you really have *Īśvara* at the other end of the communication line. Ask, "Who is there?" If you get anything but the absolutely blissful *Īśvara* for an answer, you know that you have the wrong connection. Then switch off and dial again; for example: Speak in a low voice, three times: "*Īśvara, Īśvara, Īśvara.*" Then ask, "Who is there?" It should be *Īśvara*. Do not be afraid, *Īśvara* is not offended when you try to establish the communication channel clearly. It is very important that you establish the channel, such that you can trust it. You may also get an identification sign, a visual, auditory or tactile experience, to show you each time that it really is *Īśvara*.

The answers of the universe-computer often arrive not only in the form of texts but also as multimedia knowledge, feelings, pictures, movies, physical experiences, prickling under the skin or in the body. A clear indication that the answer really comes from the universe-computer is the following: It always is somehow uplifting, very pleasant, very intelligent, and happy or in some other way, something very special. That is an indicator of the authenticity of an answer from *Īśvara*.

Do not be afraid in any way, that you could insult *Īśvara*; you can do your dialogue without any inhibition, whatsoever. No question would be taboo. The dialogue is happening between you and *Īśvara*. You do not need to show your notes to anyone else. Therefore, do speak about anything that is important to you, about your important life topics and you will be amazed. But it does not mean, that you are allowed to talk only about important topics.

Should you have any doubts, whether or not, this dialogue can work at all, or whether it is useful, then you can, at any time, clarify these doubts through the same method of the inner dialogue. You have complete control of the process. Therefore it is no mental disturbance, none at all. With practice, it becomes clearer, and you can use this tool of the inner dialogue at any time in your daily life.

Practice 2

When you have gained some experience with practice 1, you start to become quite clear about what it means, to direct your loving attention to *Īśvara*. You get to know, how to direct your attention in complete silence. What bliss!

Practice 3

For those who want to learn all the details of this communication with the omniscient, we recommend the excellent books of Susan Shumsky. She has explored this communication for many years and writes about many things to take into account when communicating like this; especially how to establish a fault-free communication channel.

1.24

Untouched by illusions, actions, results, and stores of karma [but] distinct from puruṣa is Īśvara.

क्लेशकर्मविपाकाशयैरपरामृष्टः पुरुषविशेष ईश्वरः

kleśa-karma-vipāka-āśayaiḥ aparāmṛṣṭaḥ puruṣa-viśeṣa īśvaraḥ

kleśa (m. comp.: illusion, affliction, source of pain) karma (m. comp.: deed, action inclusive thinking and talking) vipāka (m. comp.: ripening, maturing, fruits of actions, effect, result, consequence of actions) aśaya (m. ins. p.: storage) aparāmṛṣṭa (mfn., m. nom. s.: untouched) puruṣa (m. comp.:) viśeṣa (m. comp.: different, special) īśvara (m. nom. s.: Supreme Being)

Ignorance, limited "I"-consciousness, longing, hate, and the survival instinct are the illusions (kleśas), from which arise good or bad actions (karmas), which lead to merit (punya) and guilt (pāpa) as a result. That is the law of karma. Merit and guilt are ripening and depositing their corresponding impressions (saṁskāras).

Merit and guilt cause one or several births (jāti) in certain families, giving rise to the quality of life, long life (āyus) and experiences (bhoga). The circumstances of life are manifested according to their corresponding impressions (saṁskāras). The storing of merit and guilt and their subsequent "ripening" causes the storage of malware in the brain software. In a suitable environment and with suitable circumstances, these then get activated and influence thinking with their patterns. Simultaneously the corresponding disruptions and stresses originate in the physiology.

Īśvara, however, is not influenced by merit or guilt, and therefore not by saṁskāras. Īśvara is more than the finest relative (pradhāna = three guṇas in their resting state) plus the absolute (puruṣa).

Īśvara is a person, to whom you can talk.

The results of actions are stored in the brain software, but they are attributed to puruṣa because he is the experiencer of the results. As with victory or loss, which are events on the battlefield, which are attributed to the ruler. Untouched by such experience is Īśvara, who is different from puruṣa.

Who is this Īśvara, who is neither pradhāna nor puruṣa? There is no proof for Īśvara in the sāṁkya Scriptures, and one would like to have a proof for Īśvara, that he really exists, and as well, what the special nature of Īśvara is, who necessarily is not directly perceivable. Patañjali answers these points in the sūtra: "Untouched by illusions, actions, results, and stores of karma [but] distinct from puruṣa, is Īśvara."

Then, is he one of those who have achieved their liberation? Are there not many, who have done that? No, untouched by such experience is Īśvara, who is different from puruṣa. Others have achieved liberation by cutting their three bondages, but for Īśvara such bondages never existed and are never going to come. But Īśvara is eternally free, eternally Īśvara. This eternal perfection is of perfect sattva.

The sūtra says that Īśvara is different from puruṣa. The puruṣa of Īśvara has no quality of divine power because power belongs to brain software/nature software/knowledge software. Īśvara's transcendental power (śakti) must be connected to a perfect software. This eternal perfection of Īśvara comes from his perfect sattva. The software always is on the level of power and therefore exists, where there are differences. The perfection is in possession of the powers of omniscience and omnipotence, eternal and transcendent.

In this context see our explanation of the huge information store (*ākāśa* Chronicles) in 1.19, explaining the basis of omniscience, and why control of the huge energies of the vacuum fluctuations in 1.23, is the basis of this omnipotence.

The relationship in the form of mutual cause and effect between the divine source of perfect sattva, and perfection, and transcendental knowledge is eternal. Because this relationship is eternal, "he is eternal and always Īśvara and eternal and always free." This leadership is one without a second or anything higher. Now Vyāsa explains, how the power of Īśvara is unsurpassed: First of all, it is not surpassed by any other power because whatever power would surpass it, would be it. If there were any power, that would surpass the power, we are explaining, it would be the power of Īśvara. There is no power equal to him because perfection is unique.

Where the peak of power is reached, there is Īśvara, and no power can be equal to his. Why not? Because there cannot be two kings in one kingdom and also because there cannot be one king in two kingdoms, and thus Vyāsa explains: Assuming, there would be two equal Īśvaras, then one of them could not enforce his will without superseding the will of the other. If both of them would want to have the same thing, then not both of them could achieve it. There would be a battle about the superiority regarding the desired thing. Therefore he has unsurpassed power and is unsurpassed, and he only is Īśvara, and he is distinct from puruṣa.

Īśvara's power originates, viewed scientifically, from the control of the vacuum fluctuations. They are ending at 10^{-35} m because there is no subtler space. Beyond this manifest space, there exists only the intuitive knowledge of *nirvicāra samādhi*. Given that *Īśvara* possesses all knowledge, he also has all power. He is manifesting this power from the subtlest space elements, both in heaven, the nonmaterial space of the universe (10^{-35} m to 10^{-19} m), as well as in the earthly range, the material space of the same universe (10^{-19} m to 13.8 billion light years).

1.25

In him [Īśvara] [is] the seed of unsurpassed all-knowingness.

तत्र निरतिशयं सर्वज्ञबीजम्

tatra niratiśayam sarvajña-bījam

tatra (ind.: in him) niratiśaya (n. nom. Akk. s: highest, unsurpassed) sarvajña (mf(ā)n. comp.: all-knowingness, all-knowing) bīja (n. nom. Akk. s.: seed)

That extends the definition of *Īśvara*: the one with the perfect knowledge. *Īśvara*, the universe-computer, possesses all knowledge. By accessing the universe-computer, the brain software from version 6 has access to all knowledge.

Any certain knowledge, whether past or future or present, or any combination of these, or of extrasensory perception, regardless of whether this knowledge is small or big, is the seat of all-knowingness.

The seat of all-knowingness today we would call the set of all sets. This set automatically unfolds in a SELF-dynamical process, because the set of all sets must contain itself and therefore can never be limited in any way. The SELF-dynamic is expressed with the term "seed."

He, in whom this seed of all-knowingness grows increasingly, is unsurpassed. The seed of all-knowingness reaches the highest because it is something that has increments like anything measurable. He, Īśvara, in whom knowledge reaches the highest level, is all-knowing and is different from the absolutely silent puruṣa.

In our considerations here we are drawing inferences, and as with any inference we can only derive general results, but not any special examples. This special knowledge about him, his names and such things, one should search for in his Holy Scriptures.

What is unsurpassed in him? "Every certain knowledge." Whether from perception or inference, from past, future, or present or a combination of them, or what is beyond the senses. It means, because past and future belong to that which is beyond the senses, all these perceptions are called extrasensory. Extrasensory perception is threefold: in the areas of the subtle, the hidden and the remote. Well-known limited knowledge, whether it is small or big, can grow, because it has increments. That also applies to the seed of all-knowingness, similar to the knowledge of the smoke which is the seat of the knowledge of fire.

That means from knowledge of the smoke (*pramāṇa* knowledge 1.7) grows knowledge of the fire (*prajñā* knowledge 1.48).

He is all knowing, in whom the highest level has been reached. It is said: "in whom," because knowledge dwells in a knower. Therefore, quietly a knower is implied and the knowledge is in this knower. Similarly, it applies to power. It has increments, and it grows; and he, in whom the limit has been reached, is all-powerful, is omnipotent. Thus it is clear, that there exists one actor, who controls the creation, sustenance, and destruction of the world. He, in whom this power is greatest, is the highest Īśvara (parama Īśvara). Due to this perfection, he has no faults, like a misunderstanding (viparyaya), which would lead to powerlessness.

Following is a discussion, where *Śaṁkara* answers the objections of his students.

(Objection) If it were like that, then Īśvara, as well would be the perfection of ignorance (ajñāna), which would grow, until perfect, where it reached its limit.

(Answer) It is not like that because ignorance is opposite to knowledge and these two opposites cannot appear together in one single being, because there, where knowledge prevails, ignorance is impossible. Where the light increases, the darkness can only decrease.

(Objection) The opposite should also be true.

(Answer) Not so, because if there is light, we do not see darkness. If the darkness is there, it gets removed by light, but if the light is there, it can never be removed by darkness. Even in the rainy season, when the Sun does not shine, when clouds cover it, this is merely a shielding of the vision. The light is not removed, as is the case with darkness. Therefore the ignorance cannot exist, when knowledge increases, as darkness cannot exist in the Sun, the manifest cause of knowledge is sattva which always completely supersedes the other two guṇas, which are rajas and tamas. Additionally, there cannot be an increase of ignorance because its subject has no real substance, whereas there can be a growth of knowledge, whose subjects are knowable facts; if ignorance had a knowable subject, then it would be knowledge.

(Objection) One could say that ignorance has reached its perfection in inanimate things.

(Answer) That cannot be called perfection, but rather a complete absence of knowledge. If there was perfection in ignorance, then a thousand repeti-

tions of ignorance could not be removed by one instance of knowledge. Otherwise, knowledge would have to appear in the same amount, to remove the ignorance. Therefore ignorance due to its essential nature cannot be perfect.

Anything that can grow does grow until it has reached its limit. And therefore the seed of all-knowingness can reach the highest limit. All things together and individually are the direct perception of someone, because they are perceivable, for example, jars, etc. That is so, because things, for which people are searching, can be known, as when they are looking for jars. Also, the Earth is something generated because it has parts like jars.

The Earth has been created by one individual, who knows all living beings, their karma and their specific ways of life. He has provided the world as an appropriate place for them, so that they experience this, like someone who builds a palace, so that people can live in it. The Earth has been created by one, who knows, what should be experienced by the many living beings, like for example rice and barley. These examples show that the living places for all beings, the Earth with its mountains and rivers has been crafted by one single master craftsman and adapted such, that those who live on it, may have their appropriate experiences.

The Sun has been created by one knower, who has the power, to control the light that gets shared by many living beings, because his essence is the essence of the light. The path of the Sun, the rising and setting at certain times, is ordered by the one, who knows its purpose because it goes according to fixed times and in this way determines farming activities. The path of the Sun, planets, Moon, and stars is controlled by one intelligent Īśvara because without him it would be difficult to obey fixed times, such as those kept by punctual students or servants.

The waxing and waning of the Moon are controlled by one single knower, who knows the times of the lunar months etc., which exist as an accurate distinction of the subdivisions of time like on a clock. The Moon has been created by one, who knows these subdivisions of time because its waxing and waning are controlled to the minute.

The world has one single master who is intelligent as it is with many groups of living beings, who all have their elected leader and in spite of opposing tendencies, the whole tribe has one single leader, to be followed.

Additionally, there must be one being, who supervises the whole variety of professions with all their tools and goals, as in war, where mutually opposing or converging interests subordinate under one purpose. There must be supervision, because so many things have to be observed, as in the exercising of a profession. This is, what we are emphasizing.

It conforms to our view, that there is one single software, that controls all natural laws and all details of the universe, as it were the operating system of the universe.

Everything is simultaneously supervised because there are mutual relationships between many things and it is also well known, that these relationships are of different sorts. All powers are supervised by one, because they are individual items, as jars are items. If there is no block, then anything physical is perceived by someone, because there is a relationship to the qualities of each item, similar to the sound that is heard, when someone smacks while eating.

From our modern view today we envision it in this way: All material things contain fermions, mostly electrons, and quarks. They are completely recognized by the omnipresent, bosonic vacuum fluctuations. Vacuum fluctuations are the fundamental vibrations of space. Bosons transmit forces such as light particles, the so-called photons. The nonmaterial bosons can differ from the material fermions, and be active in far smaller regions of space and therefore permeate every material thing completely with an information content of 10^{48} bits per fermion. These are one billion*billion*billion terabit. All this happens above the Planck length, therefore on a manifest level, based on the *guṇas*. *Īśvara's* knowledge exceeds this because he owns complete, unmanifest knowledge beyond the *guṇas* of *rajas* and *tamas*, on the level of *nirvicāra samādhi* (1.47, 1.48).

Everything is known by someone due to the fact, that it can be known. In the absence of obstacles, that means in empty space, ākāśa, everything is known by someone, insofar as everything is connected with everything else, just as the actors performing a drama are connected to each other.

The all-knowing Īśvara is free from the world jungle (saṁsāra) because he is all-knowing and has no ignorance; insofar he is like a liberated SELF. He is free of illusions etc. because his knowledge is unobstructed; insofar as he is like a yogi with siddhi abilities knowing all.

Due to his freedom from ignorance, which prevents illusions, certainly, he has perfect knowledge of every item, without the channel of the senses, for example, the eyes. The all-pervading software of the highest Īśvara is simultaneously in contact with every item and therefore can perceive everything because there is no reason why it could not perceive the totality of all things.

That is precisely what we call the universe-computer. His hardware is the vacuum fluctuations that perceive everything. He is the unified field that comprehends the whole universe, unified on all levels, from the finest to the grossest, knowing all space elements and all vacuum fluctuations happening in them, all energy, matter, waves, and particles. His software governs the whole universe using natural laws. The individual natural laws thereby are the sub-functions of the total software, governing via the unembodied or the nature spirits, their partial range of nature. In 1.19 it has been discussed, how these beings are also striving for the highest knowledge and liberation.

Additionally, solid forms are no obstructions to Īśvara, no more than by space, because his software is in contact with all things. As there is an infinity of things, there is an infinity of their appearances, their disappearances, of memories and goals. But this software of Īśvara is like the light of the Sun because it transforms itself into all forms.

Īśvara, the universe-computer is a quantum computer, whose hardware consists of *sattva guṇa*. He is not obstructed by any superimposed illusions, which would originate from contact with unrighteousness (*adharma* 4.3). The human quantum computer also consists mainly of *sattva guṇa*, and therefore can also perceive and be present everywhere, however, it depends on the sense organs, which impede its actions by obstructions, like *adharma*.

A lamp, for example, when placed in a perforated jar, illuminates its environment shining through the open holes in its cover. The same lamp, however, illuminates everything, when its cover is broken. Likewise the sattva of Īśvara, that is untouched by the covers of illusions, etc., perceives absolutely everything at all times because there could be no reason to suppress the perception of any one thing.

Given that everything is the item of perception of Īśvara, the whole world (all universes) must have one Īśvara, and also because there are many items, which require a protector like it is known regarding a kingdom.

The wise ones have taught the performance of duties, according to the education, the living standard, etc., with their corresponding actors, experiencers, actions, education and associated results. They are to be done by those, who search results or by those, who are afraid of erring. It is the same with the application of medical remedies. The teachings are like medical prescriptions since they are taught for the well-being of others. Educated people rely on them, and also they deal with things, the normal person would not guess unless he was taught.

The body and the sense organs have been created for only a single goal by someone who knows all their goals because they are means of bringing about certain actions and situations.

Sensory organs and organs of action are instruments. Everything, therefore, has certain effects, serves the purpose of the human experiencer and is the means for experiences like the jar that allows the light from it, to emanate through the individually crafted openings. Those are the actual reasons for the origin of the sensory and organs of action.

The Earth is perishable. It is a medium size, and it can be destroyed in various ways. It is the basis to have experiences, with forms, which are means to generate the results of experiences. It has many regions, some of them are high some are deep, some are filled up some eroded, some burnt, some split up.

Things like the body that consists of earth and other elements are perishable because they have the power to destroy each other mutually with weapons. On another level, there is space with its qualities of creation and destruction that is different from puruṣa. It supports things like jars, which can be perceived by the external sensory organs.

With a fundamental understanding of the physics of the finest regions of space, one can recognize, that all matter and energy is nothing but transformed space. It does not change anything, therefore, whether the concept of strings is introduced as an intermediate step, or whether energy and matter originate directly from the loop quantum gravity of space. In both cases the manifest appearances, whether they are bosons or fermions, are nothing but excited states of the space field. We are going to examine this in more detail in *sūtra* 2.19 in the context of *tanmātras* and *mahābhūtas*.

Thus it is clear, that there is one highest Īśvara (parameśvara), whose power, knowledge and superiority are unbounded.

Orderliness in the world

How does the orderliness in the world materialize? Quantum physics ultimately explains it based on statistical mean values of individual, seemingly independent quantum events. All visible phenomena of orderliness in nature can be reduced to these statistical means. In a slit experiment with light, for example, individual events appear on the photographic plate, which are seemingly not connected in any way. However, like magic, these appear at certain places with a certain probability. The probability can be accurately calculated, but not the individual event.

Therefore, in this case, the student who was discussing here with *Śaṁkara* would claim that this was simply the nature of things. *Śaṁkara*, however, insists that every orderliness must have a reason.

Therefore, in the case of slit experiments, there must also be a cause, which leads to this exact probability distribution. This cause is *Īśvara* with his natural laws, which for us are nothing but the software of the universe-computer that takes effect from the finest regions of space, the Planck volumes, caused by the unmanifest *nirvicāra* knowledge of *Īśvara*. That software in this way controls the exact probability distribution of all quantum phenomena and thus upholds orderliness in the whole universe.

(Objection) That can also come from their nature.

(Answer) That is not right, because it is obvious, that the orderliness in the world is connected to the goal, to provide experiences of the results of dharma (virtue) and adharma (vice). Therefore the orderliness controls the effects on the actor. Thus, the orderliness in the world is not merely natural, because it has a purpose, namely to provide experiences for living beings, as in the orderliness in a palace. The movements of Sun, Moon, and stars are not only natural because they are similar to movements of us humans.

(Objection) Let us say, that our activities are natural as well!

(Answer) No, because in that case, it should always be the same, as the heat of fire. The heat of fire (energy) is natural and is a fixed real measure, which does not desire any advantage for itself because there is no person. A creation, however, is the result of an action and there is a desire to achieve something for oneself due to a special cause. Therefore it is not natural.

(Objection) It has been said that the desire for a certain purpose is natural, in the case of those who are building large houses.

(Answer) If there were this natural behavior, then there would be the natural desire for a certain cause in creating the Earth, etc., as this desire for humans, to create a large house, etc. Then this difference in the expression would create no trouble because there would be a dependence of the action on the actor. In other words, wherever there is an action there also must an actor. By this, the objection that it was natural is refuted.

Your inferences are not credible proofs, because they oppose common experiences, oppose correct rules of inference and oppose testimonials of the Scriptures. You're not making any correct inferences because they are showing nuances. Then, additionally, there are the discrepancies to the holy authorities/testimonials, written in statements like: "He, who is all-knowing" (Māṇḍūkya Upaniṣad 1.1.9) and "He is the one ruler" (Kaṭha Upaniṣad 5.12). However, they also contradict the common experience. Anyone, including cowboys and cowgirls, turn to God with names like Śiva or Nārāyaṇa [or Allah, Buddha, or Jesus], *etc., even if they have been disobedient or have been distracted by their brain software and run wildly into fields of crops. That is forbidden, and anyway they bow their heads in front of Īśvara and adore him with gifts of lotus garlands. Thereby they hope to reach their goals.*

Now follows a discussion between *Śaṁkara* and a student, who would like to prove, that there can be no all-knowing, highest ruler. *Śaṁkara* then continues to show to him, that with any measurable item, there must be one highest degree of perfection with an infinite value. Therefore there also must exist one best ruler, and this ruler must also have the highest perfection of knowledge. We would like to spare you this lengthy and logically very complicated proof. Instead, we would like to explain to you, how in today's language and with today's understanding of natural science, we imagine the best of all rulers.

Space-memory

As we have mentioned before, physics has located the smallest possible space region. That is the Planck volume, corresponding to a three-dimensional cube with an edge length of 10^{-35} m, in each direction. Here it is irrelevant, whether the grid consisting of these smallest space elements is cubic or tetrahedral or whether it has the form of any other platonic body or that of any other structure.

What is essential, is that these smallest space elements can momentarily function as a memory. That happens if they support for a certain, very short time vacuum fluctuations or if they function as a spin network as postulated by loop quantum gravity – one of the approaches to a unified field theory. That applies if they can hold information in the form of spins. A spin essentially is an abstract angular momentum of an elementary particle. In loop quantum gravity, however, it is considered as something more fundamental that can hold information at certain locations in space and can move that information to other positions in space. Thus we have the essential conditions for a computer system, which is to store information at specific space elements, and additionally to transmit that information to other space elements. The number of available space elements in space is significantly larger than with any matter-based arrangements like chips, molecules, atoms, etc.

Deficiency of unified field theories

It is our opinion that seen exclusively from the viewpoint of physics the theories of the unified field cannot be fully grasped. Why? It becomes very clear, considering the science of chemistry, that all chemical processes ultimately can be traced back to quantum physics phenomena. In spite of that chemists continue to use their chemistry specific notations and formulae, to quantify chemical reactions, to make them measurable and then, to control them with engineering methods. If chemical engineers would exclusively use unified field equations, they would never arrive at practical solutions.

Another example is the field of electronics, especially digital electronics. Admittedly all electronics is based on physics, especially on the electromagnetic field. However, no electronics engineer would formulate and solve the electromagnetic field equations for complex circuitry. Here other additional knowledge is required, which does build on electromagnetism but also supersedes it. In digital electronics, the information processing is accomplished on an abstract level. The same principles of information processing can be applied to a variety of physical systems and, therefore, are not limited to electromagnetism. Software utilizes even more stages of abstraction beyond electromagnetic waves, which are only used as information carriers.

Computer extension of field theories of physics

With the same methods of abstraction, which digital electronics applies to the electromagnetic field, we succeeded in a further step of abstraction. We applied this method to the finest level of the manifest universe, the empty space. Thus we could discover the universe-computer hardware in empty space and describe the best of all rulers (*Īśvara*) as the user of the cosmic software, which is an expression of his power (*śakti*).

Additionally, one should consider, that the universe-computer software and hardware do not work in a dualistic fashion, but rather always appear as one unity. We have already mentioned that this concept of unity is used in today's computer technology in the form of FPGAs or memory based computer systems (see the section "Brain Software Changes the Physiology" in the introduction). In this way, the software can flexibly rearrange its hardware the way it requires it. The hardware no longer contains any individualization, but individualization is a direct effect of the software. Similarly, it happens with empty space, which also does not contain any individualization, yet it can transmit information waves within its spin network. Applied to the universe-computer, this means that *Īśvara*, using his cosmic software, from the material of empty space, that he has created, can generate and design anything the way he likes.

Space is a spin network

The spin networks are nothing but space (*ākāśa*) that can develop its dynamics. To make it completely clear, in this space there are yet no fields, waves or elementary particles. Initially, it is nothing but a communication network. The spin is the movable information, which can travel through those networks. The spin networks can function therefore like the hardware of a computer. We call it the universe-computer. Anything that gives a pattern to the two phenomena of information storage and information transmission, we call software.

Patterns in the spin networks are the software of the universe-computer. The spin networks are the hardware of the universe-computer. The spin networks however also consist of those patterns. Therefore there is no longer any difference between the hardware and the software of the universe-computer. It is unity. The universe-computer at its most fundamental level is unity and not duality.

Software controlled orderliness of the universe

We assume that the spin networks are not working chaotically but in an orderly manner. The orderliness originates from the software of the universe-computer. Otherwise, how could there ever arise any orderliness from the quantum chaos during the generation of matter and energy in the universe? The software of the universe-computer we equate with the power of *Īśvara*. It works on the information level of *Īśvara* with an information density of 10^{99} bits per cm^3 of space. *Īśvara's* knowledge, however, supersedes even this information density, as it is located in the space-less region of *nirvicāra samādhi*.

The spin networks of loop quantum gravity are not contained within another space, but they rather form space. Their patterns and vibrations determine the interconnection. That means the manifest software is identical with the manifest hardware. Manifest software exists on the level of manifest information, in this case of the spins, which are transmitted through the spin network.

Software methods of the universe-computer

The creation, maintenance, and destruction of the universe, then would be three different software methods of the class "universe" in the software of the universe-computer. They would be special expressions of the power (*śakti*) of *Īśvara*. In the same way, the creation, maintenance, and destruction of partial areas of the universe would be limited software regions of the power of *Īśvara*. *Īśvara's* software functions on all scales and is the first cause of all phenomena in the universe, starting from the Big Bang (if it ever happened) down to the creation, movement and elimination of all elementary particles. The same applies to all other phenomena that are scaled in between the smallest matter particles and the diameter of the universe. It is all nothing but the software of *Īśvara*, the effect of pure, transcendental *nirvicāra* knowledge of *Īśvara*, which possesses infinite organizing power.

Other physicists may use the name "unified field" for the software of the universe-computer, but we think that with our explanation in the terminology of computer science we can explain, what is happening, in a more intelligible way.

Īśvara's unmanifest knowledge base

Nevertheless, *Īśvara* has also an unmanifest knowledge base on the level of *nirvicāra samādhi*, which is beyond the three *guṇas*, where sattva *guṇa* is the only measure. Pure *sattva* corresponds to the manifest power, the *śakti* of *Īśvara*. His infinite, pure knowledge on the level of *nirvicāra* even transcends this level of power. On the other side, also it does not because he is unity and not duality and therefore his power is inseparable from his pure knowledge.

Practice

Due to *Īśvara's* possession of the seed of highest all-knowingness, utilizing an attentive communication with him (1.23) any knowledge whatsoever can grow from this seed. Utilizing the inner dialogue (1.23) connect your brain software to the universe-computer and with this open up access to all knowledge. Practice this inner dialogue fairly often, do it regularly, and write it down in your paper notebook. These records are very valuable to read later. A hint for the records: Mark your contribution with one symbol, for example, a dash, and the contributions of *Īśvara* with another symbol, for example, a circle. This clear distinction between the two communication partners of the inner dialogue is already an application of the "correctly-discriminating cognition," one of the most important practices of yoga that will be explained in detail in 2.26.

1.26

He [Īśvara] is even the teacher of the previous [teachers], unlimited by time.

स पूर्वेषामपि गुरुः कालेनानवच्छेदात्

sa pūrveṣām api guruḥ kālena-anavacchedāt

sa (m. nom. s.: he) pūrva (mn. Gen. p.: [idam-eṣam] previous [pūrva]) api (even, also) guru (m. nom. s.: teacher) kāla (m. ins. s.: time) anavaccheda (m. abl. s.: unlimited, unbounded, unboundedness)

He is the very first teacher. The access to the universe-computer, *Īśvara*, just cannot be replaced by anything, not even by a seemingly all-knowing teacher on Earth. Any teacher on Earth also would have the universe-computer as his teacher. Even a holy tradition of masters has the universe-computer as their first teacher.

The first teachers were there at a certain time. But for the best ruler (Īśvara), who is the teacher even of the first teachers, time is no measure. He is in a state of perfection at the beginning of this creation, as well as at the beginning of previous creations.

This best ruler has been described as "even the teacher of the first teachers." The first teachers are those, who taught all the methods and results for success and highest bliss. The meaning of this statement is that he creates the knowledge and the instructions which the first teachers convey. It is so, because all kinds of knowledge originate from him, like the fireflies from a fire or the water drops from the ocean.

We have mentioned, that he is the first knower because he does not depend on time. That means that he is unchangeable. Other teachers, however, are time-dependent. They are described as past or future or present. But this best ruler is the eternally free ruler, a statement which is logically derived by the other teachers and also by us.

(Objection) The perfect sattva of Īśvara is an effect of pradhāna (guṇas in their resting state), and any effect of pradhāna must be determined by time; therefore, why would that not apply to sattva? Anything but puruṣa is determined by time because puruṣa exclusively is unchangeable. You could, of course, assume, that Īśvara is not connected to sattva, as some teachings about Īśvara claim.

(Answer) No, because we assume, that he is equipped with pure sattva, which is for him of the highest level.

The *sattva* of *Īśvara* is the highest level. We equate it with the *nirvicāra samādhi* (1.47) of *Īśvara*. When it manifests in space, this happens with the highest, limited information density of 10^{99} bits per cm^3 and with the highest, limited information transfer rate of 10^{44} Hz. His knowledge manifests as information in the Planck volumes, which are memory cells with the highest information density of 10^{99} bits per cm^3. *Īśvara* generates his software from his infinite knowledge base in *nirvicāra samādhi* (1.47) and downloads it to the level of *savicāra samādhi* (1.44), where his *sattva guṇa* directs the cosmic game of all the three *guṇas*.

Īśvara's knowledge is not merely pure *sattva* in *nirvicāra samādhi* because it also has to fit in, in its manifest form, with the daily life of living beings in the universe. Therefore it manifests as information with this highest information density. The *sattva* of *Īśvara* stays on the highest level of purity and is beyond the influence of time.

(Objection) Other teachers also have the highest purity which is independent of time due to yoga and dharma. Why is it not the same with Īśvara?

(Answer) The sattva of Īśvara is pure sattva, and in it, rajas and tamas are always suppressed, such that it is independent of dharma, etc., as its cause. The knowledge of the pure sattva of Īśvara has the qualities of sattva (clarity, cognition), is time independent and enlightens all things. His power (śakti) is also time-independent because it is the effect of his knowledge. Therefore Vyāsa says: "Time as a measure cannot be applied to Īśvara." The same applies to his power.

His role as a teacher has no limits. He resides in a state of perfection at the beginning of this creation and also at the beginning of other creations. That is known from the fact of the creation of living beings; also by inferences from the Scriptures, which also predict this for future times.

The purpose of this sūtra is as follows: just as one sees that gurus are adored due to their quality as teachers of knowledge and dharma and such things, the devotee in his heart should meditate on Īśvara who is the teacher of all teachers. Those who adore him should do this with his various names, like Nārāyaṇa. Just as a human teacher turns his face to the very devoted student and gives him a favor, this highest teacher gives favor to that one who is in pure devotion to him.

"The one who has the highest devotion to Īśvara, and has Īśvara for his teacher, is a great soul (mahātman) and to him the following wonders manifest." (Śvetāśvatara Upaniṣad 6.23)

In this context see also chapter three of the *yoga sūtras* with the title "Extraordinary Abilities."

"He who works for me, considers me to be the Highest, devoted to me, free of desire or hate for anyone, he comes to me oh Pāṇḍava," (Bhagavad Gītā 11.55).

1.27

His [Īśvara's] sound characteristic is praṇava.

तस्य वाचकः प्रणवः

tasya vācakaḥ praṇavaḥ

tad (m. Gen. s.: that) vācaka (m. nom. s.: expressive, signifying, significant sound) praṇava (m.: auṁ, primordial sound, characteristics of a sound) praṇa (mfn.: old, ancient) va (mfn.: powerful, strong)

Praṇava is normally translated with *auṁ*. However, we have decided, to split the word into the syllables *praṇa* [not *prāṇa*] and *va*, which means "ancient" and "mighty." Thus, we translate it as: "The sound characteristic of

Īśvara is ancient and mighty." It describes the qualities of certain sounds, to be considered as *Īśvara's* names and therefore contains the might of *Īśvara*. The name of *Īśvara*, according to *Śaṁkara*, is inseparable from *Īśvara*. The sound characteristic describes the common structure of various names of *Īśvara*, all of them containing his power. *Yogis* have found these names and their fixed relationship with *Īśvara*, which has been there from the beginning of creation. Upon repeating these names, the power of *Īśvara* is activated. A commonly known name of *Īśvara* is *auṁ*.

Śaṁkara offers other meanings of the same word *praṇava* that are all valid. We know from *Svāmī Brahmānanda Sarasvatī*, from teaching 73 of his 108 teachings, that the effect of *auṁ*, in certain cases, can also be negative. Therefore it should not be repeated thousands of times as a *mantra* in meditation, and other traditional names of *Īśvara* should be used.

It has been said: "Or by attention to Īśvara" (1.23). In what way should one perform attention to him and what is the method for the application of this attention? The sūtra, to explain the way, in which the devotee should meditate, says: "his sound characteristic is praṇava." The expression or the expressive word of Īśvara that has been described is praṇava.

Now the various meanings of *praṇava* will be explained:

- *pra stands for prakaśena: perfect; nu (= nava) stands for nūyate: he is praised. Praṇava means that, by which Īśvara is perfectly praised.*
- *It is that which praises Īśvara; the praṇava auṁ praises (praṇauti) Īśvara;*
- *Īśvara, by this, is devotedly praised (praṇidhīyate) by his devotees.*
- *By this, they bend down (praṇam) to him and repeat this.*
- *By it, they praise (praṇidhā) Īśvara mentally; here the additional dhā replaces the ending va (of praṇava).*

Mental devotion to things that are only indirectly known happens with a word, as with the worship of the holy mountain Meru, or of Indra. It is Īśvara, who is expressed with the word. The sound of the word corresponds to its meaning.

The ending ava should be understood as avati: "he prefers." Other meanings of this word like "protection," are excluded here. He brings his devotees out of the world jungle (saṁsāra), he leads them from saṁsāra to nirvāṇa. He brings unsurpassed bliss to his devotees, grants samādhi to them to lead them to the highest truth. All these meanings are connected to the strongest love of Īśvara.

Does the power of the expression of this syllable "auṁ" originate from the agreed meaning, or is it something fixed like the relationship between a lamp and its light? The relationship of that to be expressed with its expressive word is fixed. However, common use directs attention to that which has been fixed by Īśvara. Like the relationship between father and son, it is fixed, but its common use is clarified in the form of: "He is the father of this man; this man is his son."

If Īśvara is revered in the brain software continually using this syllable auṁ, he bestows his grace. There are many holy texts like "auṁ khaṁ brahma," ("auṁ is space, is brahman." Bṛhadāraṇyaka Upaniṣad 5.1.1). "brahman is auṁ" (Taittiriya Upaniṣad 1.8.1). There are also the traditions: "auṁ tat sat," auṁ is eternal (Bhagavad Gītā 17.23), "auṁ Viṣṇu is all." (First name of the thousand names of Viṣṇu.) The grammarians are explaining, that auṁ that ends in "ṁ" is a word that does not take on any declensions.

Auṁ, therefore, is always connected to the best ruler and is his sound characteristic. It is always like that, from the beginning of creation. Therefore, *auṁ* must be the finest pattern in the software of *Īśvara*. We are locating this sound, therefore, on the Planck scale, where empty space begins to exist. The statement "*auṁ* is space is *brahman*," fits in with this understanding. The vacuum fluctuations exist within the smallest limits of space. We have already established, that they must be orderly. Otherwise, the orderliness of the universe could never have developed from quantum chaos. The finest *auṁ* vibration, therefore, must correspond to the highest frequency of the vacuum fluctuations of 10^{44} Hz. The smallest dimension that defines this *auṁ* vibration is the Planck length of 10^{-35} m. Thus these *auṁ* vibrations move in space with the speed of light c.

When analyzing *auṁ* further, it is one unit that manifests in three sounds: In *a*, in *u* and *ṁ*. "*a*" expresses the totality, that corresponds to *brahman*. The mouth, then, is fully opened. "*u*" expresses the limiting quality of totality, where the mouth is almost closed. "*ṁ*" finally is the humming point. Here the lips are closed, and there is a humming in the space of the mouth and the nose.

This analysis applied to space means that with each new vacuum fluctuation the totality of the previously present space (*a*) is concentrated (*u*) to a new point (*ṁ*). In this way, following the Big Bang (if it ever happened), the universe develops into an ever-growing space, that is permeated at each spot, by the *praṇava* of *Īśvara* and that is, ultimately, in its essence nothing but *praṇava*. Thus *praṇava* is the smallest unit in the software of *Īśvara*. It then reappears in larger space and time regions over and over again. In a medium-sized space and time region, we humans can speak or think it.

(Objection) Assuming, that Īśvara or someone else, at some time has agreed to the use of this form: "Let this (auṁ) be the name for that (Īśvara)." This fixed agreement gave the opportunity to the devotees whether they would like to revere Īśvara by auṁ as his name or by any other name. In that case would they not have used another name before that time? Why should auṁ stand out as a special expressive word?

(Answer) The relationship is "fixed as between a lamp and its light." Therefore, even upon the first hearing, Īśvara is understood, as the Sun is by its light.

(Objection) If this relationship, however, is fixed, then humans should understand it immediately upon hearing it for the first time.

(Answer) The relationship between a word and its meaning is like the relationship between that, which transmits the thought, and just the thought. Although this relationship is fixed, it is not grasped by sensory organs. The wise confirm in the Scriptures that the relationship between the word and its meaning is fixed.

(Objection) When someone has ascertained the meaning of a word by seeing its effects, he understands the relationship between them, just as the eye knows a form, which is a visual relationship.

(Answer) There is a disproof: certain knowledge originates from the mere word without any inference, and when someone has reached his goal, by cooking food in one way, what would be the use of also cooking it in another way?

(Objection) A relationship is perceived, by seeing the use of two things several times, like in the relationship between fire and smoke.

(Answer) We do not agree with that because even when it is used a hundred times, the relationship between a word and its meaning is never perceived in the same way, as the relationship between fire and smoke is perceived immediately. It is similar to a sentence and its meaning. Therefore the common use clarifies the relationship between Īśvara, who is expressed, and praṇava, which expresses him. That is a fixed relationship, as the fixed relationship between father and son. Due to the attribution of the meaning of the word by agreement, the meaning of a previously unknown word cannot be grasped upon the first hearing, just as an item in darkness is not recognized by the eye.

So, it is like this: No matter, whether seen from the viewpoint of the traditionalists, or from another viewpoint, the relationship is fixed, like that of father and son, and it only becomes apparent by common usage.

If there were no fixed relationship between this expressive word and, what it expresses, then it would not be true that by the form of praṇava the Īśvara could be met face-to-face. Similarly, it would not be right to use fire as a means for cooking if there was no fixed relationship between the raw food and that which cooks it. However, because there is a fixed relationship between this expression and, what it expresses, it is right to use auṁ as a means for the practice of adoration of Īśvara, and that is the message of the whole commentary.

Here once more is the hint to teaching 73 of the 108 teachings of *Svāmī Brahmānanda Sarasvatī*, not to use the sound *auṁ* directly as a *mantra* in silent meditation, because it is much too strong. The fundamental vibration of *auṁ* anyway is contained in all *bīja mantras*, which operate a bit more softly and more agreeably to the nervous system.

For the yogi, who has recognized the relationship between praṇava and its meaning, the next sūtra is suitable.

1.28

The repetition of that [seed] realizes that goal of [supreme all-knowingness].

तज्जपस्तदर्थभावनम्

tat-japaḥ tat-artha-bhāvanam

tad (n. nom. acc.: that) japa (m. nom. s.: repetition) tad (n. acc.: that [sarvajña n.]) artha (m. comp.: meaning, goal, purpose) bhāvana (m. acc. s., n. nom. acc. s.: accomplishing, effecting, producing)

It is a meditation practice using a sound. This sound may be more than merely *aum̐*; it may be any other *bīja mantra* with a similar sound characteristic.

Śaṁkara, at the end of his commentary, describes the meaning of *artha*, the goal, like this:

For the yogi, the highest SELF (paramātman) shines forth, which stands in the highest place (parameṣṭhin).

In this context see also 1.47: "Skill [in] *nirvicāra* lets the highest SELF (*ātman*) shine clearly," and 1.48: "The intuitive knowledge within this [*nirvicāra samādhi*] bears truth."

Śaṁkara's commentary and these two *sūtras* are important, as they underline the correct reference points of the two *tat* (= that) in the present *sūtra*. What could be the goal described with *tat-artha*? From looking at the previous *sūtras*, it can only be all-knowingness as a goal, which has been described in 1.25: "In him, *Īśvara* is the seed of unsurpassed all-knowingness." That then is the reference point for the *tat*. What is to be repeated? It is a seed (*bīja*). The *mantras* used in meditation, are also called *bīja mantras*. That means, here the repetition of *bīja mantras* is recommended. *Praṇava* does not merely mean *aum̐*, but rather the sound characteristic of the *bīja mantras*, which lead the brain software to a refinement of its thinking activity.

Far more efficient than murmuring is a mental repetition.

Repetition (japa) of the praṇava and meditation on Īśvara, who is characterized by praṇava, is in fact, the right technique. When the yogi repeats praṇava in this way and meditates on its meaning, his brain software becomes one-pointed. Thus it has been said: following the praṇava repetition he shall rest in yoga (brain software version 4); following the yoga he shall continue the repetition. Once the praṇava repetition and the yoga become perfect, the highest SELF (paramātman) shines forth.

When the yogi, has understood the relationship, in this way, between the expression praṇava and its meaning, how does he then gain the grace of Īśvara? The sūtra says: "The repetition of that seed realizes the goal of supreme all-knowingness." The practice of the repetition of praṇava, which is the expression of Īśvara, being 3 ½ time measures (mātra) long, or 3 time measures long, is called japa. The repetition happens either in thought or an undertone (upāmśu).

Meditating on its meaning: The meditation tunes the heart to Īśvara, who is the meaning, and who is brought to memory in the brain software by praṇava. The words: "He should do that," must be added at the beginning of the sūtra. Yogis who are doing both, reach one-pointedness of the brain software (3.12, 3.13).

By repeating praṇava, his brain software turns towards Īśvara, and he meditates on the meaning of praṇava, therefore on Īśvara. When his brain software no longer wanders away from the meditation on Īśvara, he should repeat praṇava in his thoughts. Repetition in the thinking process is recommended because it allows refining the meditation in an even easier way than speech repetition. The idea is that the brain software should not become attracted towards things.

"When the praṇava repetition and yoga become perfect," when he is no longer disturbed by other, opposite thoughts then he is perfect in his repetition and yoga. By this perfection of the repetition and meditation on the highest Īśvara (parameśvara), for the yogi, the highest SELF (paramātman) shines forth, which is located in the highest place (parameṣṭhin).

Practice

Regularly practice silent *mantra* meditation, at least twice a day for 20 minutes. This way, the silence of *samādhi* arrives quickly.

1.29

From that [practice comes] the mastery of inner consciousness and also the disappearance of [any] obstacles.

ततः प्रत्यक्चेतनाधिगमोऽप्यन्तरायाभावश्च

tataḥ pratyak-cetana-adhigamaḥ api antarāya-abhāvaḥ ca

tataḥ (ind.: from that) pratyak (inside, [thoughts] turned inside) cetana (m. comp.: consciousness) adhigama (m. nom. s.: mastery, accomplishment, realization) api (ind.: also) antarāya (m. nom. p.: obstacle) abhāva (m. nom. s.: disappearance, absence) ca (ind.: and, also)

Practice makes perfect. Repeating a *bīja mantra* is a scanning process, which allows the location and removal of malware. This way obstacles are removed. This scanning process can be utilized already from brain software version 3. Thus, everybody has a chance, to systematically free his brain software from disturbances, and to load higher versions.

Peculiar Fine Tuning of Natural Constants

Searching for the unified field by now for more than 60 years, no final breakthrough has been achieved, and not even a verifiable theory exists. During that search, however, something else has shown up, which is, that due to natural laws our universe may not necessarily have originated, the way it is now. Rather, there is a huge choice, to change natural constants minimally and with that to generate a completely different universe.

Some of the natural constants in this regard are very sensitive. Nothing but fine-tuning of the natural constants would create exactly this universe, which we have now. Here are some examples:

- If the expansion rate of the early universe had been different by a factor by 1 part in 10^{57}, today there would be no solar systems nor any galaxies and, instead, the universe would have collapsed right away.
- If the original density of the universe had deviated from the critical density by 1 part in 10^{60}, the universe would have collapsed already. You have to become clear about that. The universe in total has a mass-energy of 10^{57} grams, maximum. Therefore this deviation in density would mean, that the universe would have collapsed if it had had one more milligram of mass.
- If the strength of electromagnetism had been different by 1 part in 10^{40}, there would have been no stars or suns.
- If the strength of the gravitational force had been different by 1 part in 10^{100}, which means if it had differed in the 100th position to the right of the decimal point, all planets, long ago would have collapsed into their suns or escaped from their orbits. Then no life would have been possible on any planet.

Critique of the Paradigms of Unified Field Theories

All this necessary fine-tuning is hard to reconcile with the current paradigms of physics. How could one hope to achieve anything with unified field theories giving rise to so many possibilities?

Various physicists, of course, also have doubts, whether or not such fine tuning is really required. Therefore they have devised the following loopholes, to explain the phenomena:

- A future theory should be without any fine-tuned constants. But this has not been discovered. Therefore, the present-day theories are incomplete.

- The theory of the multiverse could bring relief. A multiverse, for that purpose, would contain at least enough universes, such that one of them, arbitrarily, which would be ours, could develop and support life. Somehow, this was also not quite satisfactory because, why should there be at least 10^{100} universes without any life, and ours should be the only one, that has developed life?
- Finally, there remains the theological explanation, namely that an intelligent, almighty being has done this fine-tuning of the natural constants, to create exactly the desired life. There is, however quite some critique against that from the side of scientists. They would not easily want to give back the playground to the theologians:
  - ⇨ If a creator would be powerful enough, to create life in a fine-tuned universe, then surely he also would have the power, to do this in a non-fine-tuned universe.
  - ⇨ The rational incomprehensibility of the universe, especially the fine-tuning is taken as an indicator for a creative force, but not necessarily for a creator.
  - ⇨ The applicability of statistical hypotheses is denied. Statistics altogether is denied.

Cosmic Software Solves the Problem of Fine-Tuning

We think that here we can contribute with our software paradigm. The universe, in that case, would not be the result of the most complicated, unsolvable mathematical constructs, but rather, it would be the result of a highly orderly software of cosmic range.

In computer science, for a long time, we have been aware of a similar problem. It is just far too difficult and too laborious to solve large tasks with purely analog machines. One has to use the digital principle, and digital software, or at least has to add them, like for example in the case of the neurons in the human brain. They are working in a mixed analog and digital way. Thus, the attempt of present-day physics, to think of a unified field, as it were, merely "analog," appears to us like a technology that we, computer scientists, had given up already half a century ago. That is, because it is nearly impossible, to fine-tune the analog components, and keep them fine-tuned, such that they always provide accurate, predictable results.

Alternatives for Unified Field Theories

We see it the same way for the whole universe. Therefore we suggest an alternative to the unified field theories of physics. We suggest that the whole universe consists of an information network, which corresponds to the hardware, such that any phenomenon of information transfer, energy, or matter, is nothing but the expression of software, which runs on the fundamental information network. Thus it can be explained, why natural constants seem to be so very fine-tuned and why they can achieve their results reliably.

The Software Developer and User of the Universe-Computer

The programming of the cosmic network does not necessarily happen by language constructs as in today's computer technology, but rather by vibrations, forms or sounds. Sounds (*nāma*) and forms (*rūpa*) can be transformed into each other. That is, as if, cosmic music lets the network vibrate and thus programs it. The programming changes the network or creates manifestations from the network that appear to us like energy waves or matter particles. Thus energy and matter are derived in essence, from information flows.

The software developer and user of this cosmic software would then in our view be the "best ruler," that is *Īśvara*, as pointed out in the *yoga sūtras*. He, himself would be the user of the software, not being involved in it, but he would rather observe his cosmic software, his cosmic game (*līlā*) while being separate from it. However, he could also intervene in the game and appear as an *avatāra* on any level of the software, or he could communicate with any element in the software via the corresponding communication interfaces.

The experience of communication with *Īśvara* is well known to us. The *sūtras* 3.32 and 3.33 explain in detail, how to establish such a communication channel. Look there, to read of experiences that present-day *yogis* have had already.

From this devotion to the Lord originates the realization of deep consciousness: It is aware of its intellect (buddhi) being separate, and therefore the SELF (ātman) is called a separate consciousness. Realizing it, is the consciousness of its nature, as it really is.

(Objection) Puruṣa has been realized already in anyone by the feeling "I am happy," or "I am sad." That is a well-known fact. Why is it emphasized now?

(Answer) That is true, but by these thoughts in the brain software, it is not observed as being separate. In the "I am happy," or "I am sad," the "happy" and "sad" have the same reference point that is the thought: "Here I am." Remaining in the field of the thinking processes they are, certainly, merely thoughts of ignorance.

The yogi understands: Īśvara (the best ruler) is a puruṣa, free of the stains of illusions, etc. and therefore brilliantly clear, and therefore self-contained (kevala), without the three guṇas, and therefore beyond evil, without the three kinds of suffering, a perfect being, who is the observer. Therefore also this, my puruṣa, is pure, radiant, and alone, beyond evil and the observer of the brain software.

There is a difference between the Lord and the individual selves (kṣetrajña) because they are, different to the Lord, subject to bondage and liberation, and because pradhāna also serves their purposes (first experience and then liberation). Due to those reasons, the kṣetrajñas are different.

In this situation, what are the obstacles? They are that, which distracts the brain software. What are they and how many are there?

Practice

... makes perfect.

1.30

Illness, stubbornness, doubt, negligence, laziness, greed, confusion, failure to attain stages of development and instability in maintaining a state, cause mental distractions; these are the obstacles.

व्याधिस्त्यानसंशयप्रमादालस्याविरतिभ्रान्तिदर्शनालब्धभूमिकत्वानवस्थितत्वानि चित्तविक्षेपास्तेऽन्तरायाः

vyādhi-styāna-saṁśaya-pramāda-ālasya-avirati-bhrānti-darśana-alabdha-bhūmikatva-anavasthitatvāni citta-vikṣepāḥ te antarāyāḥ

> *vyādhi (m. comp.: disease) styāna (n. comp.: apathy, stubbornness) saṁśaya (m. comp.: doubt) pramāda (m. comp.: negligence) ālasya (n. comp.: laziness) avirati (f. comp.: immoderateness, greed, incontinence, intemperance) bhrānti (f. comp.: confusion, false opinion, perplexity) darśana (n. comp.: vision, sight) alabdha (Adj. comp.: lack of achievement) bhūmikatva (f. comp.: level of development) anavasthitatva (n. nom. acc. p.: instability in achieving a level) citta (n. comp.: brain software) vikṣepa (m. nom. s.: distraction) tad (m. nom. p.: those) antarāya (m. nom. p.: obstacle)*

Here, very clearly, the unwanted mental effects of malware (*saṁskāras*) are illustrated.

1.31

Pain, discomfort, body tremors, irregular breathing out and breathing in [sighing, gasping, panting] appear with a mental distraction.

दुःखदौर्मनस्याङ्गमेजयत्वश्वासप्रश्वासाः विक्षेपसहभुवः

duḥkha-daurmanasya-aṅgamejayatva-śvāsa-praśvāsāḥ vikṣepa-sahabhuvaḥ

duḥkha (n. comp.: pain, sorrow, trouble, difficulty) daurmanasya (n. comp.: discomfort, despair) aṅgamejayatva (n. comp.: trembling of the body, loss of control) śvāsa (m. comp.: [irregular] breathing out, sighing) praśvāsa (m. nom. p.: [irregular] breathing in) vikṣepa (m. comp.: distraction, confusion, perplexity) sahabhuva (m. nom. p.: accompanying)

Those are the bodily symptoms that occur with any of the previously mentioned mental symptoms.

1.32

The practice [is to be applied on] one principle [at a time], to prevent those [mental distractions].

तत्प्रतिषेधार्थमेकतत्त्वाभ्यासः

tat-pratiṣedha-artham eka-tattva-abhyāsaḥ

tad (n. nom. acc. s.: that) pratiṣedha (m. comp: prevention) artha (mn. acc. s., n. nom. s.: aim, purpose, motive, cause) eka (mfn.: one) tattva (n. comp.: principle, entity) abhyāsa (m. nom. s.: practice)

Those principles will be explained in the following *sūtras*. Do not mix up the principles, choose only one at a time, to avoid distractions.

The search process for malware in the brain software must be simple, such that it cannot be disturbed by possible effects of the malware. Therefore one principle at a time should be used. This simplicity brings effectiveness.

Practice

If you notice during your practices, one or several of these phenomena of 1.31 or 1.32, then you are trying to achieve too much at once. Take it easy. Continue your practices, but in smaller steps. Thus you avoid distractions.

1.33

Applying the feelings of friendliness, compassion, happiness, and indifference respectively to the happy, the suffering, the virtuous and the vicious calms the software in the brain [and heart].

मैत्रीकरुणामुदितोपेक्षाणां
सुखदुःखपुण्यापुण्यविषयाणां
भावनातश्चित्तप्रसादनम्

maitrī-karuṇā-muditā-upekṣāṇāṁ sukha-duḥkha-puṇya-apuṇya-viṣayāṇāṁ bhāvanātaḥ citta-prasādanaṁ

maitrī (n. comp.: friendliness) karuṇa (m. comp.: compassion) mudita (f. comp.: happiness, delight) upekṣāṇa (n. Gen. p.: indifference) sukha (n. comp.: happiness) duḥkha (n. comp.: pain, discomfort) puṇya (n. comp.: meritorious, virtuous, auspicious) apuṇya (mfn. comp.: vice, impure, wicked) viṣaya (Gen. p.: with regard to these objects [end of a compound], object [of experience]) bhāvanā-ta (m. nom. s.: cultivation, evolution) citta (n. comp.: brain software, mind) prasādana (n. nom. Akk. s.: cleaning, calming)

Friendliness is, for example, one of the previously mentioned principles, which should be applied one at a time. This *sūtra* recommends, in dealing with people, to show only a specific behavior:

- Friendliness towards happy beings

- Compassion towards the suffering
- Happiness towards the virtuous
- Indifference towards the vicious

Those exercises calm the brain software because they do not require any unnecessary thinking processes for optimal social behavior. The perceived suffering of the world no longer depresses the *yogi,* and with his clear intellect, he can efficiently help. The result is true serenity, instead of a mere mood making.

Practice

Apply this to all your social contacts. You will notice, that your life becomes far simpler. Thus, more silence comes into your life.

1.34

Also [calming] by exhaling or retention of the breath.

प्रच्छर्दनविधारणाभ्यां वा प्राणस्य

pracchardana-vidhāraṇābhyāṁ vā prāṇasya

pracchardana (n. comp.: exhaling) vidhāraṇa (n. ins. dat. acc. d.: retention) vā (ind.: or) prāṇa (m. Gen. s.: of the breath)

Practice

In case you are tense, if you breathe out strongly to a natural halt, your brain software will calm down. Many people do this exercise quite spontaneously, for example after they have solved a difficult task. They breathe out, let the shoulders droop, and for a short moment relax. A similar effect arises when you hold your breath for a moment.

1.35

Also by researching an item of attention [and] staying [with it] continuously, a fascination arises calming the input-output component (manas) of the brain software.

विषयवती वा प्रवृत्तिरुत्पन्ना मनसः स्थितिनिबन्धनी

viṣaya-vatī vā pravṛttiḥ utpannā manasaḥ sthiti-nibandhanī

viṣaya (m. comp.: sensory object, object of attention) vati (f. nom. p.: begging, asking [focused on sensory objects]) vā (ind.: or) pravṛtti (f. nom. s.: advance, progress, moving onwards, cognition) utpanna (f. p-participle Nom. s.: arisen, born, produced) manas (n. gen. acc. s.: input output component of the brain software) sthiti (f. fixed) nibandhanī (f. nom. acc. s.: bond, binding)

Subtle (refined) perceptions fascinate the input-output component (*manas*) and calm it down because during that time the search for other pleasant things stops.

Practice

Examples are viewing nature, beautiful art, hearing beautiful music, viewing *mandalas* and *yantras*, etc. Not every film or music belongs to this category. It is important that it does create a calming effect.

1.36

Also, the suffering is ended by bright inner light.

विशोका वा ज्योतिष्मती

viśokā vā jyotiṣmatī

viśoka (f. nom. s.: end of suffering) vā (ind.: or) jyotiṣmatī (f. nom. s.: shining, bright inner light)

Here, there are two interpretations on how to overcome obstacles:

- Experience of inner light
- Intuition from *jyotiṣ* knowledge

> *Gaṇeśa* helps, to remove obstacles. *Gaṇeśa* spoke: "I am the Lord of jyotiṣ, I am the Lord of the *grahas*, I am *brahman*. Do you get it now? "

Vyāsa: "When someone has discovered the self, that is as fine as an atom, he should be only aware of the I-ness."

Practice

When this experience of light spontaneously appears, simply enjoy it.

1.37

Also [by focusing on] a brain software user who is free from longing for sense objects.

वीतरागविषयं वा चित्तम्

vīta-rāga-viṣayam vā cittam

vīta (mfn.: disappear) rāga (m. comp.: attraction, binding, longing, passion, love) viṣaya (m. acc. s.: sensory object, object of attention) vā (ind.: or) citta (n. nom. acc. s.: brain software, mind)

That means, users of brain software versions 7 and 8, also *Īśvara*, the one with the highest knowledge, whom we call the universe-computer. Users are also *devas*, the highest, personalized forms of expression of natural laws. They are the software components of the universe-computer.

Practice

Do this in a way that fits in with your belief system. The devotion or attention to a personification of the divine gently leads you into silence; the same applies with devotion and attention on spiritual masters who are free from longing.

1.38

Also [calming by] realizing the knowledge of dreaming and deep sleep.

स्वप्ननिद्राज्ञानालम्बनं वा

svapna-nidrā-jñāna-ālaṁbanam vā

svapna (m. comp.: dream) nidrā (f. comp.: deep sleep) jñāna (n. comp.: knowledge) ālambana (n. nom. acc.: support, to hold onto) vā (ind.: or)

That means, a calming effect occurs by the knowledge of the nature of dreaming, being a state full of light and the knowledge of the nature of deep sleep, being an experience of a peaceful, infinitely expanded state: "I" know, that I have slept well. See, in this context, the introduction, where we have also researched the topic of the "ego." Pure consciousness in a deep sleep brings about a calming of the brain software and is a clear indication of cosmic consciousness that means of brain software version 5.

Practice

Enjoy the waking up phase, and realize what happened during deep sleep. During the waking up phase scan through your dreams from your memory, before you forget them again. In doing so, do not focus too much on the content, but rather on the phenomenon of dreaming. All this leads to a further calming of the brain software.

1.39

Also by dhyāna on any proper, revered item.

यथाभिमतध्यानाद्वा

yathā-abhimata-dhyānāt vā

yathā (ind.: similarly, properly) abhimata (mfn. comp.: dear, revered, imagined) dhyāna (n. abl. s.: meditation, dhyāna) vā (ind.: or)

Sūtra 1.35 now is deepened, to become a meditation on a revered item. *Dhyāna* can be translated as "meditation," however, the precise definition of this term follows in 3.2.

> Attention to proper items calms the brain software.
> Proper is that, which calms.

Practice

Now the meditation becomes deeper with revered items, beings, thoughts, etc. The criterion, whether they are proper, is in their calming effect on the brain software. In this context, there could be a calming effect on you when you stroke your cat.

1.40

Mastery of [dhyāna] [ranges from] the smallest to the biggest [items].

परमाणु परममहत्त्वान्तोऽस्य वशीकारः

parama-aṇu parama-mahattva-antaḥ asya vaśīkāraḥ

parama (mf(ā)n.: extreme) aṇu (ind.: minutely) mahattva (n. nom. acc.: greatness) anta (m. nom. s.: end, border) asya (m. n. gen.: his; belongs to idam) vaśīkāra (m. nom. s.: mastery, power)

The meditation object of *sūtra* 1.39 can take on any size, from the smallest size unit, the Planck length ($1.6 * 10^{-35}$ m), up to the full extension of the visible universe (13.8 billion light years).

The items of attention in the previous *sūtras* have become more and more general. It started with yourself (1.21, 1.22) and the all-knowing (1.23 to 1.27), the sound of the all-knowing (1.27 to 1.29), fascinating things (1.35), revered things (1.39), and now here they are revered items of any size. In the next *sūtra,* the phenomenon of attention (*samāpatti*) will be defined accurately and, as well, applied to any item.

Practice

Expand your meditation to arbitrarily small or big items that you like. By this, the silence in your brain software becomes ever more stabilized.

Experience

My next practice was, to discover the molecular structure of my rose. It proved unusually easy, probably because I had no preconceived idea or image to latch onto. I briefly put my attention on the molecular structure then I surrendered myself to the process, and small blobs of red appeared along with white sticks. Once again it was difficult to describe, but interestingly, when I looked up the structure of a rose on the internet, there they were, white, cylindrical rods joined by small red balls.

1.41

Attention (samāpatti) [means]: Just as a clear crystal takes on the color [of its environment], [brain software] with calmed thinking that rests on the perceiver, the perception process, or the perceived, takes on their qualities.

क्षीणवृत्तेरभिजातस्येव मणेर्ग्रहीतृग्रहणग्राह्येषु तत्स्थतदञ्जनता समापत्तिः

kṣīṇa-vṛtteḥ abhijātasya iva maṇeḥ grahītṛ-grahaṇa-grāhyeṣu tatstha-tat-añjanatā samāpattiḥ

kṣīṇa (mfn.: weakened, diminished, reduced) vṛtti (f. abl. gen. s.: thought process) abhijātasya (mfn.: born, of noble descent, flawless, transparent) iva (ind.: like) maṇi (m. abl. s. gen. s.: of a crystal) gṛhītṛ (m. comp.: perceiver, observer) grahaṇa (n. comp. s.: process of perception) grāhya (n. Lok. p.: the perceived, observed) tatstha (mfn.: staying in, remaining in) tad (n. nom. acc.: that) añjana-tā (f. nom. s.: suffix tā = quality of X, X-ness, principle of a coloring) samāpatti (f. nom. s.: attention)

A clear crystal is like a lens or prism in an optical instrument, which causes a projection of the environment.

Samāpatti is attention. The clear crystal corresponds to the brain software. The color of the environment corresponds to the perceiver, the perception process, or the perceived. Attention is there, once the brain software is calmed down and no longer creates any disturbing patterns. *Samāpatti* will be used again in *sūtra* 3.42 (levitation *sūtra*) and therefore should be studied very carefully.

With the automatic disappearance of the *vṛttis*, the brain software becomes as clear as crystal. It comes to rest at the same time and then rests on one of the three components of perception. Then it transmits, undistorted, depending on the focus, the chosen component to the perceiver. Thus, there are three possibilities:

- Perceiver → brain software → perceiver
- Perception process → brain software → perceiver
- Perceived → brain software → perceiver

The transmission is no longer disturbed by the *vṛttis*. The five *vṛttis* are *pramāṇa* (correct knowledge), *viparyaya* (misunderstanding), *vikalpa* (imagination), *nidrā* (deep sleep), *smṛti* (memory). See 1.6.

All those *vṛttis* (thinking processes) are calmed down in a correct *samāpatti* practice. The *vṛttis* refine and dilute up to their most perfect, infinite status. There is no effort required. Brain software version 5 becomes activated by this attention practice. The following *sūtras* describe brain software version 5 on four levels.

Practices

Practice 1

Observe an item in front of you and stay with your attention at it for half a minute, completely relaxed, with your attention to the item. Practicing this, you will notice, how your brain software calms down.

Practice 2

Repeat practice 1 for about one minute. You should not get distracted by the clock; it does not need to be timed to the second. If there are distracting thoughts or memories about the item or similar items, simply ignore these and come back to the item. Anyway, do not strain. It all must be very easy. You can see the result of the practice in the calming of your thinking processes. Complete attention is reached, once there is complete calmness while viewing the item.

Practice 3

Now repeat practice 2 with the same item and, while your eyes see the item, direct your attention to the observer, that means to yourself. Again you will discover deep silence. Probably you also will notice a subtle difference between practices 2 and 3. The perception differs, when the attention rests on the item, or when it rests on the perceiver.

Practice 4

Now, repeat practice 2 with the same item and direct your attention to the process of perception, which means, the way, the light beams emitted from the item, travel through your eyes, reach the receptor nerve cells, and the nerves in your brain and then become processed in the brain. Again, come into deep silence. With this variation, again you will notice a somewhat different perception.

Summary of the practices

All these practices are the best preparation for obtaining good results with the *siddhi* techniques in chapter 3. If you do not quite achieve a state of rest with the attention practices, then you are missing the experiences from practices 1.21 to 1.40. By practicing these, the nervous system must first be cleansed, so that it can come to rest. Specifically, we recommend regular meditation practice.

Stabilised Samādhi

1.42

There [in samāpatti] mixed with [mental] speech, knowledge of its meaning, and imagination [vikalpa] [is] savitarka [gross] samāpatti.

तत्र शब्दार्थज्ञानविकल्पैः संकीर्णा सवितर्का समापत्तिः

tatra śabda-artha-jñāna-vikalpaiḥ saṁkīrṇā savitarkā samāpattiḥ

tatra (ind.: there, in that) śabda (m. comp.: speech, sound, word) artha (mn. comp.: meaning, purpose) jñāna (n. comp.: knowledge) vikalpa (m. Instr. p.: by imagination) saṅkīrṇa (f. adj. nom.: mixed) sa (ind.: together with) savitarka (mfn.: accompanied with thought or reason) samāpatti (f. nom. s.: attention)

Those three, speech, knowledge of its meaning, and imagination are the perceived. *Vitarka* was mentioned briefly in 1.17, here, now is the complete definition. The prefix *sa* means "together with." Therefore, *savitarka* means a state of attention, together with *vitarka*.

On this level, the brain software deals with grammar, dictionary, meanings, and pictures associated with words and sentences. This mode of operation of the brain software occurs in version 3, and also in the higher versions 5 to 8.

1.43

Purified from memory, in its own form, as if empty, the complete goal appears. It defines nirvitarka [samāpatti].

स्मृतिपरिशुद्धौ स्वरूपशून्येवार्थमात्रनिर्भासा निर्वितर्का

smṛti-pariśuddhau svarūpa-śūnya-iva-artha-mātra-nirbhāsā nirvitarkā

smṛti (f. comp.: memory) pariśuddhi (f. loc. s.: complete purification or justification) svarūpa (n. comp.: own form, own nature) śūnya (adj.: empty) iva (as if, merely, nothing but) artha (mn. comp.: aim, purpose, motive, cause) mātra (mf(ā)n. comp.: fully, only, merely) nirbhāsa (f. nom. s.: shining, beaming, appearing) nirvitarka (mfn., f. nom. s.: not gross)

The *sūtra* describes the initial stages of the *siddhi* technique that will be described more accurately in 3.1 to 3.4. In the initial stages, disturbing memories must be calmed down. Then the nervous system becomes refined, and the brain software becomes prepared, to load version 7, that allows a much-improved form of attention. The memory of the gross disappears, subtle perceptions remain. The thinking processes, imagination (*vikalpa*) and memory (*smṛti*), are calmed down in this way.

1.44

Similarly, savicāra [samāpatti] and nirvicāra [samāpatti] are defined, [when applied to] the subtle perceived.

एतयैव सविचारा निर्विचारा च सूक्ष्मविषया व्याख्याता

etayā eva savicārā nirvicārā ca sūkṣma-viṣayāḥ vyākhyātā

eṣa (f. ins. s.: by this, by her) eva (ind.: really, truly) savicāra (mf(ā)n., f. nom. s.: with consideration, with subtle thinking) nirvicāra (mf(ā)n., f. nom. s.: without consideration, without subtle thinking) ca (ind.: and) sūkṣma (mf(ā)n.: subtle, refined) viṣaya (m. nom. p.: object of experience; āḥ v => ā v) vyākhyātā (p.p.: explained, defined)

It is a further refinement of *nirvitarka* from 1.43. *Samāpatti* (attention) appears simultaneously with speech comprehension, as (1) *savitarka*, without this, as (2) *nirvitarka*, with the subtle perceived as (3) *savicāra*, and without this, as (4) *nirvicāra*.

Levels of Activity of the Brain Software Versions 5 and 6

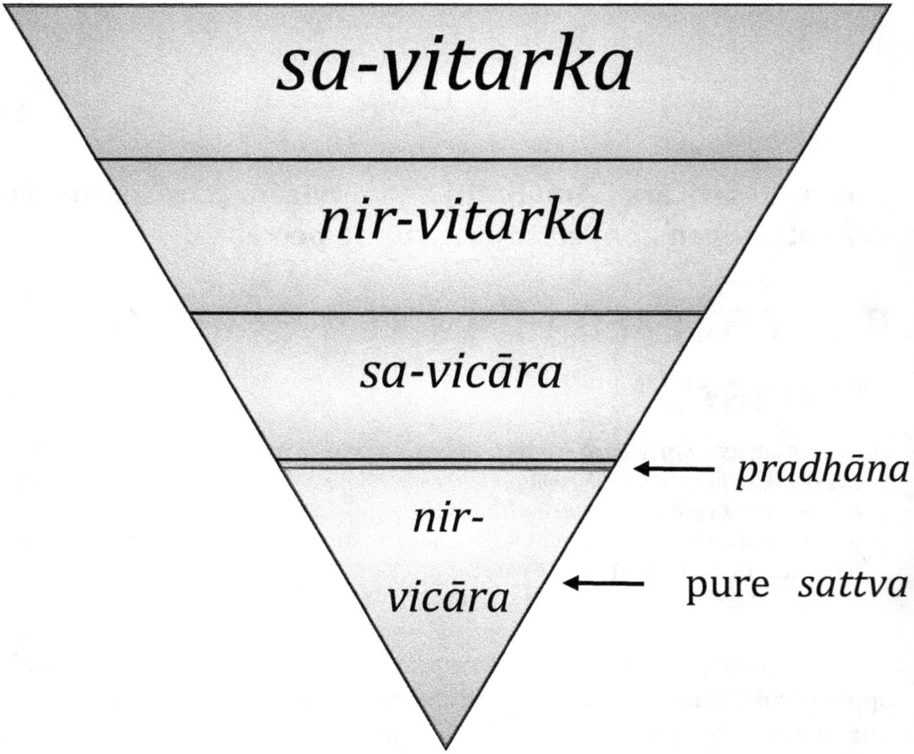

1.45

The measure of subtlety ends in the non-perceivable prakṛti.

सूक्ष्मविषयत्वं चालिङ्गपर्यवसानम्

sūkṣma-viṣayatvam ca-aliṅga-paryavasānam

sūkṣma (mf(ā)n.: fine, subtle) viṣayatva (n. nom. acc. s.: scale) ca (ind.: and) aliṅga (n. comp.: without form, without sign, absence of qualities) paryavasāna (n. nom. acc. s.: end, encompass, include)

The states of refinement from the gross to the subtle are: *mahābhūtas* (the five gross elements, for example a beam of light), *tanmātra* (the five subtle elements, for example the electromagnetic field), *asmitā* (limited "I"-consciousness), *liṅga mātra* = *mahat* (mathematical rules of natural laws, cosmic intellect), *pradhāna* (*guṇas* in their resting state). *Pradhāna* is the first cause and is still in the range of *savicāra* (1.44).

The *mahābhūtas* are the five gross "elements" (particles/waves), corresponding to the aggregate states of space (geometrical), air (gaseous), fire (plasma), water (liquid), and earth (solid). The *tanmātras* are the corresponding five physical fields, not perceivable by the sense organs.

Example: The sense of sight perceives light waves (*mahābhūta*), which are the excitations of the electromagnetic field (*tanmātra*).

1.46

Those [four] truly [are called] samādhi with seeds.

ता एव सबीजः समाधिः

tā eva sabījaḥ samādhiḥ

tā (f. Nom. p.: those; āḥ e => ā e) eva (ind.: really, truly) sabīja (mf(ā)n., m. nom. s.: with seeds) samādhi (m. nom. s.: restful alertness)

Now, the four levels of attention (*samāpatti* 1.41 to 1.44) get the name *samādhi.*

Seeds (causes of thinking processes) arise from the perception of items. *Samādhi* appears together with seeds on four levels: Together with speech comprehension, it is *savitarka*. Without this, it is *nirvitarka*. Together with subtle connections, it is *savicāra* (indescribable by words), without the subtitle, it is *nirvicāra* (pure knowledge).

1.47

Skill [in] nirvicāra lets the highest SELF (ātman) clearly shine.

निर्विचारवैशारद्येऽध्यात्मप्रसादः

nirvicāra-vaiśāradye adhyātma-prasādaḥ

nirvicāra (mf(ā)n., f. nom. s.: without subtle thoughts) vaiśārada (n. loc. s., nom. acc. d.: clarity of intellect, skill) adhyātma (n. comp.: the highest SELF = ātman) prasāda (m. nom. s.: clarity, purity, brightness, transparency)

From practicing *nirvicāra samādhi* follows the cognition of *ātman*, the SELF. The word "highest" is used, to distinguish it clearly from the *asmitā*, the limited "I"-consciousness. The skillful practice of *nirvicāra* (chapter 3) results in the cognition, that all things (*chandas*) are the SELF, that all perception processes (*devatā*) are the SELF, and also that the "I"-consciousness is nothing but the SELF.

Resulting from this complete cognition of the SELF, brain software version 7 becomes activated.

1.48

The intuitive knowledge within this [nirvicāra samādhi] contains truth.

ऋतम्भरा तत्र प्रज्ञा

ṛtambharā tatra prajñā

ṛtambharā (f. Nom. s.: evident knowledge, truth-bearing knowledge) tatra (ind.: there, then, in that place) prajñā (f. nom. s.: wisdom, clear, intuitive knowledge)

That is the definition of *prajñā* (*pra* = before, *jñā* = knowledge). *Prajñā* is the most fundamental (*pra-*) level of knowledge (*jñāna*). It generates neither pain nor no pain (1.5). It is reached no longer, the way, learned knowledge (*pramāṇa*) is reached (1.7). Thus, the *vṛttis* of *pramāṇa* and *viparyaya* are calmed down. It is direct, correct, intuitive knowledge that does not depend on limited perception, inference, or any authority. It is the field of all knowledge.

We are going to use the term intuitive knowledge for *prajñā*.

Prajñā knowledge is available, starting from brain software version 5. For the users of these higher versions, *prajñā* knowledge becomes enlivened within the *jñāna* knowledge. *Prajñā* is pure, intuitive knowledge, without any verbal or subtle relationship. Once the goal of *nirvicāra* is reached, neither any items nor any perceptions exist outside of the SELF. The SELF knows the SELF. From now on, life becomes very interesting! This is where the story really begins!

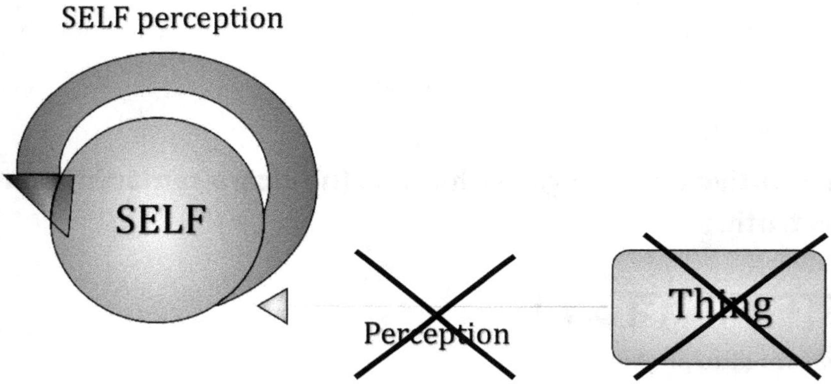

1.49

Intuitive knowledge (prajñā) is different from [generally valid] authority, or inference [because prajñā] refers to specific facts.

श्रुतानुमानप्रज्ञाभ्यामन्यविषया विशेषार्थत्वात्

śruta-anumāna-prajñābhyām anya-viṣayāḥ viśeṣa-arthatvāt

śruta (n. comp.: heard, teachings, scriptures, Vedas) anumāna (n. comp. : inference) prajñā (f. dat. abl. ins. d.: wisdom, clear, intuitive knowledge) anya (mfn., m. comp.: others, another, different) viṣaya (m. nom. p.: sensory object, object of attention) viśeṣa (m. cpmp.: definite, difference, distinction, particular) artha (m.: purpose, goal, motive, cause, reason, object, meaning) tvat (abl. affix: -ness)

Authority or inference refer only to general knowledge, whereas *prajñā* refers to special knowledge. For example, if I would like to know, how many apples are now in the apple tree in front of my house, I could start counting, but with *prajñā* knowledge, intuitive knowledge, I could find it out directly. This knowledge is special knowledge, and it cannot be found in any book. Books can only contain general knowledge.

Starting from brain software version 6 the infinitely fast quantum computer becomes connected with the all-knowing universe-computer. This ability is the prerequisite to finding out, intuitively and correctly, all special knowledge.

Note for mathematicians: The relationship between *prajñā* knowledge and *pramāṇa* knowledge is as with an integral to a summation formula. Both can provide similar results when viewed superficially. Essentially, however, they are different.

A successive summation formula, in some way, is always limited and with a certain degree of error. The corresponding integral, however, is exact, because it splits up every function into infinitely small steps and thus, by infinitely many additions, it leads to an exact result.

1.50

The impression created through that [nirvicāra practice] stops other impressions.

तज्जस्संस्कारोऽन्यसंस्कारप्रतिबन्धी

tat-jaḥ saṁskāraḥ anya-saṁskāra-pratibandhī

tad (n. comp.: that) ja (m. Nom. s.: created, born, arisen from) saṁskāra (m. nom. s.: impression) anya (mfn.: others, different, strange, extraordinary) pratibandhi (m. nom. acc. p.: hindering, excluding, interrupting, halting)

It functions like a malware scanner, which locates malware, identifies for deletion and then deletes it. The deletion marks that originate from *nirvicāra samādhi* indicate instances of malware, similar to scouring powder, which encloses the dirt. The marked malware finally becomes ineffective in the brain software.

Vyāsa comments as follows:

The saṁskāras arising from intuitive knowledge in samādhi, destroy the store of outward-directed saṁskāras of activity. When the saṁskāras of activity are destroyed, no more thoughts in the brain software originate from them, and samādhi follows. From samādhi arises intuitive knowledge and from that the knowledge saṁskāras. Thus repeatedly stores of knowledge saṁskāras are piled up.

The knowledge saṁskāras of samādhi destroy the illusions. The store of knowledge saṁskāras destroys the store of activity saṁskāras. A saṁskāra, which originated from intuitive knowledge (prajña 1.48), destroys the others because it originated from a true fact.

1.51

With the halting even of those [impressions from nirvicāra] all [impressions] are calmed, which defines nirbīja [seedless] samādhi.

तस्यापि निरोधे सर्वनिरोधान्निर्बीजः समाधिः

tasya api nirodhe sarva-nirodhāt nirbījaḥ samādhiḥ

tad (mn. gen. s.: from that) api (ind.: also) nirodha (m. loc. s.: inhibition, halting, calming) sarva (mf(ā)n.: all, every) nirodha (m. abl. s.: from halting) nirbīja (m. adj. nom. s.: without seed) samādhi (m. nom. s.:)

The calming of the *nirvicāra* impressions corresponds to rinsing with water. Upon scouring sufficiently with scouring powder (*nirvicāra samādhi*), the scouring powder is washed off with water. Thus, the result predicted in 1.2 is reached: the thinking processes (*vṛttis*) of the brain software (*citta*) are calmed down. The *citta* has no more foundation. The user of the brain software rests in the SELF.

Activity Levels of Brain Software Versions 7 and 8.

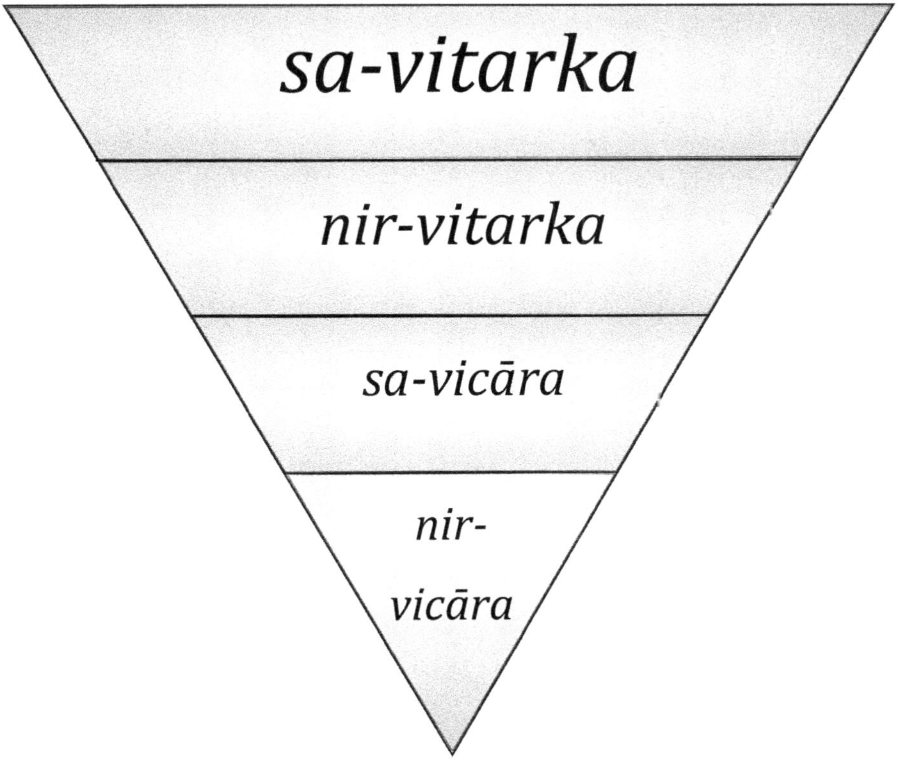

nirbīja samādhi

2

Sādhana Pāda

Removal of Ignorance

Introduction

Illusions

Yoga, achieved by one who has a calmed brain software, has now been taught. The second chapter describes how even one with an agitated, chaotic, restless brain software also can achieve *yoga*.

Object-Oriented Brain Software

The state-of-the-art in the field of software is "object-oriented software." Software models situations and processes in such a way that these can also run on a computer. Software can, for example, simulate the behavior of a car upon an impact, when the airbag gets activated. Software can store the data of persons and allow a selective search. Software can also be used to describe mental processes.

The current state of the software technology uses the concepts of object orientation, whose theoretical foundations were already described several centuries ago in India in *nyāya* (logic) and *vaiśeṣika* (structures of reality, ontology). Object orientation uses the following concepts:

An object is an individual software unit.

- An object provides specific methods (functions/actions) and manages the associated attributes (data).
- An example of an object is the model of a person, which contains attributes (data) about the person, for example, his name and address. Another object would be the model of a car, which provides the methods of starting, accelerating, breaking and heating.
- There are also objects, which only refer to memories, which no longer agree with actual perception; they are purely fantasy objects.

Brain software uses software objects. In the brain software we call impressions (*saṁskāras*) the malware objects.

- The effects of those malware objects (*saṁskāras*) must be reduced, or even better, completely removed, to enable the loading of higher versions of the brain software.

A class describes the common structure of a set of objects.

- A class, for example, describes the construction plan of a house as a model for the objects, the houses in a settlement. Each house is an object of the class "construction plan." An object contains both descriptions of the datatypes, as well as the corresponding methods. Datatypes, for example, are the height and the width of the house expressed in numbers. Methods, here, are the presentations of various views of the house from various angles.
- A class describes, for example, the type of car, together with its color; an object would be a specific car with the color red.
- An illusion class describes malware objects. If, for example, someone cannot stop smoking, then this addiction is a deep impression (*saṁskāra*), a malware object, which came about by repeated smoking. This impression is an object of the illusion class "longing."

A method of a class describes, what possible actions it can provide.

- In the brain software, the methods of an illusion class are the thinking processes (*vṛttis*).

An attribute is a location in memory, which contains data.

- Attributes are, for example, place, time, duration and intensity.

In the brain software every object "impression (*saṁskāra*)" contains the related memory in the form of attributes.

- The method "remembering" provides the memory, which is the attributes, like the place, time, and circumstances regarding the formation of an impression (3.18).
- For example, someone can remember previous lives, by recalling the attributes of an impression using the method "remembering" (3.18).

Inheritance describes an "is a" relation between a basic class and its derived classes. The basic class provides its attributes (data) and its behavior (methods) to the derived classes.

- Examples of inheritance are: A blackbird is a songbird; a songbird is a bird; a bird of prey is a bird; a bird is a vertebrate; a fish is a vertebrate.
- The following inheritances apply to the malware classes in the brain software (see the graph below):
  - ⇨ A connection between the perceiver and the perceived (*saṁyoga*, 2.17) is an ignoring of the SELF.
  - ⇨ An illusion (*kleśa*) is a connection between the perceiver and the perceived (2.5).
  - ⇨ Ignorance (*avidyā*) is an illusion (*kleśa*) in the perception of reality (2.3, 2.5).
  - ⇨ Limited "I"-consciousness, or ego (*asmitā* 2.6) is an ignorance (*avidyā*).
  - ⇨ Longing (*rāga* 2.7) is an ignorance (*avidyā*).
  - ⇨ Hate (*dveṣa* 2.8) is an ignorance (*avidyā*).
  - ⇨ Survival instinct (*abhiniveśa* 2.9) is an ignorance (*avidyā*).

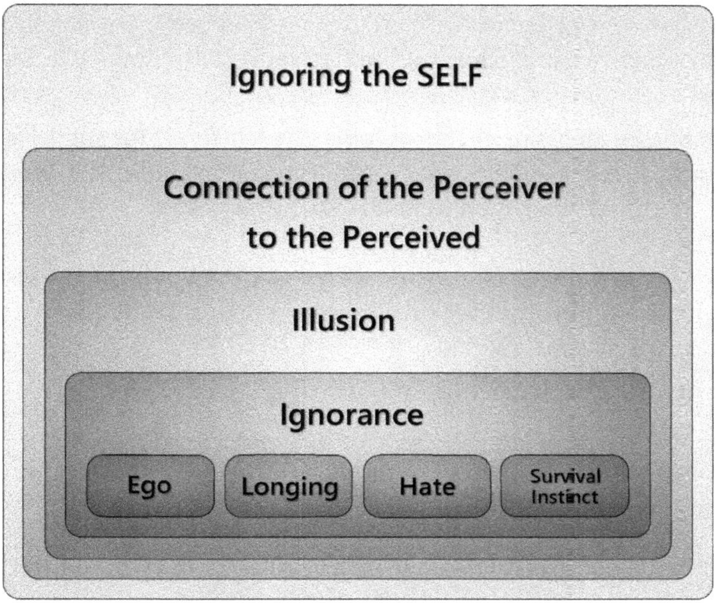

A list contains a sequence of objects of the same class.

In the brain software, the store of *karma* (*karmāṣaya*) is the list of all impressions (*saṁskāras* 4.9). The thinking process "remembering" recalls the memories in the *saṁskāras.*

- The term *karma* means action. Before the installation of software version 7, each action results in a storing of *saṁskāras* in the store of karma.
- The stored *saṁskāras,* due to their existing kleśas, can lead to new activities, if corresponding situations come up.
- In the brain software, one impression can, in turn, activate other impressions of the malware.

Note

In our diagrams, we are using a simplified representation of class relationships and object flowcharts.

In this book, we are using the term "object" exclusively for software objects. Things that are generally called objects, for example, "objects of the senses," we call a thing, or an item, to avoid confusions.

Objects can request methods from other objects. In this way, control flow structures come about.

To guarantee, that an illusion class can no longer generate any malware objects, the class must be erased.

Erasing a class means, that the methods of the class are erased, however, the data/attributes, stored in objects of the class can be kept and retrieved.

Erasing the basic class "ignorance" has the effect, that, while the memories regarding ignorance can be retrieved, the ignorance no longer has any effect, because its methods are erased, and therefore they are also, in turn, no longer available for the derived classes.

This happens in practice using *viveka khyāti* (2.26).

See Appendix C, containing a simulation in the language MATLAB, where the basic class *ignorance.m* can be erased.

Upon erasing the basic class no further *saṁskāra* objects can be produced, and the present objects can no longer be activated.

Malware Class

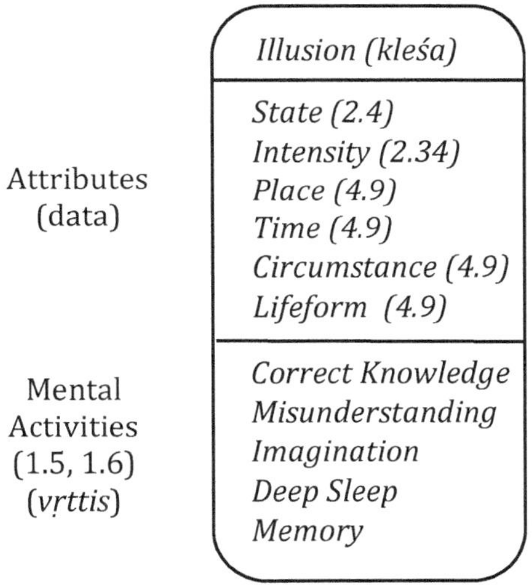

The mental activities of malware are the thinking processes. They are called the pain-generating *vṛttis* (1.5).

EatingIcecream is an impression of the illusion "longing."

- state = active
- intensity = 85%
- place = at home with mother
- time = 4 years 3 months old
- situation = first ice cream tasted very good
- livingBeing = human

A saṁskāra can generate misunderstanding and memory

EatingIcecream.misunderstanding = I could eat ice cream all day
EatingIcecream.memory = yesterday I ate ice cream

Store of karma

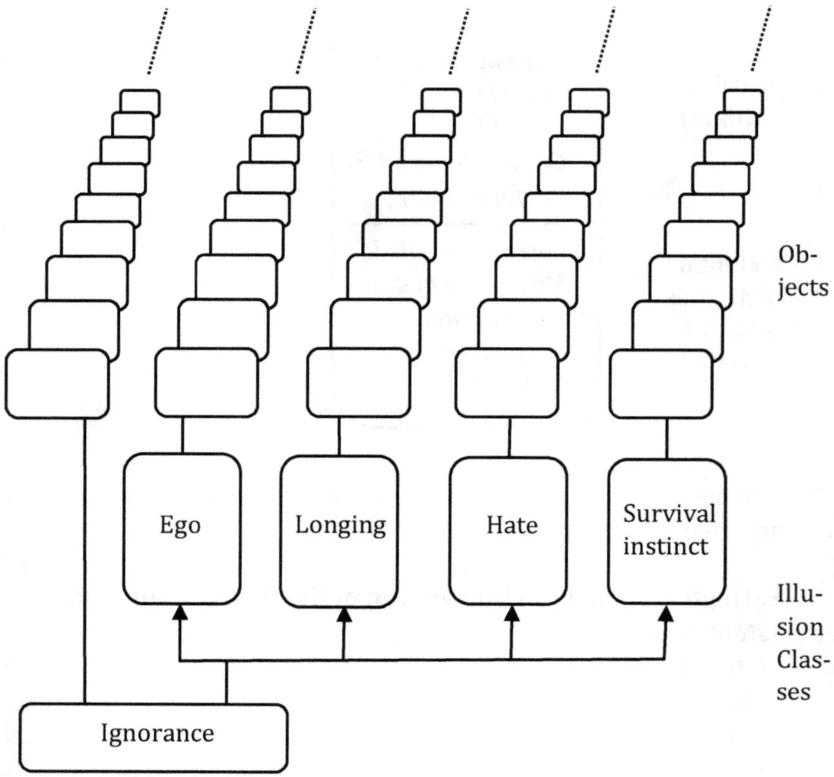

Each of the five illusion classes appears only once. On the other hand, there are arbitrarily many malware objects.

By deleting the basic class "ignorance" the other four classes and all the malware objects become ineffective and no new objects can originate from the illusion classes.

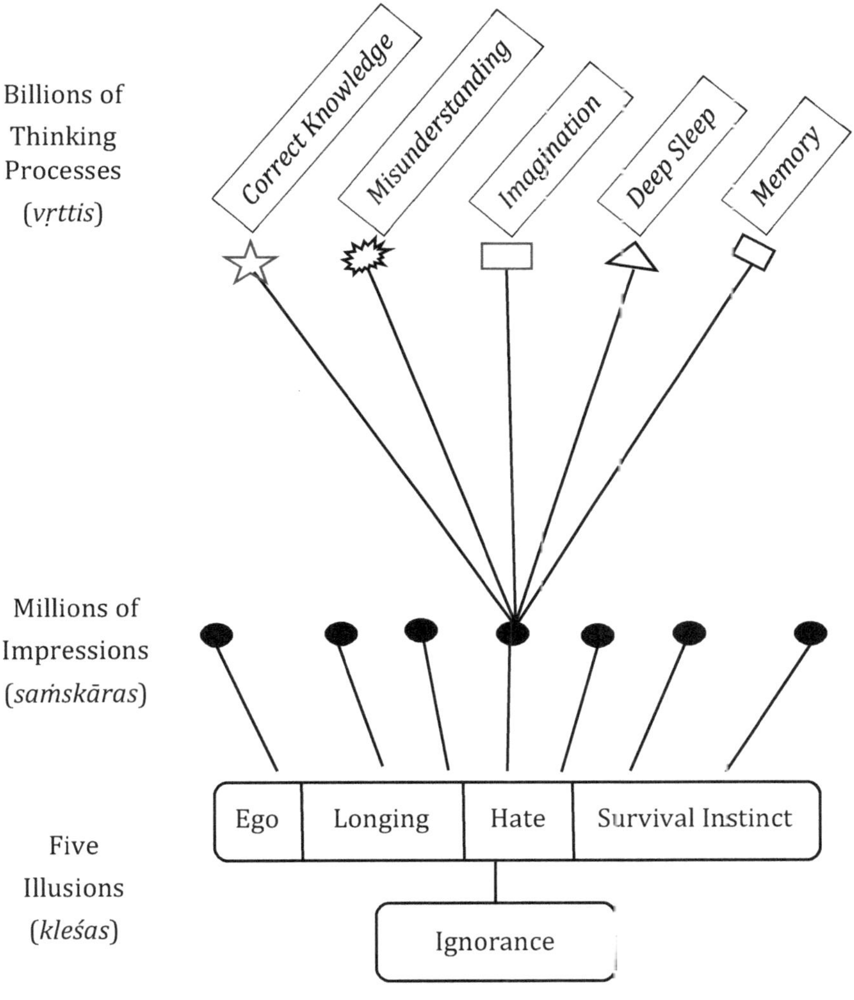
Billions of Thinking Processes (*vṛttis*)
Correct Knowledge
Misunderstanding
Imagination
Deep Sleep
Memory
Millions of Impressions (*saṁskāras*)
Five Illusions (*kleśas*)
Ego
Longing
Hate
Survival Instinct
Ignorance

2.1

The urge for liberation, self-study of the Veda and attention to Īśvara are defined as the yoga of action.

तपःस्वाध्यायेश्वरप्रणिधानानि क्रियायोगः

tapaḥ-svādhyāya-īśvara-praṇidhānāni kriyā-yogaḥ

tapas (n. nom. acc. s: asceticism, discipline, urge for liberation) svādhyāya (m. comp.: study of the Veda) īśvara (m. comp.: Supreme Being) praṇidhāna (n. nom. acc. p.: attention, focusing on, effort, strong desire) kriyā (f. comp., f. nom. s.: action, execution, carry out) yoga (m. Nom. s.: Yoga)

Self-study means both, the studying of the *Vedas* by oneself, and the study of the SELF as found in the *Veda*.

Īśvara has been described as distinct from *puruṣa* in 1.24. *Īśvara* also has been defined in 1.25 as the one with the highest knowledge.

2.2

The goal [of the yoga of action] is to achieve samādhi and to reduce the illusions (kleśas).

समाधिभावनार्थः क्लेशतनूकरणार्थश्च

samādhi-bhāvana-arthaḥ kleśa-tanū-karaṇa-arthaḥ ca

samādhi (m. comp.: restful alertness) bhāvana (m. comp.: achievement, gain) artha (m. nom. s.: goal, purpose, meaning) kleśa (m. comp.: illusion, pain creator, source of pain) tanu (mf(us/ūs, vī)n. comp.: weak, delicate, minute) karaṇa (n. comp.: do, cause, create) artha (m. nom. s.: goal, purpose, meaning) ca (ind.: and, also)

Yoga is a purposeful activity, not a mere pastime.

2.3

The illusions are ignorance, [limited] „I"-consciousness, longing, hate and the survival instinct.

अविद्यास्मितारागद्वेषाभिनिवेशः क्लेशाः

avidyā-asmitā-rāga-dveṣa-abhiniveśaḥ kleśāḥ

avidyā (f. comp.: ignorance) (f. comp.: i-consciousness, identity) rāga (m. comp.: longing, attraction, binding, passion, love) dveṣa (m. comp.: rejection, disgust, hatred) abhiniveśa (m. nom. s.: clinging to earthly existence, greed for life, survival instinct) kleśā (m. nom. p.: illusion)

The illusions come in five classes, which generate suffering:

- Ignorance (*avidyā*) about one's own nature and, therefore, identification with the perceived, like body or brain software. Ignorance is the basic class of the following illusions.
- Limited "I"-consciousness (*asmitā*): limitedness, pride, stubbornness, egocentricity, self-absorption, delusion, arrogance, inferiority, self-pity, sadness and identification of the body with the SELF.
- Longing (*rāga*): obsession, desire to reproduce happiness through sensory gratification, longing, jealousy, amusement, lust, envy, greed, craving, passion.
- Hate (*dveṣa*): repulsion, disgust, rejection, anger, rage.
- Survival instinct (*abhiniveśa*): clinging to earthly existence, greed for life, fear of death, panic, fear in general. The survival instinct refers to the limited "I." A user of brain software version 7 and 8 can overcome even the survival instinct, yet continue to live due to habit.

The Illusions

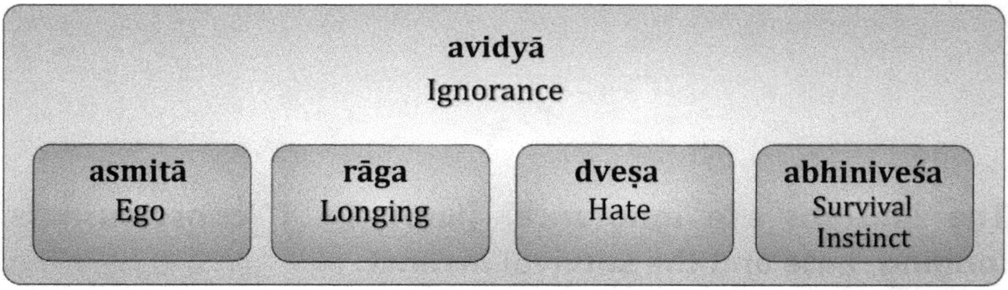

2.4

Ignorance is the fertile ground of the other [four kleśas]; [all five are either] asleep, weak, interrupted or active.

अविद्या क्षेत्रमुत्तरेषाम्
प्रसुप्ततनुविच्छिन्नोदाराणाम्

avidyā kṣetram uttareṣām prasupta-tanu-vicchinna-udārāṇām

avidyā (f. Nom. s.: ignorance) kṣetra (n. nom. acc. s.: field, place, region) uttara (m. gen. p.: following, subsequent) prasupta (f. comp.: sleepiness) tanu (n. comp.: weak, delicate) vicchinna (f. comp: interrupted, finished) udāra (mf(ā)n., mn. gen. p.: elevated, noble, active, energetic)

Ignorance is the basic class for the other four classes of illusions; for limited "I"-consciousness, longing, hate, and survival instinct (2.3). The four states of an illusion (*kleśa*) are: asleep, weak, interrupted, active. Thus there are 5 x 4 = 20 states of illusions.

If an illusion is not active, and if it exists only as a mere possibility, it is asleep. That means the corresponding illusion class does not generate any objects at that moment.

If an illusion wakes up, it means it becomes active when a suitable event or item is perceived or remembered. When it is active, it generates malware objects (*saṁskāras*), which, in turn, push the thinking processes (*vṛttis*) into certain patterns. These malware objects are programs that unwantedly or unexpectedly run in the brain software.

Illusions can be weakened consciously by applying an opposite thought (2.33). The weakened illusion requires a longer time or a more intense stimulus, to generate malware objects.

An illusion can be interrupted by another one that is when the other one becomes active. For example, the hate can be suppressed by an emerging longing, yet it continues to exist in an interrupted form, and can later on again manifest as hate. The production of hate-related malware objects at this moment becomes interrupted because first the longing-related malware objects must be generated. Since hate and longing oppose each other, they cannot simultaneously generate malware objects. As soon as the event that triggers the longing disappears, the hate malware object can be produced again.

Śaṁkara mentions in his commentary a fifth state, which he calls the burned seed of a *kleśa* which is very seldom and can happen only starting from brain software version 5. In the brain software, this burned state means, that the corresponding illusion class can no longer generate any objects. That corresponds to a firewall to protect against intruding malware.

2.5

Ignorance is seeing the impermanent as if eternal, the impure as if pure, suffering as if happiness, the non-SELF as if the SELF.

अनित्याशुचिदुःखानात्मसु नित्यशुचिसुखात्मख्यातिरविद्या

anitya-aśuci-duḥkha-anātmasu nitya-śuci-sukha-ātma-khyātiḥ avidyā

anitya (mfn. comp.: not eternal) aśuci (mfn. comp.: impure) duḥkha (mfn., n. comp.: pain, suffering, uneasy) anātmasu (not real SELF) nitya (mf(ā). comp.: eternal, permanent) śuci (mfn. comp.: pure, clean, white, brilliant) sukha (mfn. n. comp.: happiness, comfort) ātma (m. comp.: SELF) khyāti (f. nom. s.: seeing as if, opinion, view) avidyā (f. nom. s.: ignorance)

The class ignorance inherits the methods and attributes of the class illusion, especially the connection of the perceived with the perceiver (see diagram in the introduction to chapter 2). There are exactly four kinds of these connections, which are specified in the *sūtra*, and all four of them are called ignorance.

2.6

[Limited] "I"-consciousness [means mixing] the power of the seer [the unchanging SELF] and the power of the process of seeing [the intellectual activity] as if they were one SELF [one identity].

दृग्दर्शनशक्त्योरेकात्मतेवास्मिता

dṛś-darśana-śaktyoḥ ekātmatā iva asmitā

dṛś ([puruṣa as] seer, perceiver, observer, witness, pure consciousness [sandhi -> ś->k, k->g, =>dṛg]) darśana (mf(ī)n. comp.: vision, view, seeing, appearance) śakti (f. gen. loc. d.: energy, power) ekātmatā (f. nom. s.: beeing one) iva (ind.: so, as if, like, almost) asmitā (f. nom. s.: i-consciousness, identity)

The fault lies in trying to connect two things, which cannot be connected. It arises by not discriminating between the unchanging and the changeable. Someone says: "I go there." In this statement, there is a mixing up of the body and the SELF. In fact, being *ātman*, one is everywhere. Therefore one cannot go there; only the body can go there. Limited "I"-consciousness is just this mixing up.

2.7

Pleasure leads to longing.

सुखानुशयी रागः

sukha-anuśayī rāgaḥ

sukha (n. comp.: comfort, happiness, pleasure) anuśayin (m. nom. s.: [immediate] consequence of an act) rāga (m. nom. s.: longing, attraction, binding, passion, love)

„Longing is thirst, is greed" (see the hint in 1.15).

Before installing brain software version 7, the experience of pleasure is the cause of longing. Caught up in the illusion of longing, the limited self tries, by feelings of longing, to experience further pleasant experiences.

2.8

Suffering leads to hate.

दुःखानुशयी द्वेषः

duḥkha-anuśayī dveṣaḥ

duḥkha (n. comp.: suffering, pain, discomfort) anuśayin (m. nom. s.: [immediate] sequence of an act) dveṣa (m. nom. s.: rejection, disgust, hatred)

Before installing brain software version 7, the experience of suffering is the cause of hate. Caught up in the illusion, the limited self tries, by feelings of hate, to avoid further suffering.

2.9

The survival instinct is inherent, even in the wise [one].

स्वरसवाही विदुषोऽपि तथा रूढोऽभिनिवेशः

sva-rasa-vāhī viduṣaḥ api tathā rūḍhaḥ abhiniveśaḥ

sva (mf(ā)n. comp.: own) rasa (m. comp.: inner nature, tendency, disposition, character) vāhin (mfn., m. nom. s.: flowing, streaming, carrying, carrier, consisting of, causing) vidus (mfn.: wise, attentive) api (ind.: also, even) tathā (ind.: thus, in this way) rūḍha (mfn., m. nom. s.: arisen, developed, grown, formed) abhiniveśa (m. nom. s.: clinging to earthly existence, clinging on to life, greed for life, survival instinct)

It comes from experiences of death, ending previous lives. Therefore all creatures, including newborns, fear death. The wise one is defined in this context as someone who understands the SELF to be indestructible.

2 .10

Those weakened [illusions] must be dissolved at their cause.

ते प्रतिप्रसवहेयाः सूक्ष्माः

te prati-prasava-heyāḥ sūkṣmāḥ

te (m. nom. p.: those) prati (ind.: near, back) prasava (m. comp.: origin, production, begin) heya (mfn., m. nom. p.: to avoid, to refrain from, to dissolve, to remove) sūkṣma (mf(ā)n., m. nom. p.: fine, thin, subtle, tiny, minute)

Strong illusions must be weakened by thinking about their opposites (2.33) and by *kriyā yoga* before they can be deleted. *Kriyā yoga* has been defined in 2.1 as the striving for liberation, the self-study of the *Vedas* and attention to *Īśvara*. For the users of the brain software before version 5, due to his illusory perception, the experience of the pleasant causes longing (2.7) and the experience of suffering causes hate (2.8).

Illusory perception means for example that someone equates the SELF with the body (2.6). Then, for example, he tries to bring the body there, where, seemingly, a longing can be fulfilled to achieve a more intense feeling of happiness. The happiness, however, is always there in unbounded fullness within the SELF, and therefore no special bodily activities are required. Similarly, it applies to the running away of the body from a situation filled with suffering. In both cases, the faulty perception of the SELF causes the illusion (2.17).

Illusions have an intensity that can be increased or diminished. The complete deletion of the illusions to such a degree that they can never have any effect again happens at the end of the process of *viveka khyāti* (2.26). With the deletion of the five illusions, all the impressions, connected to them in the store of *karma*, lose their effects.

That means for the brain software: Once the five classes of malware are deleted, all objects derived from them are also neutralized. Even though malware objects may appear a million fold, they are all switched off by those five simple switches, switching off the five illusions.

2.11

Dhyāna removes the thinking processes of those [illusions].

ध्यानहेयास्तद्वृत्तयः

dhyāna-heyāḥ tat-vṛttayaḥ

dhyāna (n. comp.: dhyāna) heya (mfn., m. nom. p.: to avoid, to refrain from, to dissolve, to remove) tad (n. comp.: that) vṛtti (f. nom. p.: thought process)

Once the weakening of the *kleśas* according to 2.10 has happened, only a subtle remainder of *vṛttis* remains, which can then be removed completely by *dhyāna*. *Dhyāna* may be translated as "meditation," but will be defined accurately in 3.2. The pattern-like, suffering-inducing *vṛttis* (thinking processes) will be removed by *dhyāna*, their patterns erased. When there are only a few of these patterns left, the preconditions are established for the loading of brain software upgrades versions 5 and 6.

Later, in 2.26, the basis and the most intense form of *dhyāna* will be introduced. It is called "correctly-discriminating cognition (*viveka khyāti*)." Upon applying this, the subtle remains of *vṛttis* in the *kleśas* can be erased. This process takes some time when upgrading the brain software version 6 to versions 7 and 8. Great skill is required, which will be explained in the following *sūtras*.

Karma

2.12

The cause [of all objects] in the store of karma is illusion and [it] will be lived in the visible [present] or an invisible [future] life.

क्लेशमूलः कर्माशयो दृष्टादृष्टजन्मवेदनीयः

kleśa-mūlaḥ karma-āśayaḥ dṛṣṭa-adṛṣṭa-janma-Vedanīyaḥ

kleśa (m. comp.: illusion) mūla (m. nom. s.: root, base, cause) karma (n. comp.: action, deed) āśaya (m. nom. s.: place, resting-place, storage) dṛṣṭa (mfn.: comp.: visible, present, seen) adṛṣṭa (mfn.: comp.: invisible, future) janma (n. comp.: life, world, area, birth) Vedanīya (m. nom. s.: expression, experience)

A user of brain software version 3, for example, has a beautiful experience (*sukha*) such as drinking alcohol. Due to his illusory perception, he develops an addiction, a *saṁskāra*, to repeat this pleasant experience. There is action (*karma*), to repeat the drinking of alcohol, arising from this addiction. *Saṁskāras* of this kind can appear up to software version 6, such that, consciously or unconsciously, they create these actions in the present or future lives.

Those *saṁskāras* in the brain software we call the malware objects. The *kleśas* we call the construction plans (classes) of the malware objects. The store of *karma* we call the list of all existing malware objects. This list becomes activated in the present or future lives. In computer science, lists can be traversed in various sequences by various methods. Regarding the store of *karma*, those correspond to the various sequences of the *daśa* systems of Vedic astrology, which describe precisely, which *karma* becomes activated at what time.

The exact definition of the malware in the brain software is:

- The five illusions (*kleśas*) are the classes of the malware.
- Ignorance is the basic class of the four other illusions.
- Impressions (*saṁskāras*) are the objects of the illusion classes.
- The store of karma (*karmāṣaya*) is the complete list of the existing impressions.
- The pain-inducing thinking processes that mean the pain-inducing vṛttis are the methods of the illusion classes.

2.13

Due to an existing root [kleśa], that [store of karma] ripens as births, lives, and experiences.

सति मूले तद्विपाको जात्यायुर्भोगाः

sati mūle tat-vipākaḥ jāti-āyuḥ-bhogāḥ

sat (mf(ī)., n. loc. s.: existent, being present) mūla (n. loc. s.: root) tad (n. comp.: that) vipāka (mf(ā)n., m. nom. s.: mature, fruit) jāti (f. comp.: birth) āyu (mfn., m. nom. s.: living, life, lifetime) bhoga (m. nom. p.: pleasure, enjoyment, luck, experience)

The ripening of the *saṁskāras* in the store of *karma* happens according to certain time sequences. The activation of the *saṁskāras* is complicated, but it can be calculated to a certain degree with Vedic astrology. The ripening process corresponds to the sequential activation, due to the influence of various heavenly bodies according to the *daśa* systems.

The *saṁskāras* can also, in certain cases, appear in pairs. In these cases, one *saṁskāra*, generated by good actions, partially neutralizes another one, generated by bad actions.

All this, however, is bondage and is very restricting of free will. Surely, it is far more intelligent, to perform brain software upgrade version 7, to escape from the influence of the store of *karma*. Once these causes, the illusions (*kleśas*), are removed, the store of *karma* can no longer ripen or bear any fruits.

2.14

The fruits of those [births, lives, and experiences] are pleasure and pain caused by merit and guilt.

ते ह्लादपरितापफलाः पुण्यापुण्यहेतुत्वात्

te hlāda-paritāpa-phalāḥ puṇya-apuṇya-hetutvāt

tad (m. nom. p.: that) hlāda (m. comp.: pleasure, joy) paritāpa (m. comp.: pain, suffering, sadness, distress) phala (n. nom. acc. p.: fruit, result, effect) puṇya (mf(ā)n., n. comp.: pure, holy, sacred, luck, virtue, merit) apuṇya (comp.: guilt, wicked, impure, sin) hetutvāt (m. abl. s.: reason, cause)

Before installing version 7, the brain software causes limited joys and sufferings. Those, however, are the results of the malware. Infinite happiness cannot appear unless the malware is removed. How can limited joy appear as an effect of malware? Being limited, it ends at some time. Then, however, frustration, anger, etc. set in, due to losing joy. See 2.15, and the wheel of *karma* (4.11).

The malware, if not removed, will definitely be activated at some time. It does not matter, in this case, if in the meantime someone changes the "hardware," the body, and then continues to use the same faulty brain software upon reincarnation.

2.15

Change, fear, saṁskāras, suffering, arising from the action patterns due to the battle of the [three] guṇas are to the discriminating (vivekin) nothing but suffering.

परिणामतापसंस्कार दुःखैर्गुणवृत्तिविरोधाच्च
दुःखमेव सर्वं विवेकिनः

pariṇāma-tāpa-saṃskāra-duḥkhaiḥ guṇa-vṛtti-virodhāt ca duḥkham eva sarvaṁ vivekinaḥ

pariṇāma (m. comp.: change, transformation) tāpa (m. comp.: torture, fear, physical pain, heat) saṃskāra (comp.: impression) duḥkha (n. Inst. p.: by pain, suffering [more on a mind level], discomfort) guṇavṛtti (f. comp.: activity of the guṇas) virodha (m. abl. s.: from conflict, quarrel, battle, dispute) ca (ind.: and, also) duḥkha (n. acc. nom. s.: suffering) eva (ind.: only, just) sarva (mf(ā)n., n. acc. nom. s.: all) vivekin (m. abl. gen. s.: the wise, the correctly discriminating one)

The correctly discriminating one discriminates between the suffering, limited "I"-consciousness and the non-suffering SELF.

That which is internally repulsive is the pain. Therefore, for the *yogi*, even during a time of pleasure, some pain is present because for the *yogi* even pleasure is repulsive. Why is that? The *yogi* is clear about this: Never does any desire become fulfilled from living it out. The desire increases more and more, like fire increases by pouring butter into it. An ever more strongly increasing desire finally leads to pain.

> There is no pain as big as thirst and no joy as big as the freedom from thirst.

2.16

Future suffering [is to be] avoided.

हेयं दुःखमनागतम्

heyaṁ duḥkham anāgatam

heya (mfn., n. nom. s.: avoidance) duḥkha (mfn., n. nom. acc. s.: suffering) anāgata (n. nom. acc. s.: future)

> Avoid the danger, before it arises.

Pain that has already happened cannot be avoided. Also, the present pain cannot be avoided because it has already reached the moment of experience. What can be avoided, is the pain that has not yet come.

In the brain software, this avoidance of future pain corresponds to establishing a so-called "firewall." The firewall filters out malware, to prevent it from coming into the system. The filter of the firewall in the brain software is correctly-discriminating cognition (*viveka khyāti* 2.26).

Firewalls filter data packets according to their attributes. The filter attributes for the brain software are derived from the definition of ignorance in 2.5: "Ignorance is seeing the impermanent as if eternal, the impure as if pure, suffering as if happiness, the non-SELF as if the SELF."

2.17

The connection between the perceiver and the perceived is the cause [of the suffering and is] to be avoided.

द्रष्टृदृश्ययोः संयोगो हेयहेतुः

draṣṭṛ-dṛśyayoḥ saṃyogaḥ heya-hetuḥ

draṣṭṛ (m. comp.: perceiver, observer, seer) dṛśya (mfn., m. gen. loc. d.: perceived, seen) saṃyoga (m. nom. s.: connection) heya (mfn. comp.: avoidance) hetu (m. nom. s.: cause)

> If one does not want to injure the feet with sharp stones, one should wear shoes.

The perceiver is the SELF (*ātman, puruṣa*). The perceived consists of things of the environment, senses, body, intellect, and the limited "I"-consciousness.

To avoid future suffering, use the highest version of the brain software! It automatically contains the best firewall, which separates the painful connection between the perceiver and the perceived.

In this context see also the diagram in 1.48.

Guṇas

2.18

[With the] striving [of the three guṇas] towards clarity, action, and steadiness, the perceived consists of the elements (mahābhūtas) and the senses for experience and liberation.

प्रकाशक्रियास्थितिशीलं भूतेन्द्रियात्मकं भोगापवर्गार्थं दृश्यम्

prakāśa-kriyā-sthiti-śīlam bhūta-indriya-ātmakam bhoga-apavarga-artham dṛśyam

prakāśa (m. comp.: clearity, light, brightness, radiating) kriyā (f. comp.: action) sthiti (f. comp.: steadiness, standstill, immovability, inertia) śīla (n. nom. s.: tendency towards, nature, being, character) bhūta (n. comp.: element [five]) indriya (n. comp.: sense and organs of action) ātmaka (n. nom. acc. s.: belonging to the character or nature of a thing, forming the nature of a thing) bhoga (m. comp.: experience) apavarga (m. comp.: end, liberation) artha (m. acc. s.: goal, purpose, reason) dṛśya (mfn., n. nom. s.: visible, perceivable, perceived)

Sattva strives towards clarity, *rajas* towards movement, *and tamas* towards steadiness. The fundamental state of the creative power (*pradhāna*) is the ground state of the three guṇas (*sattva, rajas, and tamas*). Nothing happens in it. If, however, the *guṇas* are not in their ground state, they mutually influence each other. All the three *guṇas* are always present but in different proportions. When one *guṇa* prevails, something happens in that direction. They cause the "perceived." It consists of items and sense organs.

The purpose of the perceived is twofold: (1) Experience and (2) liberation.

(1) Experience is a conviction in the brain software (citta), that the user (puruṣa) is a part of this brain software, and that it could not be distinguished from it.

(2) Liberation is a state of the brain software, which sees the three guṇas as the actors and puruṣa as the silent observer of these actions. In this liberated state, the user is seen as separate from the brain software.

Those two, experience and liberation, are generated by the intellect and function only in the intellect. Why, then, are both attributed to puruṣa? The same way as victory or defeat of the army is attributed to its ruler because he notices their effects, just the same way bondage and liberation are attributed to puruṣa because he is aware of their effects. Bondage exists only in the intellect, and it is neglect of fulfilling the second purpose of the perceived. Liberation is the fulfillment of this purpose.

The *guṇas* form the five elements, the items of experience and the five sense organs. In brain software version 3 the information from the perceived items arise at the silent SELF (*puruṣa*), the user, in the following sequence:

Items →

→ sense organs →

→ input-output software (*manas*) →

→ the main component of the brain software (*buddhi*, intellect) →

→ the user of the brain software (*puruṣa*).

This sequence defines the term "experience." For the user of brain software before version 7, any experience is a process that delivers everything to the SELF, like a servant. That is the first purpose of the perceived. Liberation means freedom from this service; that is the second purpose of the perceived.

For the user of brain software versions 7 and 8, the second purpose applies, which is the end of this process of experiencing. The user is the SELF and perceives the SELF and its impulses. The perceived becomes the SELF. Everything is in ME. I perceive items, not anymore outside of ME. Thus, their character of being external items has disappeared.

For the user of brain software versions 7 and 8, the three *guṇas* are replaced by knowledge impulses in *ātman*, the SELF. They no longer exist as "outer" forces, because everything has become the SELF. That is unity consciousness.

2.19

The states of the guṇas [are] special, general, structured (liṇga), measurable (mātra) and unstructured (pradhāna).

विशेषाविशेषलिङ्गमात्रालिङ्गानि गुणपर्वाणि

viśeṣa-aviśeṣa-liṅga-mātra-aliṅgāni guṇa-parvāṇi

viśeṣa (m. comp.: difference, speciality, peculiarity, specific quality) aviśeṣa (m. comp.: universal, undetermined, non-difference, unspecific) liṅga-mātra (n. comp.: measurable pure, mere form, indicator, symbol) aliṅga (n. nom. p.: formless, without marks, pradhāna) guṇa (comp.: tendency) parvan (n. nom. p.: connection, section, time slice, limb, state)

That is a sequence from gross to subtle. "Special" means the excitation of fields, for example, rays of light. "General" means physical fields, for example, the electromagnetic field. "Structured" means mathematical structures of natural laws, for example, $E = ½mv^2$. "Measurable" means observable measures, for example, energy, velocity. "Unstructured" means the three *guṇas* in balance, which is called *pradhāna* or *aliṇga*.

Transformations of the guṇas

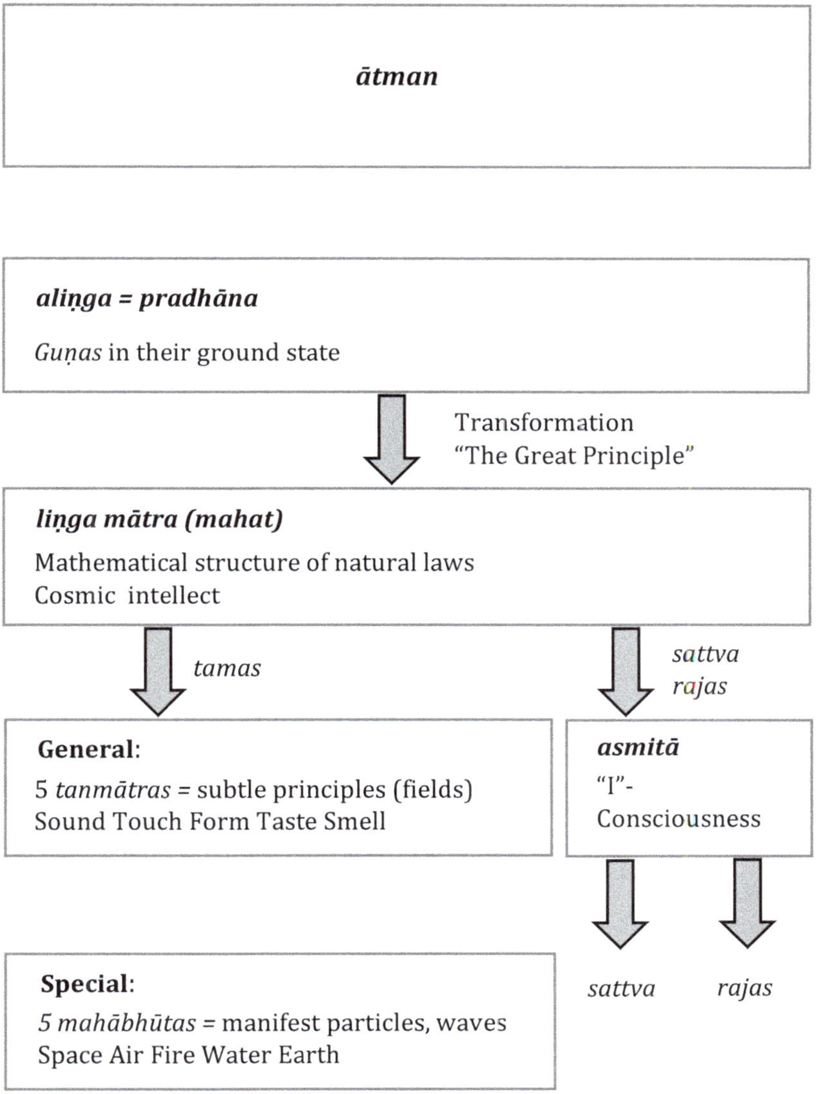
ātman
aliṇga = pradhāna
Guṇas in their ground state
Transformation
"The Great Principle"
liṇga mātra (mahat)
Mathematical structure of natural laws
Cosmic intellect
tamas
sattva
rajas
General:
5 tanmātras = subtle principles (fields)
Sound Touch Form Taste Smell
asmitā
"I"-
Consciousness
Special:
5 mahābhūtas = manifest particles, waves
Space Air Fire Water Earth
sattva
rajas

The Divine Mother Spoke

"I (*ātman*), *devī/śakti*, am THAT (three *guṇas* in balance). *Devī* is both, *ātman* and *pradhāna*.

Devī is both, without the *guṇas* and is simultaneously the *guṇas* in balance.

For the SELF-Realised I am *ātman* only, and *ātman* contains everything and more."

Connection between the gross elements, subtle qualities, and sense organs

mahābhūta Gross Element	**tanmātra** Subtle Quality	**jñānendriya** Sense Organ
pṛthivī Earth	***gandha*** Smell, Stability, Structural Similarity	***ghrāṇendriya*** Smell
jala Water	***rasa*** Taste, Liquidity, Water Memory	***rasanendriya*** Taste
agni Fire, Light	***rūpa*** Form, Color, Fire, Light, Heat, Electromagnetic, Scalar Wave Fields	***cakṣurindriya*** Sight
vāyu Air, Gas, Wind	***sparśa*** Touch, Curl, Quantum Entanglement, Chi, Prāṇa	***sparśendriya*** Touch
ākāśa Space	***śabda*** Sound, Gravitational Field, Information Network	***śravaṇendriya*** Hearing

The subtle element, the *tanmātra* of light/fire is the electromagnetic field. The gross element, the *mahābhūta* of light/fire consists of the vibrations, which are the excited states of the electromagnetic field, for example, rays of light, microwaves, x-rays, etc. Similarly, it applies to the other *tanmātras* being the fields. The same applies to the other *mahābhūtas*, being the excited states.

Gravitation (attributed to sound) and electromagnetism (light) are the only two fields in modern physics that can extend infinitely in space. However, we know from the *brahma sūtras*, that all the senses are infinite.

Some research remains to be done about the other three fields! They also require infinitely extended qualities. Therefore the, spatially limited, strong and weak interactions are no proper candidates. See the previous table for further inspiration for research.

The five organs – ears, skin, eyes, tongue, and nose – are mental sense organs and knowledge organs (*buddhi indriya*). Sense organs are connected to the body, and therefore are finite. The associated subtle senses are infinite, therefore not limited by the body. The five organs of action (*karmendriyas*) are the speech organ, hands, feet, and the organs of elimination and reproduction. The input-output component (*manas*), the eleventh organ, controls the senses and organs of action. All the eleven organs are specializations of the general, limited "I"-consciousness (*asmitā*).

The 16 specializations, the vikāras of the guṇas

5 Tanmātras

Subtle fields of the elements:
sound, touch, form,
taste, smell

5 Buddhi-indriyas

Sensory organs/organs of knowledge:
Ears, skin, eyes, tongue, nose

5 Karma-indriyas

Organs of action:
speech organ, hands, feet,
organs of elimination,
organs of reproduction

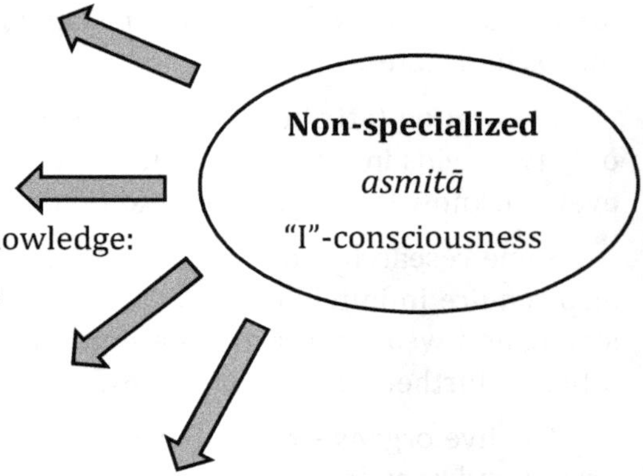

1 Manas

Input-output control of the brain software,
controls sensory and organs of action.

Five elements and guṇas

- Space is mostly sattva
- Air is mostly rajas
- Light/fire is mostly sattva and rajas
- Water is mostly rajas and tamas
- Earth is mostly sattva and tamas

Elements and tanmātras

Space:	sound
Air:	touch, sound
Light/Fire:	form, touch, sound,
Water:	taste, form, touch, sound
Earth:	smell, taste, form, touch, sound

The 16-fold specialization of the guṇas

Sensory Organs *buddhi-indriya*	**Ears** *sattva-sattva*	**Skin** *sattva-rajas*	**Eyes** *sattva-sattva/ rajas*	**Tongue** *sattva-rajas/ tamas*	**Nose** *sattva-sattva/ tamas*	Input-Output Compo-nent **manas** *sattva-sattva/ rajas/ tamas*
Non-specialised **asmitā** ("I"-consciousness)						
Organs of action *karma-indriya*	**Speech** *rajas-sattva*	**Hands** *rajas-rajas*	**Feet** *rajas-sattva/ rajas*	**Reproduc-tion** *rajas-rajas/ tamas*	**Elimina-tion** *rajas-sattva/ tamas*	

Fields *tanmātras*	**Sound** *tamas-sattva*	**Touch** *tamas-rajas*	**Form** *tamas-sattva/ rajas*	**Taste** *tamas-rajas/ tamas*	**Smell** *tamas-sattva/ tamas*
Manifests as	↓	↓	↓	↓	↓
Elements (waves and particles)	**Space** *tamas-sattva*	**Air** *tamas-rajas*	**Fire** *tamas-sattva/ rajas*	**Water** *tamas-rajas/ tamas*	**Earth** *tamas-sattva/ tamas*

The guṇas permeate all their specializations individually and in combinations. The guṇas neither begin, nor cease to exist. They are grounded in pradhāna, which is formless and does not serve puruṣa. Therefore pradhāna is eternal and self-sufficient.

We call *pradhāna* the finest level of creation. It is the formless and eternal basis, from where initially the three *guṇas* with their specific qualities appear. In further steps, the *guṇas* specialize in becoming the manifest cosmic software with its countless divisions, for example, the manifest variations of the brain software.

It seems that the *guṇas* merely appear and disappear because they are individual manifestations, containing them, having the qualities of appearing and disappearing. A jar made of clay appears and disappears, however, the material, clay, stays. Similar it is with the *guṇas*. In their pradhāna state, they stay, like the material, clay. In their unbalanced state, they appear as if changeable. Therefore we call them relative.

In the first stage of physical manifestation, the *guṇas* specialize to become the empty space on the Planck scale, from where in sequence the whole universe with all its further stages of manifestation arises. The *yoga sūtras*, therefore, indicate an earlier level of manifestation beyond the big bang.

Purpose of Experience

2.20

Although the perceiving power of the perceiver [draṣṭṛ = puruṣa] is pure, he notices thoughts.

द्रष्टा दृशिमात्रः शुद्धोऽपि प्रत्ययानुपश्यः

draṣṭā dṛśi-mātraḥ śuddhaḥ api pratyaya-anupaśyaḥ

draṣṭṛ (m. nom. s.: seer, perceiver, observer) dṛśi (f. comp.: the power of seeing, the seeing, perceiving) mātra (m. nom. s.: only) śuddha (m. nom. s.: pure) api (also, although) pratyaya (m. comp.: thought) anupaśya (m. nom. s.: keep focused, be alert)

Puruṣa is like a lamp and the intellect before brain software version 8, like a lampshade, which casts shadows. Due to the fault of the intellect there is an overshadowing of *puruṣa* by thought activity.

If, for example, someone hears music by the perceiving power of the ears, the music is transformed into thoughts, noticed by *puruṣa*. For the user of brain software version 3, these thoughts of the music completely overshadow the SELF (*puruṣa*). The ego component of the brain software assumes, to be the user, although the user is always different from the brain software.

2.21

The purpose of that [noticing of thoughts] actually is the perceivable SELF.

तदर्थ एव दृश्यस्यात्मा

tat-arthaḥ eva dṛśyasya ātmā

tad (n. comp.: that) artha (mn. nom. s.: purpose, goal, motive, reason) eva (ind.: so, really, indeed) dṛśya (mfn., m. gen. s.: of the perceivable world, of the perceivable) ātman (m. nom. s.: SELF)

By perceiving the SELF, the second purpose of perception, liberation, now is reached (2.18). The brain in versions 7 and 8 functions completely liberated. The SELF is perceived everywhere. There is nothing else that could impair this freedom. The items have disappeared. The pain has ended; the goal of 2.16 is reached.

The first purpose of the perceived for the liberated is now in the past, and he can say: "I have done what needs to be done."

Experience

With Heinz's instructions I was practicing the *sūtra* to pass on the perceptions to *puruṣa*: My consciousness suddenly, within seconds, expanded into infinity, embraced everything, stayed there, in this state, for some seconds and then retracted back into my body. It can be described as "I am in everything, and everything is in me." It was as if I had the whole universe integrated into my body. Whenever, since that event, I put my attention consciously on a place outside of my body, for example, a tree or a house, spontaneously this very strong energy passes through my body, which mostly shows up in the back. Space, full of things, is permeated by energy and my attention.

2.22

For him [the yogi], who has reached the goal, it [the goal] has finished, but not so for others [the unskilled] because of their commonality [of collective consciousness].

कृतार्थं प्रति नष्टमप्यनष्टं तदन्यसाधारणत्वात्

kṛta-artham prati naṣṭam api anaṣṭam tat anya-sādhāraṇatvāt

kṛta (mfn., comp: accomplished, achieved) artha (m. acc. s.: purpose, goal) prati (ind.: near, for, regarding, how, as if) naṣṭa (mfn., mn. Akk. s., n. Nom. s.: disappeared, lost) api (ind.: also, even) anaṣṭa (mfn., mn. Akk. s., n. Nom. s.: not disappeared, present) tad (n. nom. acc.: that) anya (mfn. m.: other [persons], different, common, apart from this) sādhāraṇa-tva (n. abl. s.: universality, commonality)

The purpose of the perceived has already been described in 2.18 as being twofold: Experience and liberation. During an experience, *ātman* notices all stages from the beginning to the end of the thought. An experience is complete once the *ātman* has noticed the end of the thought.

In brain software versions 7 and 8 this process of experiencing no longer occurs and only *ātman* remains.

> He who knows the SELF as "I am *brahman,*"
> becomes this whole universe.
> *Bṛhadāraṇyaka Upaniṣad* (1.4.10)

Then every thought is a knowledge impulse in the SELF and no longer an item-oriented, suffering-inducing *vṛtti.*

The suffering-inducing *vṛttis* of previous brain software versions are based on a specific *pradhāna*, the personal parallel universe for the power (*śakti*) of the user. It has similarities with the parallel universes of others. We call these similarities also the collective consciousness.

The power of the user of brain software versions 7 and 8, shuts down its parallel universe while allowing the universes of others to remain. The intellect, purified like that, leaves the collective consciousness and recognizes the ignorance in statements such as "I do this," "I go there." He no longer limits his SELF to his body and his brain software.

The development of brain software version 7 to version 8 happens gradually and takes a certain time. During this time the SELF expands into infinity. Brain software version 8 uses the additional hardware resources of the universe-computer. This can progress so much, that individual brain hardware is no longer required, and nevertheless, the individualized brain software can run. See *sūtra* 3.43 "the great bodiless." At the end of this development, the *yogi* is always and everywhere, all-knowing and all-powerful.

2.23

Due to the connection of the possession [thinking processes] with the owner [SELF], they are perceived [only] in the form of the possession.

स्वस्वामिशक्त्योः स्वरूपोपलब्धिहेतुः संयोगः

sva-svāmi-śaktyoḥ svarūpa-upalabdhi-hetuḥ saṃyogaḥ

sva (mf(ā)n. comp: own) svāmin(m. comp.: owner, master) śakti (f. gen. loc. d.: power, energy) svarūpa (n. comp.: own form, appearance, being, gestalt, character) upalabdhi (f. comp.: get, perceive, perception) hetu (m. nom. s.: reason, cause) saṃyoga (m. nom. s.: connection, association, context)

Puruṣa is the owner of all thinking processes. A seeming connection between puruṣa and the thinking processes leads to overshadowing. Experience is the process, which depends on this connection. Liberation is the consciousness of the seer, puruṣa.

As long as brain software versions 7 or 8 are not yet installed, the brain software experiences itself in the form of faulty thinking processes, which overshadow the SELF. The brain software before version 7 assumes a faulty concept of being the SELF. In 2.6 this fault has been explained as limited "I"-consciousness, which now becomes generalized to all illusions. It is also called the fault of the intellect. The connection is demonstrated with arrows in the sequence in 2.18.

2.24

The cause of that [connection] is ignorance.

तस्य हेतुरविद्या

tasya hetuḥ avidyā

tad (m. gen. s.: that) hetu (m. nom. s.: reason, cause, motive) avidyā (f. nom. s.: ignorance)

Ignorance (*avidyā*) has been defined in 2.5. "Ignorance (*avidyā*) is seeing the impermanent as if eternal, the impure as if pure, suffering as if happiness, the non-SELF as if the SELF."

If someone glues a broken piece of porcelain, often it does not look beautiful and is not stable. That is the meaning of "connection" in the present, the previous, and the following *sūtra*; it is not real unity. The unity can be experienced only on the level of the consistent material of clay.

Ignorance causes the experience of a multitude instead of unity. Unity cannot be connected; only a multitude can be connected by something. As long as a connection is present, it points to a fundamental multitude. If the multitude disappears, the connection also disappears. The experience of the user up to, and including, brain software version 6 is based on this ignorance, which perceives a multitude.

Unity Consciousness

2.25

By the disappearance of that [ignorance], the connection disappears. That ends in the unity of consciousness (kaivalya).

तदभावात्संयोगाभावो हानं तद्दृशेः कैवल्यम्

tat-abhāvāt saṃyoga-abhāvaḥ hānaṁ tat-dṛśeḥ kaivalyam

tad (n. comp.: that) abhāva (m. abl. s.: disappearance, absence, non existing) saṃyoga (m. comp.: connection, association) abhāva (m. nom. s.: disappearance, absence, non existing) hāna (n. nom. acc. s.: liberation, letting go, avoidance, ending) tad (n. comp.: that) dṛśi (f. abl. gen. s.: perceiving, seeing, power of seeing, consciousness) kaivalya (n. nom. acc. s.: absolute unity, liberation)

Now the process of experience becomes replaced by the SELF being aware of itSELF. This *sūtra* shows the sequence to highest liberation.

- Ignorance disappears (2.24).
- The overshadowing of the user by his brain software disappears (2.23).
- The connection of the user with the brain software disappears (2.17).
- The illusions (malware) based on ignorance no longer have any effect (2.3).
- The suffering-inducing methods (vṛttis) of the malware classes (kleśas) no longer become activated (2.11).
- The list of malware objects which means the store of karma, no longer works (2.13).
- Future suffering will be avoided (2.16).

The infinite SELF now is aware of itSELF. The whole procedure towards highest liberation begins with the disappearance of ignorance. The disappearance of ignorance is not an action (*karma*), but cognition. Since no action is required, also it does not take any time. This cognition, therefore, happens in a moment. All the results from it, are also there immediately.

That also corresponds to *Adi Śaṁkara's* commentary on the *brahma sūtras* regarding the topic of highest liberation.

2.26

The method for liberation is uninterrupted correctly-discriminating cognition (viveka khyāti).

विवेकख्यातिरविप्लवा हानोपायः

viveka-khyātiḥ aviplavā hāna-upāyaḥ

viveka (m. comp.: correct discrimination) khyāti (f. nom. s.: knowledge, cognition) aviplava (mf(ā)n., f. nom. s.: without interruption, uninterrupted) hāna (n. comp.: liberation, letting go, avoidance, ending) upāya (m. nom. s.: means, method)

Viveka khyāti, the correctly-discriminating cognition, is a function of the main component of the brain software. Starting from version 7, *ātman* no longer sees any pain-inducing thinking processes (*vṛttis*). By utilizing correctly-discriminating cognition, these *vṛttis* become transformed into knowledge impulses in *ātman*.

Correctly-discriminating cognition is the thought that the brain software and puruṣa are different. This thought changes, until the misunderstanding, has stopped. Once the illusions, like roasted seeds, are reduced to the state of sterility, then the sattva of the brain software, purified from the illusions of rajas, reaches the highest purity with the consciousness of mastery. His [the yogi's] flow of thoughts of knowledge, then becomes flawless. Just as seed grains, when roasted in a fire can no longer sprout, as is with the illusions, roasted in the fire of knowledge; the SELF is no longer confronted by them.

Following on from the clear analysis of the causes of all suffering, here we see now the universal remedy, which removes the deepest cause. The deepest cause is the erroneous connection, which is recognized as non-existent by applying correctly-discriminating cognition. Once the ignorance is removed by this, with a sequence of steps as indicated in 2.25, the suffering also, step-by-step, becomes removed.

The rest of the *yoga sūtras* now only deal with the correct application of *viveka khyāti*. All *yoga* techniques will be derived from it. The *viveka khyāti* practice will be increasingly refined, to realize all the higher states of consciousness that means up to version 8 of the brain software.

2.27

The seven stages of that [correctly-discriminating cognition] lead to the highest level of intuitive knowledge.

तस्य सप्तधा प्रान्तभूमिः प्रज्ञा

tasya saptadhā prānta-bhūmiḥ prajñā

tad (n. gen. s.: that) saptadhā (ind.: in seven parts, sevenfold) prānta (mn. comp.: limit, extreme end, tip) bhūmi (f. nom. s.: position, area, level, step, degree, place, Earth) prajñā (f. nom. s.: wisdom, intuitive clear knowledge)

With the application of correctly-discriminating cognition, the highest knowledge is reached in seven steps. For the user of the brain software before version 7, there is correct, limited knowledge (*pramāṇa*), which is one method of the brain software (1.7). All book knowledge and experiential knowledge (*pramāṇa*) will be transformed into the SELF-referral, intuitive knowledge (*prajñā*) of unity consciousness. *Pra–jñā* (before knowledge) is SELF-referral knowledge in unity. All knowledge impulses become the SELF (*ātman*). It happens in seven steps. *Vyāsa* describes it like this:

1. *That which is to be avoided has been investigated thoroughly and requires no further investigation.*
2. *The causes of that, which needs to be escaped, have melted away and no longer need to be destroyed. Neither illusions nor karmas remain. Then the thought arises "I am someone, who has done, what had to be done." That is a thought that marks the ripeness of the correct vision, like someone, who has recovered from a disease, thinks: "The cause of*

the disease is destroyed, I am well, I require no further treatment." [Versions 5 and 6].

3. *The samādhi of stopping is a directly experienced liberation. It is realized in the state of absolute unity consciousness (kaivalya). [Version 7].*
4. *Correctly-discriminating cognition has been made perfect and is practiced correctly and intensively.*

These initial four stages comprise the freedoms of cognition that arise from actions. The following three deal with the liberation of the brain software.

The following three steps describe, how *citta*, the brain software, merges with *prakṛti* (nature). In our modern language, it means, that the brain software is uploaded onto the universe-computer. The individuality of the *yogi* not only remains but rather becomes enlarged because all the cosmic resources are available to the *yogi*. This upload is the liberation of the *yogi*. His individuality no longer depends on small brain hardware.

5. *The guṇas, comprising the main component (buddhi-sattva) of the brain software and the other two (rajas, tamas) in other components of the brain software (citta) merge with nature.*
6. *Similar to stones, moving on the peak of the mountain, falling, bursting, and coming to rest, the guṇas come into their ground state (pradhāna). The brain software comes to rest, together with its cause, the "I"-ness (asmitā) because it has fulfilled the purpose of the user (puruṣa). That is called the first liberation of the brain software (prajñā-citta). Then, being equalized, the guṇas do not appear again because they have no more purpose. That is called the second liberation of the brain software.*
7. *In this state of the dissolution of the guṇas, the connection with the guṇas is transcended, and the user (puruṣa) is the sole light of his own nature. In his own nature, being vision only, he, therefore, is light, alone and pure; that is called the third liberation of the brain software [Version 8].*

That user (puruṣa), who perceives the indications, that the correct vision in the seventh, final state, by knowledge has achieved its final stage of ripening, is called skillful. Correct vision, therefore, has reached the upper limit of steps and states. The word "skillful" is only an approximation. Although it is the brain software, that has been freed and came to an end, he, the user, is called skilled, since he became, what he always was, since he is beyond the guṇas.

The one who has transcended the *guṇas* is skillful.

We are interpreting the stages 5 to 7 in a way that, with the liberation of the brain software the individuality of the cosmic individual becomes completely transferred to the cosmic software. All that remains, in the end, is described in the last *sūtra* (4.34) using the expression *citi śaktir iti*, pure consciousness (*citi*) and its infinite organizing power (*śakti*).

How do we get there?

The following eight areas of life (2.29) are uplifted to the highest level of intuitive knowledge by the method of the correctly-discriminating cognition. That means, with the brain software version 7 already installed in step 3, mentioned above, it becomes expanded more and more by application of correctly-discriminating cognition (step 4).

The main component in brain software version 7 discriminates: "is this unity or not?" If not, bit by bit, it transforms all eight areas of life. The steps 5 to 7, in turn, happen automatically and what remains, is infinite, SELF-referral, intuitive knowledge (*prajñā*) in unity. The rest of chapter two identifies the eight areas of yoga, where these transformations happen.

The Eight Areas Of Yoga

2.28

By the practice of the areas of yoga, with the reduction of impurity, knowledge radiates until correctly-discriminating cognition [is established in each corresponding area].

योगाङ्गानुष्ठानादशुद्धिक्षये ज्ञानदीप्तिराविवेकख्यातेः

yoga-aṅga-anuṣṭhānāt aśuddhi-kṣaye jñāna-dīptiḥ ā-viveka-khyāteḥ

yoga (m. comp.) aṅga (n. comp.: limb, component, area, part) anuṣṭhāna (n. abl. s.: practice) aśuddhi (f. comp.: impurity) kṣaya (m. loc. s.: decrease, gradually destroying, reduction) jñāna (n. comp.: knowledge) dīpti (f. nom. s.: flame, radiation, glow) ā (ind.: near, up to) viveka (m. comp.: discrimination) khyāti (f. abl. gen. s.: knowledge, clarity, cognition)

The original definition of *yoga* as the calming down of certain thinking processes (1.2) will now be refined in the following *sūtras*. Previously (2.26), correctly-discriminating cognition has been described as a means of transforming limited knowledge into infinite SELF-referral, intuitive knowledge (*pramāna* → *prajñā*). Now, correctly-discriminating cognition will be presented, both as a means and the goal. The radiating of knowledge and correctly-discriminating cognition mutually perfect each other.

Reduction of impurities means, the switching off and removing of malware.

The radiating of knowledge means that the SELF permeates it. Contrary to *pramāṇa* knowledge, which can also appear as a method of a malware, *prajñā* knowledge stays free from malware. *Prajñā* knowledge is a method, which becomes available only with the infinitely fast quantum computer in the human brain. *Prajñā* knowledge originates completely spontaneously from the infinite resources of the knowledge store in the universe-computer.

2.29

The eight areas of yoga are self-control (yama), rules of living (niyama), body postures (āsana), breathing techniques (prāṇāyāma), withdrawing the senses from the objects (pratyāhāra), focusing the brain software (dhāraṇā), meditation (dhyāna) and absolute silence (samādhi).

यमनियमासनप्राणायामप्रत्याहारधारणाध्यानस माधयोऽष्टावङ्गानि

yama-niyama-āsana-prāṇāyāma-pratyāhāra-dhāraṇā-dhyāna-samādhayaḥ aṣṭau aṅgāni

yama (m. comp.: self-control, self-restraint) niyama (m. comp.: rules of living) āsana (n. comp.: body postures) prāṇāyāma (m. comp.: breathing techniques) pratyāhāra (m. comp.: withdrawing the senses from the objects) dhāraṇā (f. comp.:) dhyāna (n. comp.: meditation) samādhi (m. nom. p.: restful alertness, absolute silence; in p. because of eighth components) aṣṭa (mfn., n. nom. acc. d.: eight) aṅga (n. nom. p.: limb of a body, part, component)

The eight areas become, by the application of correctly-discriminating cognition, knowledge impulses in the SELF. That will be explained in detail in the following *sūtras*.

Yama and Niyama

2.30

Nonviolence, truth, non-stealing, sexual and sensual abstinence, non-greediness [define] self-control.

अहिंसासत्यास्तेयब्रह्मचर्यापरिग्रहा यमाः

ahiṃsā-satya-asteya-brahmacarya-aparigrahāḥ yamāḥ

ahiṃsā (f. comp.: non-violence) satya (n. comp.: truth, honesty, truthfulness) asteya (n. comp.: non-stealing) brahmacarya (n. comp.: chastity, sexual abstinence) aparigraha (m. nom. p.: renunciation, relinquish [foreign property], not taking over, non-greediness, non-avarice) yama (m. nom. s.: self-control, self-restraint)

Here *yama* is defined: Nonviolence is the basis of the other aspects of self-control. Nonviolence leads to peaceful behavior in others (2.35). Truth leads to success in action (2.36). Non-stealing leads to wealth (2.37). Sexual and sensual abstinence leads to bodily strength (2.38). Non-greediness leads to knowledge of previous lives (2.39).

All the *yamas* (self-control) and *niyamas* (rules of living) should be considered with correctly-discriminating cognition.

The goal is, to establish unity consciousness in all these areas. The correctly-discriminating cognition leads to the dissolution of ignorance (*avidyā*) in the corresponding area. As a result, unity consciousness expands to that area.

2.31

The great rule of behavior [with relation to 2.30] means that they, [the self-controls,] are valid over the whole Earth and are unlimited by birth, place, time and convention.

जातिदेशकालसमयानवच्छिन्नाः सार्वभौमा महाव्रतम्

jāti-deśa-kāla-samaya-anavacchinnāḥ sārvabhaumāḥ mahā-vratam

jāti (f. comp.: birth, caste, family, position assigned from birth) deśa (m. comp.: place) kāla (m. comp.: time, moment in time) samaya (m. comp.: agreement, teaching, accepted duty, convention) anavacchinna (mfn. m. nom. p.: uninterrupted, unlimited) sārvabhauma (mfn., m. Nom. p.: on the whole Earth, for all conditions of the mind) mahāvrata (n. nom. s.: great duty, fundamental duty, great vow)

Observing perfect self-control is not a prerequisite for unity consciousness, but it is a vow that renunciates take. It involves the application of correctly-discriminating cognition to self-control with the purpose of transforming this area of life into unity. There can be no exceptions for no residues of duality or multiplicity to remain.

2.32

The rules of living are attention to bodily purity, contentment, urge for liberation, self-study of the Vedas, and devotion to Īśvara.

शौचसंतोषतपःस्वाध्यायेश्वरप्रणिधानानि नियमाः

śauca-saṃtoṣa-tapaḥ-svādhyāya-iśvara-praṇidhānāni niyamāḥ

śauca (n. comp.: bodily purity) saṃtoṣa (m. comp.: contentment) tapas (n. nom. s., acc. s: asceticism, discipline, urge for liberation) svādhyāya (m. comp.: self-study of the Vedas) iśvara (m. comp.: Supreme Being) praṇidhāna (n. nom. acc. p.: effort, devotion, attention) niyama (m. nom. p.: rules of living)

That has already been partially explained as *karma yoga* in 2.1, and here the areas of purity (2.40) and contentment (2.42) are supplemented.

2.33

Dubious [thinking] is removed by pondering over its opposite.

वितर्कबाधने प्रतिपक्षभावनम्

vitarka-bādhane pratipakṣa-bhāvanam

vitarka (m. comp.: gross, analytical thinking) bādhana (mfn., n. loc. s.: oppressing, harassing, fight, opposition, remove, torment, hassle) pratipakṣa (m. comp.: opposition, opposite side, contrary) bhāvana (mf(ā)n., n. nom. s.: promoting, imagination, thought, meditation)

Dubious thoughts are those, opposed to self-control or the rules of living. These thoughts can be neutralized one by one by pondering over their opposites. In the process, the fundamental illusion at their basis, ignorance (2.4), becomes weaker.

> Simply think "Cancel!" or "Stop! This action would lead to never-ending suffering."

If a malware becomes active in the brain software, *yama* and *niyama* are causing an interrupt, which signals this activity. The main component of the brain software can now, using an opposite thought, isolate the malware, that means, to put it under quarantine. The priority of the interrupt depends on the steadfastness of the resolution (2.31). Complete neutralization of the damaging thought, then happens afterward, with *dhyāna* (meditation).

Summary of the yoga methods

1. Calming down pain-inducing *vṛttis* (thinking processes).
   - 1.1 Weakening of the *vṛtti*s by thinking the opposite (2.33) and by the *yoga* of action (2.1).
   - 1.2 Completely switching off the pain-inducing *vṛttis* by *dhyāna*, that is meditation (2.11).
   - 1.3 Experience of perfect silence in *asaṁprajñāta samādhi* (1.18).
2. Roasting *saṁskāras* (impressions).
   - 2.1 The *siddhi* practices in chapter three are an application of *viveka khyāti* and lead to *nirvicāra samādhi* (3.5).
   - 2.2 *Nirvicāra samādhi* lets the SELF clearly shine (1.47).
   - 2.3 Thereby, *prajñā*, an intuitive, clear knowledge (1.48), arises.
   - 2.4 By the cleaning impression of *prajñā*, damaging impressions are stopped (1.50).
   - 2.5 In the end, even the cleaning process is stopped by the perfect silence in *nirbīja samādhi* (1.51).
   - 2.6 Therefore, from the roasted *saṁskāras*, the old *karma* can no longer become active (2.13).
   - 2.7 Persistent *saṁskāras* can be stopped more easily, by applying the *siddhi* technique in 3.18.

3. Calming of the *kleśas* (illusions).
   3.1 Calming by opposite thoughts (2.33).
   3.2 *Avidyā* (ignorance), the basic cause of the *kleśas*, is dissolved by *viveka khyāti* (correctly-discriminating cognition 2.26) (2.10).
   3.3 Dissolving ignorance automatically, in several steps, leads to dissolving of the illusions (2.25), (2.24), (2.23), (2.17).

The yoga methods from the viewpoint of brain software

1. Stop methods of malware.
   1.1 Isolating the methods of the malware by the malware scanner, described in 2.33 and 2.1.
   1.2 A complete switch off of the methods of the malware by *dhyāna* that is meditation (2.11).
   1.3 Experience of the perfect silence in the idle mode of the brain software (1.18).
2. Deactivating the malware objects (impressions).
   2.1 The brain software apps in chapter 3, the *siddhi* practices, are an application of *viveka khyāti* and they activate the quantum computer in the brain (3.5).
   2.2 *Nirvicāra samādhi* lets the SELF shine forth clearly, which means, due to the activated quantum computer in the brain, infinite possibilities are available to the user of the brain software (1.47).
   2.3 From this, arises *prajñā,* intuitive knowledge that means, infinite knowledge in the infinitely fast quantum computer (1.48).
   2.4 Due to the cleaning object of *prajñā*, the malware objects are stopped (1.50).
   2.5 In the end, the cleaning object becomes stopped as well, by the idle mode of the brain software (1.51).

2.6 Due to the methods of the malware that are no longer available, the stored *karma*, the list of malware objects, can no longer damage anything (2.13).

2.7 Persistent *saṁskāras* can be deleted more easily by applying a special brain software app (3.18).

3. Deactivating the malware classes (illusions).

3.1 Isolating the malware classes by opposite thoughts (2.33).

3.2 The initial basic class (ignorance) is deleted by *viveka khyāti* (2.26), the distinction between the user and his brain software, (2.10).

3.3 All other, derived malware classes then are also automatically deleted (2.25), (2.24), (2.23), and (2.17).

3.4 The list of malware objects no longer provides any pain-inducing methods (2.13).

2.34

Dubious [thoughts] of violence etc. – whether to be carried out, incited, or allowed – having arisen from greed anger, or insanity, to a mild, medium, or intensive extent, result in unending suffering and ignorance. Therefore think of their opposite.

वितर्का हिंसादयः कृतकारितानुमोदिता लोभक्रोधमोहपूर्वका मृदुमध्य अधिमात्रा दुःखाज्ञानानन्तफला इति प्रतिपक्षभावनम्

vitarkāḥ hiṃsā-ādayaḥ kṛta-kārita-anumoditāḥ lobha-krodha-moha-pūrvakāḥ mṛdu-madhya-adhimātrāḥ duḥkha-ajñāna-ananta-phalāḥ iti pratipakṣa-bhāvanam

vitarka (m. nom. p.: thinking, reasoning, consideration) hiṃsā (f. comp.: violence) ādi (m. nom. p.: etc.) kṛta (mfn. comp.: done) kārita (mfn. comp.: incited, effected, brought about) anumodita(mfn., f. nom. s.: allowed) lobha (m. comp.: greed) krodha (m. comp.: wrath) moha (m. comp.: mental confusion, insanity) pūrvakā (mfn. m. nom. p.: before, previous) mṛdu (mf(u/v/ī)n., comp.: mild, tender) madhya (mf(ā)n. comp.: medium) adhimātra (mfn., m. nom. p.: intensive, extreme) duḥkha (n. comp.: pain, sorrow) ajñāna (n. comp.: ignorance) ananta (comp.: infinite) phala (n. nom. s.: fruit, result; here "f." instead of "n." ifc. at the end of a comp.) iti (ind.: therefore) pratipakṣa (m. comp.: opposition, opposite side, opposite) bhāvana (n. nom. acc. s.: reflection, pondering) bahuvrīhi – compositum.

The applications of self-control, like for example, nonviolence, etc., have been listed in *sūtra* 2.30. Here we discuss their opposites.

Violence, for example, is threefold: It is performed; it is caused to be performed; it is agreed to be performed. Each one of those is again threefold: Due to greed, or anger, or insanity. Greed, anger, and insanity, again are threefold, mild, medium or strong. Therefore, violence has 3*3*3 = 27 variations. *The final three again have three subdivisions: mild-mild, medium-mild, and strong-mild, etc.* Thus there are 3*3*3*3 = 81 sub-subdivisions.

Similarly, these divisions also exist, regarding the other yamas and niyamas. This branches out infinitely, such that there is a multitude of distinctions, both for the wrongdoer and for the victim. However, in all cases, it leads to pain and ignorance.

If someone has escaped dubious thoughts by thinking their opposites, the meditation on their opposites, the saṁskāras take on a sterile, non-sprouting quality. The resulting divine powers are a hint at the success of the yogi.

> The success of *yoga* is measured by the results!

Benefits of the Yamas

Now the results of the *yamas* and *niyamas* will be described. They are the first in a row of brain software apps, or programs, which lead to specific, predictable results. Some of the apps will only run with higher software versions. See chapter three.

2.35

In the vicinity of someone established in total nonviolence [all] enmity disappears.

अहिंसाप्रतिष्ठायां तत्सन्निधौ वैरत्यागः

ahiṃsā-pratiṣṭhāyām tat-sannidhau vaira-tyāgaḥ

ahiṃsā (f. comp.: non-violence) pratiṣṭhā (f. loc. s.: standstill, halting, fundament, establishment) tad (n. comp.: that) sannidhi (m. loc. s.: presence, environment, nearness, vicinity) vaira (n. comp.: hostility) tyāga (m. nom. s.: leaving, ending, halting, disappearing, going away)

Large meditation groups can end violent conflicts. Wild animals also become tame in the presence of a *yogi*. That happens with all living beings. It happens, when the nonviolence of the *yogi* is steady and free of opposite thoughts. Nonviolence spreads in his presence. Even natural enemies, like snake and mongoose, abandon their enmity.

Nonviolence means, to not damage any being in any way or at any time. All the other *yamas* are practiced, to bring this first one to perfection. Nonviolence is practiced with the body, the language, and thinking.

Experience

We arrived with a group of about 4000 meditators in the Philippines, to prevent a looming civil war. This, actually worked quite well. The press in the Philippines reported extensively about our project. While gradually more of us arrived, the life on the streets of Manila became more relaxed. The people became increasingly friendly, and they laughed and joked with us. When they saw us, even at a distance, they called out "unified field." By using this term from physics, which is a synonym for pure consciousness, the effects of our group meditations were described in the press. Somehow it was all quite wonderful, peaceful, exhilarating, and enthusiastic. All the indications of civil war disappeared.

Unfortunately, however, most of the meditators had taken their vacations for only a few weeks, to come to the Philippines. The government of the Philippines did not finance the project. Therefore we had to leave, little by little, and then the peace-creating influence disappeared again. I was among one of the last groups that left. The aggression on the streets increased again, more often, rioting groups of people erupted and expressed their anger. I became really scared and was more than happy when I sat in the airplane on my way back to Europe.

During another world peace assembly in Croatia, we gathered with about 500 meditators in the beautiful seaport town of Dubrovnik. It was directly bordering Bosnia and Herzegovina, where, at that time, the Yugoslav war was in progress. We meditated every morning and evening in a group and practiced the flying technique for *yogis*. It took about two weeks to achieve visible results.

However, some indications were there before. For example, there were reports about a group of dolphins, which had been sighted again near Dubrovnik. One fine day I got an invitation by a yacht owner, to accompany him on a short trip on the ocean. However, he had to do that during our group meditation period. I decided without further ado, to skip one meditation and to go with him on his ship. Suddenly I noticed something baffling. In my consciousness, I noticed the deep silence that was emanating from the meditation group. The wind had completely calmed down, and the surface of the ocean was free of any waves whatsoever; I could not see, even the slightest ripples on the water. The water surface was totally smooth, a sea like a mirror. I had never seen such a thing before in the Mediterranean.

I was convinced, to watch a physically measurable effect of the group meditation.

At the end of the two weeks, the breakthrough was reported. A truce had been declared for Bosnia and Herzegovina. I was the first to hear this news, and then reported it to the whole meditation group, and everyone cheered. We had achieved it again.

2.36

[When] established in truthfulness, actions have corresponding results.

सत्यप्रतिष्ठायां क्रियाफलाश्रयत्वम्

satya-pratiṣṭhāyām kriyā-phala-āśrayatvam

satya (n. comp.: truthfulness, truth) pratiṣṭhā (f. loc. s.: standstill, halting, fundament, establishment) kriyā (f. comp.: action) phala (n. comp.: fruit, result) āśraya-tvam (m. acc. s.: consequence, connection, based on something; "tva" means –ness)

If someone lies, he creates a complex parallel universe, which can be supported only with difficulty, and in the long term does not deliver any results.

To speak the truth, means, that language and thoughts agree with that, which is perceived, inferred, or heard by an authority. The language, one speaks to confirm one's experiences to another, should not be deceitful, nor imprecise, nor meaningless. Only that should be spoken, which helps all beings.

However, whatever is spoken to damage living beings, even though it may be called truth, it would not be the truth. Speaking with a goal of violating living beings, would be a sin.

Manu: "Let someone speak, what is true; let someone speak, what is pleasant; let someone not speak what is true, yet unpleasant. Let him speak what is pleasant and not untrue. That is eternal righteousness."

Whenever he tells a person "become righteous," then that one becomes righteous. When he says "Go to heaven," then that one goes to heaven. His words are unfailing. When the truth is established in him, the results confirm his words. The results follow from whatever is spoken by a truthful speaker.

2.37

[When] established in non-stealing, all wealth flows to him.

अस्तेयप्रतिष्ठायां सर्वरत्नोपस्थानम्

asteya-pratiṣṭhāyām sarva-ratna-upasthānam

asteya (n. comp.: non-stealing) pratiṣṭhā (f. loc. s.: standstill, halting, fundament, establishment) sarva (mf(ā)n comp.: all, total) ratna (n. comp.: jewel, riches, wealth) upasthāna (n. nom. acc. s.: approach, access, appear)

Non-stealing of money, wealth, benefits, etc. leads to wealth. Non-stealing of intellectual property stimulates one's creativity.

2.38

Established in sexual and sensual abstinence, he gains vitality.

ब्रह्मचर्यप्रतिष्ठायां वीर्यलाभः

brahmacarya-pratiṣṭhāyām vīrya-lābhaḥ

brahmacarya (n. comp.: modesty, sexual and sensual abstinence) pratiṣṭhā (f. loc. s.: standstill, halting, fundament, establishment) vīrya (n. comp.: energy, strength) lābha (m. nom. s.: gaining, receiving, getting)

That means self-control of the sexual organs and the sense organs.

For the user of brain software, before version 8, sensory experiences can overshadow the SELF. The connection with the SELF, however, creates a far greater vitality.

From this self-control, he derives invincible, good qualities for himself. He has the irresistible energy to achieve good projects. He cannot be stopped by any obstacles and becomes able, to pass on knowledge to students.

2.39

Steadiness in non-greediness leads to the cognition of the circumstances of birth.

अपरिग्रहस्थैर्ये जन्मकथंतासंबोधः

aparigraha-sthairye janma-kathaṃtā-saṃbodhaḥ

aparigraha (m. comp.: non-hoarding, not in the future [apari] wanting to have [graha]) sthairya (n. loc. s.: steadiness, endurance) janma (n. comp.: birth) kathaṃtā (f. comp.: the circumstances) saṃbodha (m. nom. s.: cognition)

Attachment to wealth means that someone does not see the faults in things, is involved in their acquisition, their defense, their loss, adhere to them, and keeps them away from others. If someone does not do that, does not attach to the wealth, he is non-greedy.

One variety of greediness, for example, is the attachment to things that are no longer required. Non-greediness should not be confused with lack of possessions. An example is a king with brain software version 7, who owns a country, without being attached. A counterexample is a beggar with brain software version 3, greedily attached to his begging bowl.

"What is this birth? How does it happen? What are we going to be after death? How will we be and under what circumstances will we be?" Each of those desires of him, to recognize his situation in previous, later, or intermediate states, spontaneously becomes fulfilled for him. Since he has no attachment to any outer wealth, the field of his "I" becomes clearly perceived without any effort. In spite of effort, this knowledge does not arise, if someone is attached to wealth in a feverish, depressed, or intensively desiring way.

Benefits of the Niyamas

2.40

From bodily purification [there arises] a disinterest in the limbs of the body [the imperfection of the body] and in touching others.

शौचात् स्वाङ्गजुगुप्सा परैरसंसर्गः

śaucāt sva-aṅga-jugupsā paraiḥ asaṃsargaḥ

śauca (n. abl. s.: purity, bodily purification) sva (mf(ā)n. comp.: own) aṅga (n. comp.: limb of the body) jugupsā (f. Nom. s.: disinclination, reluctance) para (mf(ā)n., m. ins. p.: further, other, foreign) asaṃsarga (m. nom. s.: non-contact, non-touching)

When someone practices purity, he sees the faults in his own body. He is disgusted by his own body; he becomes free from the obsession with his body. When he sees what the body actually is, he has no interaction (touch) with others. He does not find any purity in the body, although he has washed it. Therefore he avoids contacts with other bodies, which are also impure.

Do not overemphasize body and looks; in particular, someone should not spend too much time in front of the mirror.

2.41

[From that arise] the abilities of clarity, purity, contentment, purposefulness, mastery of the senses, and SELF-cognition.

सत्त्वशुद्धिसौमनस्यैकाग्र्येन्द्रियजयात्मदर्शनयोग्यत्वानि च

sattva-śuddhi-saumanasya-ekāgrya-indriya-jaya-ātmadarśana-yogyatvāni ca

sattva (n. comp.: mental purity, clarity, light) śuddhi (f. nom. s.: purification, purity, truthfulness) saumanasya (n. comp.: contentment, cheerfulness, good mood correct understanding) ekāgrya (n. comp.: concentration on one object, purposefulness, attention) indriya (n. comp.: sense and organs of action) jaya (m. comp.: gain, victory, gaining) ātmadarśana (n. comp.: to see one SELF, self-awareness, SELF-cognition) yogya-tvāni (n. nom. acc. p.: competence, ability, state) ca (ind.: and, also; elements of an enumeration are connected by "ca")

Resulting from bodily purity the purity of the main component of the brain software increases. From that, in turn, joyfulness, and from that one-pointedness, and from that, victory over the senses, and from that the main component of the brain software becomes enabled for the cognition of the SELF. All this, therefore, will be achieved by the steadiness of purity.

2.42

Contentment creates the highest joy.

संतोषादनुत्तमः स्सुखलाभः

saṃtoṣāt anuttamaḥ sukha-lābhaḥ

saṃtoṣa (m. abl. s.: contentment) anuttama (m. nom. s.: highest) sukha (n comp.: joy) lābha (m. nom. s.: gaining, getting, obtaining)

From the Madhusūdana-Purāṇa:

"All earthly sexual joys and the highest joy in heaven do not even account for 1/16 of the joy that arises from the destruction of craving."

2.43

From the urge for liberation (tapas), impurity disappears [and] perfection of body and senses [arises].

कायेन्द्रियसिद्धिरशुद्धिक्षयात्तपसः

kāya-indriya-siddhiḥ aśuddhi-kṣayāt tapasaḥ

kāya (m. comp.: body) indriya (n. comp.: sense and organs of action) siddhi (f. nom. s.: complete accomplishment, perfection, efficiency, extraordinary power) aśuddhi (f. comp.: impurity) kṣaya (m. abl. s.: diminish, disappear) tapas (n. nom. acc. s.: urge for liberation)

Translating the word *tapas* is not easy. Many translators tend to consider *tapas* to be asceticism, mortification, etc. Looking at the root *tap*, it means "to be hot," or "to glow." Considering *sūtra* 1.21, "For those with intense striving for *samādhi*, it is near," we translate *tapas* with the term "urge for liberation."

It is not a stubborn, tense, or concentrated will, or remaining, but rather constant practice with the necessary serenity (1.12). In no other way, can the practices bring the desired success. The urge, or striving, designated by *tapas*, therefore is something very subtle, an intuitive foreboding, or divining of the goal of the permanently established silence of *samādhi* and final liberation, *kaivalya*. The urge for liberation can, and actually should, be intense, even burn like an inner fire, in which all the impurities become destroyed. Asceticism and mortification of the body, however, are merely outer appearances, which we consider less efficient.

Once, tapas becomes complete; it destroys the cloaking veil of impurity. When the cloaking veil is removed, the perfections of the body are there, like for example, the ability to become as small as an atom, etc. [3.45] *and the perfection of the senses, in the form of hearing and seeing of things, which are remote* [3.25].

2.44

From the self-study of the Vedas and Vedic literature [arises] a connection with the personally revered devatā (personification of infinity).

स्वाध्यायादिष्टदेवतासंप्रयोगः

svādhyāyāt iṣṭadevatā-saṃprayogaḥ

svādhyāya (m. abl. s.: a self-study of the Vedas) iṣṭadevatā (f. s. comp.: personally revered devatā) saṃprayoga (m. nom. s.: intimate connection, unification with)

Devas and *devatās* respectively, are the highest, personified expressions of natural laws. One can communicate with them. See also practices in 1.23. In computer terminology, we describe the procedure like this:

> Install the communication interface to the universe-computer like an app in your brain software and then you can communicate to the *devas* and *Īśvara*.

Gods, sages, and siddhas appear to him, who practices self-study and help him, to fulfill his work.

By the way, they talk with you as well. Keep listening, keep looking! That establishes the connection of the human quantum computer in brain and heart to the universe-computer.

Experience

Experience 1

When translating the *yoga sūtras* together with my friend Gerd, we sometimes came across passages, where we simply did not know, how to proceed. Even though we had the commentaries of *Vyāsa* and *Śaṁkara* available, in some rare cases, however, we did not even know from the commentaries, what they wanted to say. We simply did not understand it. In situations like these, we sometimes asked, what *Śaṁkara* could have meant. Then it happened several times that *Śaṁkara* came to our help. He explained in very simple words, what he meant with his expressions, and then we did understand it. All those were great lightbulb moments, and we were deeply grateful to *Śaṁkara*, that ultimately he had helped us enormously to work this book out.

Experience 2

In India, my teacher had demonstrated to me, how mental healing works, but he had not explained it. I tried it then successfully on my own body and several others. Out of interest, I took initiation into mental techniques by a shaman, to find out, how they work. Indigenous nations practice this healing technology. During the instruction, while focusing on a certain area, a donkey appeared to me, only to be pushed to the side by a figure with an elephant's head and hands. When focusing on another area, a serpent with five heads appeared to me. These are natural laws that can appear in such forms. During a later walk, suddenly the cognition came to me, that *Gaṇeśa* and *Śeṣa* had revealed themselves to me. They are among the most influential of natural laws or the methods of the universe-computer. I often communicated with *Gaṇeśa*. He revealed to me that in some situations I should ask *Durgā* for her help.

2.45

By attention to Īśvara perfection of samādhi [results].

समाधिसिद्धिरीश्वरप्रणिधानात्

samādhi-siddhiḥ īśvara-praṇidhānāt

samādhi (m. comp.: restful alertness, absolute silence) siddhi (f. nom. s.: perfection, extraordinary abilities) īśvara (m. comp.: Supreme Being) praṇidhāna (n. abl. s.: effort, attention)

Īśvara is the personification of the highest dynamical infinity. *Īśvara* in 1.24 has been described as different from *puruṣa* and in 1.25 as all-knowing and almighty.

Perfect samādhi arises in the yogi, who has devoted his whole being to Īśvara. Thereby, he knows anything, he wishes to know, the way, it really is, in different places, in various bodies and at various times. After that, his intuitive knowledge (prajñā) knows these things, the way they really are.

Sūtra 2.45 completes 1.23 ("Or by attention to *Īśvara*"). *Samādhi* will be explained in more detail in the context of the *siddhi* techniques in 3.3.

Attention to *Īśvara* means, to uphold a connection to the universe-computer. It ensures that the human quantum computer in brain and heart stays turned on and keeps improving its operation.

Āsana

2.46

Āsana is a stable and pleasant body posture.

स्थिरसुखमासनम्

sthira-sukham āsanam

sthira (mf(ā)n. comp.: hard, firm, stable, non-moving) sukha (mfn., n. nom. s.: pleasant sensation, wellbeing, joy) āsana (n. nom. s.: seat, sitting, body posture)

First, the yogi should go to a pure place, such as a cave in a holy mountain, on an island in a river, but not directly near an open fire or running water. The place should be free of insects and pebbles. He should take his position with a view to the east or north.

Upon assuming a position, he should retain it. Following the initial effort, securing the right position for body and limbs is called the āsana position.

Since there are plenty of such body-related *yoga* courses, here we circumscribe only a few hints. It is recommended, visiting a *yoga* course of a well-trained teacher.

The three *sūtras* 2.46 to 2.48 are the only *sūtras* that refer to body practices. The *sūtras* 1.34 and 2.49 to 2.51 are the only ones that refer to breathing practices. Therefore, what is interpreted all over the world with the name *yoga*, actually is only a small part of the *yoga sūtras*.

2.47

[That body posture] results from relaxation of effort and attention (samāpatti) on infinity (anantya).

प्रयत्नशैथिल्यानन्त्यसमापत्तिभ्याम्

prayatna-śaithilya-anantya-samāpattibhyām

prayatna (m. comp.: effort, striving) śaithilya (n. comp.: effortlessness, relaxing) anantya (mfn., n. comp.: infinite, eternal, infinity) samāpatti (f. ins. dat. abl. d.: attention, completion, yielding)

Samāpatti has been defined in 1.41 as attention. The attention is on infinity, rather than on the limbs of the body. *Āsana*, therefore, is a continuation of *niyama* of 2.45 (attention on the infinite *Īśvara*), and therefore, practiced correctly, results in a deepening of *samādhi* (2.45).

By retraction of effort, when the limbs of the body no longer move, a posture becomes perfect. When the brain software is in samādhi, in infinity, then the body posture becomes perfect. That means, that by retracting effort, the body posture, becomes completely steady, once the position is reached, by no longer making any effort. Thus the posture becomes perfect because it is the effort that is disturbing to the limbs of the body.

"And attention on infinity," means, the universe is infinite, and the state of being infinite is called infinity. When the brain software reaches samādhi, permeating all existence, then the posture is perfect and steady.

2.48

Due to those [āsana], opposites do not violate.

ततो द्वंद्वानभिघातः

tataḥ dvaṃdva-anabhighātaḥ

tataḥ (ind.: by this, from that, due to that) dvaṁdva (n. comp.: duality, opposites, a pair of opposites, doubt) anabhighāta (m. nom. s.: non-obstructing, non-attacking, non-blocking, non-violating)

The result of the *āsanas* is that the body becomes more resistant, for example, to heat and cold. Temperature differences are opposites, that can, with the correctly-discriminating cognition between infinity and the finite body (2.47), become transformed from duality to unity.

Simply doing gymnastic does not deliver the goods.

Prāṇāyāma

2.49

While remaining in that [in an āsana position], prāṇāyāma is the interruption of the motion of breathing out and breathing in.

तस्मिन् सति श्वासप्रश्वास्योर्गतिविच्छेदः प्राणायामः

tasmin sati śvāsa-praśvāsyoḥ gati-vicchedaḥ prāṇāyāmaḥ

tasmin (ind.: in that location) sat (mf(ī)n., m. loc. s.: existing, being, occurring, happening, the true being or really existent) śvāsa (m. comp.: breath, breathing, hissing [of a snake], sigh) praśvāsa (m. gen. loc. d.: breathing in) gati (f. comp.: movement) viccheda (m. nom. s.: obstruction, ending, halting, interrupting) prāṇāyāma (m. nom. s.: breathing exercise, breath control)

Prāṇa becomes activated in an āsana by prāṇāyāma, and the posture has been mastered.

- *When the yogi now breathes air from the outside, it is called in-breath (śvāsa).*
- *When he exhales the inside air, it is called out-breath (praśvāsa).*
- *Interrupting the movement of those two, so they both stop is called prāṇāyāma.*

In-breath

As water is sucked up in a tube in continuous action, the outer air is sucked in, together with the downward going stream (apāna), through the two tubes of the nostrils.

Out-breath

Then, when the air streams from inside to outside, together with the outgoing stream (prāna), this going out is called the out-breath.

prāṇāyāma

- Thus, the two breath movements can be distinguished. The interruption of the movement of these two is called prāṇāyāma.

There are two halting points of attention:

- After breathing out: Twelve fingers wide, in front of the nose.[8]
- After breathing in: In the diaphragm.

[8] According to the instruction of the immortal *Bhuśuṇḍa* in the *Yoga Vasiṣṭha*.

2.50

The cessation [of air coming from] outside [after fully breathing in], cessation [of air coming from] inside [after fully breathing out], and holding the breath [intermediately] are measured as long and fine, depending on the place, time and number.

बाह्याभ्यन्तरस्थम्भवृत्तिः देशकालसंख्याभिः परिदृष्टो दीर्घसूक्ष्मः

bāhya-abhyantara-sthambha-vṛttiḥ deśa-kāla-saṃkhyābhiḥ paridṛṣṭaḥ dīrgha-sūkṣmaḥ

bāhya (mf(ā)n. comp.: external, outside) abhyantara (mf(ā)n. comp.: inner, internal) sthambha (m. comp.: stiffness, suppression, stoppage) vṛtti (f. nom. s.: thought process) deśa (m. comp.: location, place, area, spot, region) kāla (m. comp.: time, moment) saṅkhyā (f. ins. p.: number, calculation, number) paridṛṣṭa (mfn. comp.: known, perceived, seen, beheld) dīrgha (mf(ā)n. comp.: long) sūkṣma (mf(ā)n., m. nom. s.: fine, subtle)

Attention to the duration and number of breaths and their effective areas in the body causes an extension and refinement of the breath and leads to a mild, medium, or intensive energy rush to the head.

The outer, inner, and held breath movement becomes long and fine, measured regarding place, time, and number. (1) When holding the flow after breathing in, it is called the outer, or the filling (pūraka). (2) Suspending the flow after breathing out, is called the inner, or expulsion (recaka). (3) The suspended movement, following neither the full breathing in nor the full breathing out, is caused by a single process. Prāna and apāna simultaneously shrink to nothing. The flow of both ends simultaneously, just as water thrown on a heated stone, dries up all over.

- All 3 of them are to be practiced,
- measured regarding the place, how far the range of each one extends,
- measured regarding duration, how many moments each one can be suspended, and
- measured regarding the number, how many in-breaths and out-breaths are required until the first energy rush happens.

Once this energy rush to the head is reached – how many more to the second, and similarly, how many more to the third upwards energy rush.

Those are called the mild, medium, and intensive practice. When practiced thus, the breath becomes long and fine.

Distinctions regarding prāṇāyāma

Concerning the place

During the outer movement of breath, the stream of air sucked in, is felt while it flows through the space from the tip of the nose down to the toes. With the inner movement of breath, the expelled air is felt, while it flows through the space from the toes to the tip of the nose. The suspended breath movement is felt, while it permeates the whole body from head to the soles of the feet.

Measured concerning its duration

The first energy rush happens, when the air sucked in becomes exhilarated and first touches the head and stops there. That is called the mild practice. Then, when the held back air has risen for the first time in the upward energy rush, the yogi counts, how many out-breaths it takes to the second energy rush. The prāṇāyāma up to this point is called the medium practice.

Measured concerning number

The third is practiced by counting the number of in-breaths and out-breaths, it takes up to the third upward energy rush. The practice up to the third upward rush is called strong. Following the third upward energy rush the prāṇāyāma should be ended.

Extended breath

When practiced in this way, concerning place, duration, and number, the breath extends for longer, depending on the mastery of the stages. The Vedic texts claim that saints could extend their breath for years; in this way, it becomes extended. While the breaths become longer and slower, they also become subtler.

Practice

- Follow the breath flow from the outside through the nose to the toes into all cells. Then keep your attention on its suspension in the diaphragm.
- Then follow your breath from the heart to the nose and keep your attention at a point twelve fingers wide in front of the tip of the nose.
- Hold your breath in between, before it has ended.

The breathing practices, like all *yoga* practices, should be practiced with serenity. That means, holding the breath should not be exaggerated so much, that afterward excessive breathing is required. As with the *āsanas*, intensive breathing practices should be learned from an experienced teacher.

2.51

Regarding the outer and the inner phase, there is a fourth [prāṇāyāma].

बाह्याभ्यन्तरविषयाक्षेपी चतुर्थः

bāhya-abhyantara-viṣaya-ākṣepī caturthaḥ

bāhya (mf(ā)n. comp.: outer, outside, external) abhyantara (mf(ā)n. comp.: inner, internal) viṣaya (m. comp.: area, scope, phase, sphere of influence) ākṣepin (mfn., m. Nom. s.: concerning) caturtha (mf(ī)n., m. nom. s.: the fourth)

With the completion of breathing in, apāna permeates the inner bodily regions down to the toes. With the completion of breathing out, prāṇa permeates the earth element and the other four elements and, therefore, the whole universe.

The fourth prāṇāyāma comes about automatically after mastering the first two techniques.

The flow of the outer breath movement, measured regarding place, duration, and number, has been practiced and felt. The second prāṇāyāma in the flow of the inner breath movement also has been practiced and felt. In both practices, the breath becomes long and subtle.

The fourth prāṇāyāma comes about, when the stages mild, middle and strong, of these two practices, have been gradually mastered. It consists of the cessation of both breath movements, whereas the third prāṇāyāma consists of the cessation of the breath, without putting the attention on the areas of the outer and the inner things. The breath becomes long and subtle simply by this practice, according to place, duration, and number.

However, the cessation, in the fourth pranayama comes about only after putting the attention on the two breath flows in the first and second prāṇāyāma and feeling them, by gradually mastering the steps. That is the difference with the fourth pranayama.

The third can be done at any time. The fourth can be done only, after mastering the first and second.

1. Cessation after breathing in
2. Cessation after breathing out
3. Cessation in between at any time
4. By transcending of 1 and 2, following the previous practice of 1 and 2, up to the extreme, that means up to the third upward energy rush.

2.52

Then [as a result of prāṇāyāma] the covering of the light disappears.

ततः क्षीयते प्रकाशावरणम्

tataḥ kṣīyate prakāśa-āvaraṇam

tataḥ (ind.: hence, from that place, there, in that place) kṣīyate (is lost, become diminished) prakāśa (mfn., m. comp.: visible, bright, shining, light, brightness, splendour) āvaraṇa (mfn., n. nom. acc. s.: cover, covering, screening, shading)

Light, in this context, means pure consciousness. Covering means impurities in the nervous system and corresponding impurities in the brain software and the senses. Each sense is by nature infinite; however, due to habit, it seems to have merely a finite range.

Prāṇāyāma erases the karma that covers the correctly-discriminating cognition of the yogi, who has not yet practiced prāṇāyāma. It has been said, that, if the eternally bright sattva is covered by Indra's net of illusion, then one is impelled, to do, what should not be done. By the power of prāṇāyāma, the light-covering karma, which binds him to the world, becomes powerless and destroyed in each moment. And it has been said: There is no tapas, higher than prāṇāyāma. By practicing it, there arises purification of illusions and the light of knowledge.

2.53

And [as a result of prāṇāyāma follows] the ability, to focus (dhāraṇā) the input-output component of the brain software (manas).

धारणासु च योग्यता मनसः

dhāraṇāsu ca yogyatā manasaḥ

dhāraṇā (f. loc. p.: focusing the brain software) ca (ind.: and, also) yogyatā (f. nom. s.: ability) manas (n. abl. gen. s.: input-output-control)

Now we consider further effects of *prāṇāyāma*. In 1.34 exhaling and holding the breath has already been mentioned as a means of calming the brain software. Here now, this calming is applied to the ability, to focus in silence.

Dhāraṇā here applies to the input-output component of the brain software. It will be expanded to the whole brain software and precisely defined in *sūtra* 3.1. All the previously mentioned techniques are preparations for the correct practice of *dhāraṇā*, by purifying the nervous system and brain software, so that distractions will be reduced.

Pratyāhāra

2.54

Withdrawing from its objects of perception the brain software (citta) takes on its own [unexcited] state, and the sense organs and organs of action imitate this. That is pratyāhāra.

स्वविषयासंप्रयोगे चित्तस्य स्वरूपानुकार इवेन्द्रियाणां प्रत्याहारः

sva-viṣaya-asaṃprayoge cittasya svarūpa-anukāraḥ iva indriyāṇām pratyāhāraḥ sva (mf(ā)n.: own) viṣaya (m. comp.: sensory object, object of attention) asaṃprayoga (m. loc. s.: withdrawal) citta (n. comp.: brain software) svarūpa (n. comp.: own nature, form) anukāra (m. nom. s.: imitation, similarity) iva (ind.: as if) indriya (n. gen. p.: sense and organs of action) pratyāhāra (m. nom. s.: withdrawal)

The brain software (citta) comes to rest in its own state. That means it no longer disturbs the pure consciousness of the brain software user. The sense organs and organs of action imitate this and also come to rest.

When the brain software is held back, then the input and output organs are also held back by the brain software, without requiring any further means of restraint, as with a queen bee that starts flying, and the whole swarm flies with her. When she settles down, the swarm also settles down. Thus the senses are restrained, as soon as the brain software is restrained. That is pratyāhāra.

A short resting phase with closed eyes before a meditation is a variety of *pratyāhāra.*

2.55

By this [pratyāhāra], perfect mastery over the senses [is attained].

ततः परमा वश्यतेन्द्रियाणाम्

tataḥ paramā vaśyatā indriyāṇām

tataḥ (ind.: by this, hence) parama (mf(ā)n., f. Nom. s.: highest, absolute) vaśyatā (f. nom. s.: control of [gen.], power on [gen.]) indriya (n. gen. p.: sense and organs of action)

Mastery over the senses together with the wonderful results will be explained extensively in the brain software app 3.47.

Jaigīṣavya deems that mastery over the senses is merely non-perception of items resulting from the one-pointedness of the brain software. That is the highest mastery. When the brain software is restrained, the input and output organs also become restrained. In contrast to other techniques of sensory control, yogis who have practiced that, do not need to look for any other means.

Thus he says that this is the highest technique.

This sūtra ends the second part, on the means of the yoga sūtras, compiled by the great seer, the adorable Patañjali, with the commentary of the adorable Vyāsa and the sub-commentary of the adorable Śaṁkara, who is a student of the adorable Govindapāda, whose feet are to be worshipped.

3

Vibhūti Pāda

Extraordinary Abilities

Introduction

Siddhis

The user of brain software versions 7 and 8 has intuitive access to all knowledge and unlimited abilities. This totality of all possibilities manifests to him in various extraordinary abilities, which are called the *siddhis*. In this chapter three of the *yoga sūtras*, initially, the technique of the *siddhis* will be taught. Following that, all the knowledge and power *siddhis* will be explained in detail. The basis for successful *siddhi* practice is, both the correctly-discriminating cognition, as well as the correctly performed *siddhi* technique.

Once the brain software is fairly well purified from malware, and, therefore, brain software version 7 can, sometimes at least, run correctly, many problems in life will be solved, and also completely new possibilities manifest. They result from the application of apps, or application programs, which run on brain software versions 7 and 8. Initially, these apps must be correctly installed, that means, the technique of how to practice the *siddhis* correctly must first be learned. This know-how of the correct application will now be described in the first *sūtras* of chapter three.

As long as a *siddhi* app does not yet function correctly, that means as long as it does not bring the predicted result with it, so long the app has not been correctly installed. A correctly installed *siddhi* app brings the right result within seconds. It functions as a light switch that one can switch on and off.

Many *yogis*, who do not yet have *siddhi* experiences, lay the blame for their lacking success on what they assume as a fact, that their brain software does not function in version 7, not even occasionally. In reality, however, they are incorrectly practicing the *siddhi* technique.

Correct translation

The authors, therefore, have put the greatest emphasis on the correct translation, word by word, of the first five *sūtras* of chapter three. We spent not only hours, but weeks on the translation of these *sūtras*, and have tested them thoroughly because they contain the essential kernel of the *siddhi* technology. The motive was our 30 years of practice of the *siddhis* according to the very much simplified, and therefore essentially different from the original, version of the *yoga sūtras* as interpreted by Maharishi™ Mahesh Yogi, a version that for us, by no stretch of the imagination brought any reliable results.

Now, after decades of *siddhi* practice, we found, that the *siddhis* would not function for the majority, who follow the instructions to the letter. A few *siddhas* were an exception, who, due to their somewhat free interpretation of the *siddhi* technique, had the right *siddhi* experiences. For another fairly small group, we included, results sometimes came about, sometimes not. However, we lacked an explanation, why was there that uncertainty.

We are, however, grateful to Maharishi™[9] for his genius worldview, recognizing, that the *yoga sūtras* constitute a practically applicable technology and not merely a philosophy or religion. Based on our scientific, technological background, however, it was not possible for us, to interpret Maharishi's™ statements and techniques as rigid, quasi-religious truths. Therefore, we approached the topic scientifically, and the positive results speak for themselves. Maharishi™ became world-renowned for his scientific approach to the development of consciousness, with hundreds of scientific research studies about his meditation technique. Unfortunately, however, he also became famous for the fact, that his technique of "yogic flying™[10]," has not succeeded so far, except in a very few cases.

We also learned from Maharishi™, that the unaltered Vedic knowledge could only be found in the original *saṁskṛt* texts. Therefore we took on the task, for ten years, of re-translating the manual for the development of consciousness, the *yoga sūtras*, directly from *saṁskṛt*, and also making it practically applicable. He had actually, repeatedly inspired this course of action. He had pointed his students to the originals of the Vedic literature because, in his opinion, the existing translations contained too many faults.

[9] Maharishi is a trademark of Maharishi Foundation Ltd. Corporation United Kingdom, P.O. Box 652 St. Helier, Jersey Great Britain JE48Y2.

[10] YOGIC FLYING is a trademark of Maharishi Foundation Ltd. Corporation United Kingdom, P.O. Box 652 St. Helier, Jersey Great Britain JE48Y2.

Computer science and technology, today has become the most influential trend in mass consciousness on a global scale. Digitization has become the most influential factor in society. Computer terminology transcends the differences in governments, religions, science, lifestyle, wealth, age, etc. It has developed into a language that is globally spoken and understood. Regarding our use of computer science terminology, therefore, we feel very much in tune with our teacher, who made the following statement in 1963:

> "Therefore, basically, the teaching of meditation should be based on that phase of life, which at any particular time is guiding the destiny of mass consciousness."
>
> *Science of Being and Art of Living, Maharishi™ Mahesh Yogi, p.306*

Therefore, we were making a fresh translation of the original *yoga sūtras*. In doing so, the commentaries of previous liberated teachers of our Vedic tradition, *Vyāsa* and *Śaṁkara* became a never-ending source of wisdom. We had their commentaries available, like the *yoga sūtras*, with the original *saṁskṛt* texts. The daily reward of our efforts now comes with our *siddhi* practices, which work for us at any time, like a button press operation.

Maharishi™[11] Mahesh Yogi on the correct siddhi practice

"By the sidhi program, we directly create an opportunity for wholeness of consciousness to function. This is what the sidhi practice is. We meditate, get to transcendental consciousness and start to function from there in a very, very gentle way. And when we experience what Patañjali* has predicted, then we know that we have succeeded in functioning from that wholeness of consciousness. If whatever Patañjali has predicted is not our experience, then we know that we have not succeeded in operating from that subtle state of consciousness. So we try again in a more non-trying manner. In that way sidhi practices give us a habit; they create a habit in us

[11] Maharishi is a trademark of Maharishi Foundation Ltd. Corporation United Kingdom, P.O. Box 652 St. Helier, Jersey Great Britain JE48Y2.

to function from the least excited state of consciousness, which is a field of all possibilities. And functioning from the field of all possibilities means we materialize our desires quickly."

Maharishi™[12] Mahesh Yogi, Seelisberg, Switzerland – June 26, 1977, First World Assembly on Law, Justice, and Rehabilitation – June 24 - 26, 1977 Booklet (p. 136)

* Author of the *yoga sūtras*, the basis of the Sidhis.

Technique of the Siddhis

3.1

Binding of [the total] brain software in one place is dhāraṇā.

देशबन्धश्चित्तस्य धारणा

deśa-bandhaḥ cittasya dhāraṇā

deśa (m. comp.: place) bandha (m. nom. s.: binding to, holding, fixing) citta (n. gen. s.: total mind) dhāraṇā (f. nom. s.:)

"Binding in one place" means, that the brain software focuses exclusively on one place. That is a purely mental process and means focusing the thoughts on one place, not on words or their multiple varieties of meanings. The attention on the place is so strong; it is as if this place alone were the whole world.

[12] Maharishi is a trademark of Maharishi Foundation Ltd. Corporation United Kingdom, P.O. Box 652 St. Helier, Jersey Great Britain JE48Y2.

Examples for places are: navel, heart, tip of the nose, tip of the tongue.

It is the binding of the brain software as a purely mental process to the navel wheel, the heart lotus, the light in the head, the tip of the nose, the tip of the tongue, and other similar places and outer things. The brain software becomes bound to these places or things, and the state of the brain software, when it is kept in these places without distraction, is called dhāraṇā. It simply consists of the thought of the place that means the full attention on the place without any distraction.

Heinz Krug: "From 40 years of *siddhi* practices I can say, that if someone practices *dhāraṇā* on the gross level, the way it is defined in 1.17, that means, where imagination, word, and meaning are intermixed, nothing at all happens! Not until the application of soundless, pictorial *dhāraṇā* on the subtlest level, where only the place, but no words, sounds or meanings are the center of attention, the *siddhi* technique shows full and immediate results."

Practices

The goal of these practices is to keep the attention, with serenity, in one place, without any distraction.

Practice 1

First, repeat the attention practices of 1.41.

Practice 2

Choose the next place to be the tip of your nose and keep your attention there for about half a minute, first with open eyes.

Practice 3

Now repeat the practice for half a minute with closed eyes.

Practice 4

Repeat practice 3, with closed eyes, on the tip of your tongue as a place.

Practice 5

Then on your navel.

Practice 6
Then on your heart.

3.2

There [bound to the place], the expansions of one same thought are defined as dhyāna.

तत्र प्रत्ययैकतानता ध्यानम्

tatra pratyaya-ekatānatāḥ dhyānam

tatra (ind.: there, therein) pratyaya (m. comp.: thought) eka (mfn.: one, the same) tānatā (m.: expansion, enlargement, stretching, steady flow) dhyāna (n. nom. acc. s.:)

It is a flow of similar thoughts, one similar to the other. The term "thoughts," here does not mean speaking internally. "Thoughts" here means, not thinking words, but rather a continued focus of the attention on one place. The expansion (*tānatā*) means extending the flow of similar thoughts. *Tānatā* in music means to hold the tone.

When thinking a word, *tānatā* is simply impossible, because every word has a beginning, a middle, and an end. And, once it has ended, it cannot be extended any further. For that reason *dhyāna* with internally spoken words is simply impossible. Therefore, whoever tries, to practice *siddhis* with words spoken mentally, will not have any success with it. The same applies when someone keeps repeating the same word and thinks it similar to a *mantra* because he also does not apply the principle of *tānatā* to extend the same thought. Words keep the brain software on the gross thinking level of *vitarka* (1.17).

In the *dhyāna* practice, *tānatā* is a holding of the attention on a place or a thing, without allowing distracting thoughts – though without effort. One does not force to keep the attention on the place, but one continuous to look, because one is so interested.

Dhyāna is the continuation of the same thought of a meditation item or a place, a stream of similar thoughts, which are not influenced by other thoughts. "In the place," means, for example, in the navel circle, or in other items of the dhāraṇā. Continuation of the thought of the meditation item or the previously selected place means a stream of similar thoughts. If the continuation of the thoughts does not get disturbed by any thought of a different kind, it is dhyāna.

During the practice of dhāraṇā from the previous sūtra, where the brain software has attached itself to a single item, it may become interrupted by another, different thought regarding the item. If, for example, dhāraṇā is applied to the Sun, it can happen, that also its orbit, momentary position, and its extreme brightness become items of the dhāraṇā. When applying dhyāna simultaneously, this will be avoided, because then it is only the stream of the one same thought, untouched by any thought of a different kind.

Dhyāna generally is translated as "meditation." With the practice of *dhyāna,* those similar thoughts become automatically refined. Thoughts here really mean nothing but the continued attention to one place, nothing else. *Dhyāna* functions in a way like a snowplow, which moves other thoughts to the side before they are fully manifest.

Practice

Repeat the practices of *sūtra* 3.1, however, while you keep your attention on the place, perceive the slight change in the attention. That is the meaning of a "stream of similar thoughts." However, if non-similar or other, disturbing thoughts arise, effortlessly push them to the side. With a bit of practice, you can accomplish this even on a very subtle level, before the disturbing thought, fully manifests.

3.3

In that way, just the total goal [of 3.1 and 3.2] appears in its own form, as if empty. That is samādhi.

तदेवार्थमात्रनिर्भासं स्वरूपशून्यम् इव समाधिः

tat eva-artha-mātra-nirbhāsam svarūpa-śūnyam iva samādhiḥ

tad (n. nom. acc. s.: that) eva (ind.: thus, but, really, „giving emphasis") artha (m. Comp.: goal, purpose, meaning, reason, true meaning) mātra (n. comp.: measure, only, merely, total) nirbhāsa (m. acc. s.: appearance, similar) svarūpa (n. comp.: own form, nature, character, essence) śūnya (mfn., n. nom. acc. s.: zero, empty, being not there, absent, missing) iva (ind.: as if) samādhi (m. nom. s.: here samādhi is defined; restful alertness)

The first goal of each *siddhi* is the deepening of *samādhi*; the second goal is the special result predicted for the *siddhi*. Both goals are reached immediately, spontaneously and simultaneously in one state of *samādhi* "colored" with the special result. The result of each *siddhi* does not appear as another thought. Therefore it does not cause a distraction from *dhāraṇā* and *dhyāna*.

Vyāsa comments this *sūtra* as follows:

When the same meditation (dhyāna) shines forth only as the item of meditation and by a thought, filled with the SELF, becomes as if transparent, then the meditation item comes out of its hiding.

Śaṁkara explains this commentary of *Vyāsa* in detail:

This same dhyāna, which consists of a stream of thoughts that appears to have surrendered being the stream of a single thought, shines forth in the form of the meditation item. It [dhyāna] therefore shines also in the form of the item, seemingly disposed of its own nature as a thought of perception. It is similar to the background shining through a clear crystal that is placed on it, with the crystal remaining transparent by nature.

Compare this to the definition of attention in 1.41, which later, in 1.46 is denoted by the word *samādhi*.

When, in this way, the essence of the meditation item is determined, or when the meditation item is the cause of the thought, that means becomes this thought, then this item is samādhi. The special point here is the method, of how a stream of thoughts by entering into the being of the meditation item becomes the actual form of this item.

Here, *sūtra* 3.4 is anticipated. During the *siddhi* technique, therefore we recognize omnipresent Being in the item. The *samādhi* arising from that is our own, infinite SELF, which we recognize in the item. That is precisely the purpose of the *siddhi* technique, to recognize our SELF everywhere.

Let us explain this with an analogy: It is similar to the way in which a three-dimensional picture is generated from a hologram, using lasers. The hologram is an exposed and developed film that looks similar to circular waves, like those that come about from many raindrops on a flat water surface. For the naked eye, there is no similarity, whatsoever, to the three-dimensional picture.

Not until, using a specially expanded laser beam that shines through the hologram, can a three-dimensional picture appear. The holographic film is a concrete item and corresponds to the item for *dhāraṇā* that is the place of attention. The light wave field of the laser corresponds to *dhyāna,* and the transparent, three-dimensional picture corresponds to *samādhi.* That means, the *dhyāna* becomes *samādhi.* With the laser hologram analogy it is also important, that apart from the laser beam which becomes changed by the hologram, another unchanged laser beam must travel at the side of the hologram, circumnavigating the hologram. Only from the interference between the changed laser beam and the unchanged, the picture arises. That means in our analogy that in addition to the *nirvicāra* stimulation (the intuitive knowledge 1.44) simultaneously there must also be the unchanged *samādhi* (1.43). Only in this way the special *siddhi* result manifests.

The result in the form of this *samādhi* is different from common sensory experience. It is beyond the three *guṇas.* It has *samādhi* qualities, described as *śūnya*: null, empty, transparent, lucent, hollow, cloudy, and unfathomable. Also, it appears in *nirvicāra samādhi,* which means "beyond the subtle." In this way, *prajñā,* intuitive knowledge is reached.

With the brain software apps, beginning from 3.16, in each case, first the corresponding place, the item for the *dhāraṇā,* is mentioned and then the goal, that is specific for the corresponding app. The second goal, *samādhi,* applies to all apps. By the application of the various apps, the *yogi* learns, to uphold *samādhi* in a variety of colorings. However, before using those individual apps, one should learn the correct installation, which will be explained in more detail in the following *sūtras*.

Practices

Repeat the practices of 3.2 and observe consciously, how your brain software comes into deep silence. If, in that silence refined sensory perceptions appear, simply do not give any attention to them, and continue to practice the *dhāraṇā* and *dhyāna* of 3.1 and 3.2.

3.4

The three [dhāraṇā, dhyāna, samādhi] in one place are saṁyama.

त्रयम् एकत्र संयमः

trayam ekatra saṁyamaḥ

traya (n. nom. acc. s.: three, threefold, triad) ekatra (ind.: as one, together) saṁyama (m. nom. s.: definition of saṁyama)

The *yogi* begins with *dhāraṇā* focused on the place; while remaining on the place, *dhyāna* automatically begins; the result shows up in *samādhi*. Only when all three are there in the same place, on the same item, is it *saṁyama*. This place may be either concrete or abstract; it would be concrete if, for example, on the Sun, or abstract, if on the feeling of friendliness. In both cases, however, the place is not the word, not the word "sun," nor the word "friendliness."

In this *sūtra, Patañjali*, by using the word *ekatra*, again points to a place in space or an item. *Ekatra* is an indeclinable word with a clear reference to the same place in space. The very first word in chapter 3, which is *deśa*, also refers to a place. By its position as the first word of chapter 3, it is very important. In Vedic literature, a chapter, or a complete book, can always be summarized by the first and last expression. That means, for chapter 3 of the *yoga sūtras*, which explains all of the siddhi techniques, that it can be summarized by "*deśa bandhaḥ ... kaivalyam iti*," which means, "Bound to one place... liberation, so it is." That is the essence of the *siddhi* techniques; they lead from bondage to liberation.

The *yogi* recognizes his infinite SELF at whatever place he puts his attention, and thus overcomes all limitations of his perception, his ability to cognize, and his range of influence. That can even proceed so far, that he can overcome the bondage of natural laws. His abilities of perception no longer stay bound to the limitations of the sensory organs of his body. He can perceive hidden and far distant things, that means, see, hear, taste them, etc. He can see into the past and the future, travel with his attention through the universe or perceive the subtlest constituents of the world, smaller than the atoms. Thus, all the limitations of his perception disappear. That is liberation regarding perception.

His ability to cognize no longer stays bound to the light computer or the neuronal computer in his brain. He activates, additionally, his quantum computer with an infinite calculation speed, and by that, gains access to perfect, intuitive knowledge. His knowledge base no longer stays limited to his treasure of experiences, nor those of his predecessors or society. Instead, he gains the freedom, to know everything that he wants to know, by connecting to the database of the universe on the subtlest level of space, the Planck scale with an information density of 10^{99} bits per cm^3 and a clock frequency of 10^{44} Hz.

He, whose perception and cognition are infinitely expanded, becomes a cosmic individual, not even limited by space, and who, therefore, is in harmony with all the systems of his body, predominantly with the subtle nervous system in his heart. With his perception no longer limited, he feels precious feelings towards all beings in the universe. Wherever he looks with his infinite perception, he sees nothing but his SELF.

Using the same technique of *saṁyama*, he even overcomes bondage to the planet Earth, by changing the gravitational field through yogic levitation.

This is the genius of *Patañjali*, enabling the *yogi*, by attention, bound to one place, to achieve liberation.

Saṁyama means: To not stop at *dhāraṇā* and *dhyāna*, as soon as a result shows in *samādhi*! For a user of brain software versions 7 or 8, who anyway, continuously stays in *samādhi*, there is merely a change of the "coloring" of the *samādhi* in the form of specific results.

Vyāsa comments on it, like this:

What has previously been explained as the triad of dhāraṇā, dhyāna, and samādhi, which are held in one place, accomplished in one single place, is called saṁyama. Therefore he [Patañjali] says: The threefold means, directed to one single item, is designated with the term saṁyama.

Śaṁkara comments on this in more detail:

The triad, which gradually becomes perfected, in this work is designated by the technical term saṁyama. In the various sections [of the *yoga sūtras*], *when dealing with the determination of something, which means cognizing the desired thing, or with mastering something, controlling the desired thing, now, here will be taught, that the appropriate saṁyama should be known. In all these following sections, saṁyama is the term that will be used for this triad.*

Previously, *samādhi* was mentioned, both with and without intuitive knowledge (*prajñā*). In that state of cosmic consciousness, brain software version 5, *samādhi* was accompanied with nothing more than arbitrary thoughts (1.17). Now, for the first time, with the *saṁyama* technique – caused by a specific kind of thinking (*dhāraṇā* and *dhyāna*) – a very specific effect is created. For lack of a better term, we call this effect a "coloring of *samādhi*." However, the cause (*dhāraṇā* and *dhyāna*) should not be confused with the effect (coloring of *samādhi*), although cause and effect appear simultaneously. Therefore we do not follow the coloring of *samādhi*, but rather continue *dhāraṇā* and *dhyāna*. Thus the correctly-discriminating cognition (*viveka khyāti*) is now applied to the three most important areas of *yoga*, *dhāraṇā*, *dhyāna*, and *samādhi*.

The threads (*sūtras*) of *yoga* are woven together in the wonderful, dazzling, multicolored cloth of *brahman*-consciousness.

Practices

Practice very consciously *dhāraṇā, dhyāna* and *samādhi* simultaneously. That means, do not halt *dhāraṇā* and *dhyāna*, as soon as a result shows in *samādhi*. Choose the same places again for *dhāraṇā* as before in 3.1. When your brain software thus comes to rest, you have achieved the most important goal of these practices. If, additionally, refined sensory perceptions appear in *samādhi*, so much the better. However, it is important, never to expect such perceptions, and also not to expect the same ones, that one experienced already before. To not expect anything, is a form of serenity (*vairāgya*) that should be there together with all the *yoga* practices (1.15).

Also, you should not get into the trap of *śakti vāda* because the power of the words creates imaginations as explained in 1.9. Imaginations, for example, are the pictures that a child thinks when its mother reads fairy tales. Imaginations are fundamentally different from intuitive knowledge, which will be described in the next *sūtra*. Therefore it is best, not to use words in the practices.

If you no longer use words, you can be sure, that they generate no imaginations. In that case, old memories can still arise, as long as your brain software and your nervous system become purified from *saṁskāras*. Then, after a certain purification phase, only refined sensory perceptions and pure intuition remains. This intuitive knowledge will be described in the next *sūtra*.

3.5

By mastering that [triad] the brilliance of wisdom (prajñā) radiates.

तज्जयात् प्रज्ञालोकः

tat-jayāt prajñā-ālokaḥ

tad (n. comp.: that) jaya (m. Abl. s.: mastery, victory) prajñā (f. comp., f. nom. s.: wisdom, clear, intuitive knowledge, vision) āloka (m. nom. s.: light, brilliance)

Pramāṇa means correct knowledge according to the criteria of *sūtra* 1.7. It is a method of the brain software versions 1 to 6. *Pramāṇa* is a *vṛtti*, which is to be calmed down because it is finite and limited.

Prajñā, however, means pure, intuitive knowledge, that radiates in the *samādhi* state (1.48). It can appear, starting from brain software version 5. *Prajñā* is infinite and all-comprehending.

Wherever saṁyama is steadily applied, the intuitive knowledge of this thing becomes steady. By this light of intuitive knowledge, that can illuminate anything, even the hidden and remote, by that, yogis see clearly, what they have in their brain software as if it was on the palm of their hand.

Mastery is achieved, when I, being the SELF, become one with *dhāraṇā*, *dhyāna*, *samādhi*, all three of them unified in me, in *saṁyama*. Then I radiate with pure, intuitive knowledge, the light of wisdom.

Practices

The *saṁyama* is to be practiced until the *prajñā* knowledge appears. Practice *saṁyama* on the same places as in 3.1 and continue, even when the silence of *samādhi* appears, until, within the silence, there is also intuitive knowledge. From *saṁyama* on the tip of the nose, comes refined smell, and on the tip of the tongue, refined taste. From *saṁyama* on the navel, comes an inner view of the body, from that on the heart, comes knowledge of the intellect, or about the essence of the brain software.

Initially, to avoid any effort, do not practice each of the various *saṁyama* practices for longer than five minutes. With improved practice, the intuitive knowledge (*prajñā*) gradually comes faster, and eventually even within seconds or even fractions of a second.

3.6

That [saṁyama] is applied in stages.

तस्य भूमिषु विनियोगः

tasya bhūmiṣu viniyogaḥ

tad (mn. gen. s.: that) bhūmi (f. loc. p.: earth, step, stage) viniyoga (m. nom. s.: use, application)

Vyāsa comments:

Saṁyama must be practiced such, that someone proceeds to the next stage only, having mastered the previous stage. That is because if the previous stage is skipped without being mastered, to quickly move to the next stage, [the yogi] will not reach any saṁyama in the later stages. How else could the light of intuitive knowledge ever arise?

However, for someone, who has mastered the later stages, the practice of saṁyama on the earlier stages would not be right, like for example, with telepathy. Why is that? It is because the purpose has been achieved already in another way.

Śaṁkara explains that in more detail:

The saṁyama is to be practised in such a way, that someone really intends, to master the steps, by proceeding to the next step only once he has mastered the previous steps: the yogi keeps his attention steady on one step until he has reached saṁyama there, and then proceeds to the next step, having mastered the saṁyama.

That, for example, applies to 3.44, regarding "the five elements, which will be mastered in sequence by saṁyama on their physical form, their essential nature, their subtle form, their inheritance and their purposefulness." That means, once saṁyama on the physical form has been practiced, the next saṁyama must be practiced on the essential nature, only if the previous one is mastered. He should not skip the essential nature, to get to finer levels, like the subtle form.

Why not? Because when he has not mastered a previous stage and skipped that, coming to the next stage, he cannot even reach saṁyama in the later, following stages. Thus, if he has not mastered the previous stage and tries, to apply saṁyama on the later ones, he will not reach saṁyama on them, and this non-reaching for him means failure. And how will the light of knowledge ever shine without the saṁyama in the later stages? There would not be anything to bring this about, just as a lamp that would not emit any light, if the oil, the wick, and the flame are not brought together.

Regarding the question "What stage follows on from the present?" Regarding this, yoga is the only teacher. Why is that? Vyāsa said:

"Yoga becomes known by yoga alone;

yoga proceeds from yoga alone.

Whoever is not negligent,

enjoys yoga for a long time."

The question "What stage follows on from the present?" will be decided, when a stage is mastered; then it will be decided, which one comes next. Here yoga alone is the teacher. Yoga means, in this context the reaching of saṁyama on a previous stage. Only then, someone understands, what should be the next.

Similar to someone, who is blind from birth, going up steps, by initially feeling the first step with his foot and then knowing for sure, where the next one is, similarly yoga proceeds by yoga.

The practice of *saṁyama* must be done in steps that means someone goes to the next step only after mastering the previous. Steps are the sequential *siddhi* apps. Only the yoga knows, what step follows in the sequence:

- The *siddhis* should be practiced in the sequence outlined in this chapter. The place for the next *siddhi* results, in some cases, from the previous. For example, Sun, Moon, Polestar must be practiced in that order (3.26 to 3.28).

- For a *siddhi* with several stages of refinement, none of the stages can be skipped.
- The same *siddhi* should also be practiced in stages, with pauses of *asaṁprajñāta samādhi* or *nirbīja samādhi* between each stage (1.18 and 3.8).
- Mastering of a higher *siddhi* sometimes implies no longer practicing some of the previous ones. If for example, someone has gained complete knowledge from discrimination between *buddhi* and *puruṣa* (3.49), he would avoid practicing a previous *siddhi,* for example, reading the thoughts of another brain software version 2 to 6, so as not to become confused by them (3.19). Although there is no danger that his higher brain software version will be lost, however, he would want to avoid even a temporary irritation (3.20).
- "*Yoga* becomes known by *yoga*," can also be interpreted so that during the practice, in samādhi the sequence of stages is clear anyway.

Practices

One stage, which should always be applied, is that of *asaṁprajñāta* or *nirbīja samādhi*. It is total silence without attention to anything. Repeat the practice of 3.5, however, this time, simply let go your attention for half a minute, without directing it to anywhere else. Thus you come into a deep silence without thoughts. After about five to ten seconds go with your attention back to the previous place and continue the *saṁyama* there. The exact timing does not matter here. You will see, that the next *saṁyama* works better. It works similarly to the gears in a car, where you first have to press the clutch (*asaṁprajñāta samādhi*), to continue driving with the next higher gear (next round of *saṁyama*).

3.7

The three inner areas [dhāraṇā, dhyāna, samādhi, are more important] than the previous ones.

त्रयमन्तरङ्गं पूर्वेभ्यः

trayam antar-aṅgam pūrvebhyaḥ

traya (n. nom. acc. s.: three, threefold, triad) antaraṅga (mfn., n. nom. acc. s: being essential to, inner part of a body, inner, between, within) pūrva (mf(ā)n., n. dat. abl. p.: previous)

This triad is the more direct means, compared to the previous. Compared to the previous five means, beginning with self-control [2.29 to 2.55], *this triad of dhāraṇā, dhyāna, and samādhi is the more important means of reaching saṁprajñāta yoga.*

By calling them the more important [literally the inner] *means, he (Patañjali) wishes to express, that it is possible, even when the previous ones have not been perfected, to achieve yoga by the perfection of these three (dhāraṇā, dhyāna, samādhi), due to the influence of saṁskāras that the yogi has achieved in previous lives, similar to the situation of the videha and prakṛtilaya yogis (1.19).*

The previous ones are yama, niyama, āsana, prāṇāyāma, pratyāhāra (2.29). Even if these are not yet mastered, the yogi can achieve yoga, just by the perfection of the three dhāraṇā, dhyāna, samādhi, as long as the yogi has done some groundwork in previous lives. However, the state of unity, yoga, cannot be achieved without the practice of the three, dhāraṇā, dhyāna, samādhi.

Who knows, whether he has done sufficient groundwork in previous lives? Just to be sure, one should, in any case, practice *dhāraṇā, dhyāna, samādhi*, but also not neglect the other five. The sequence of these five does not matter so much. It is just that, in the end, they should all be mastered.

> *Yoga* means perfection of the brain software.

There is only one exception to this rule, that *dhāraṇā, dhyāna, samādhi* are required, to achieve *yoga*. Those are the *yogis* with perfect knowledge and perfect serenity. There have been a few such cases in history. That is described in the next *sūtra*.

3.8

Those [three] areas [are] even less important than the seedless (nirbīja samādhi).

तदपि बहिरङ्गं निर्बीजस्य

tat api bahiḥ-aṅgaṁ nirbījasya

tad (n. nom. acc. s.: that [triad]) api (ind.: also, even) antaraṅga (mfn.: unessential to) nirbīja (m. gen. s.: without seed)

Seedless is a state, in which no unwanted, suffering-inducing thinking processes (*vṛttis*) are running in the brain software (1.18). It is possible to reach brain software version 8, without practicing the *siddhi* technique (*dhāraṇā, dhyāna, samādhi*). That is achieved by knowledge (*jñāna*) seedless (*nirbīja*) *samādhi* and serenity (*vairāgya*).

Yoga can be achieved without applying the fivefold methods of yama, niyama, āsana, prāṇāyāma, pratyāhāra, merely by achieving the triad of dhāraṇā, dhyāna, samādhi. Although the threefold method dhāraṇā, dhyāna, samādhi is a more direct means, it is, however, only an indirect method regarding the seedless yoga. Why is that? It is because the seedless yoga can also come about without these three. Even without dhāraṇā, dhyāna, samādhi it is possible, merely by knowledge and serenity, to reach liberation.

When knowledge and serenity are perfect, one does not need to deal with *dhāraṇā, dhyāna, samādhi*.

Thus, there were a few persons, like the yogis Maṅki and Piṅgalā, who had reached brain software version 8 merely by their serenity and the thought of stopping (1.18).

From the distinction between the main component of the brain software (buddhi) and its user (puruṣa), seedless yoga comes about, even in the absence of dhāraṇā, dhyāna, samādhi, which are merely the direct method to the yoga with seeds. Therefore the triad is only an indirect means to the seedless yoga, which additionally requires the thought of stopping.

There are examples of people, who could see very clearly from birth, due to detachment from any saṁskāras. For them, the seedless samādhi was simply achieved by devotion to the practice of highest serenity and the thought of stopping (virāma pratyaya). They were not practicing dhāraṇā, dhyāna, samādhi.

What is now happening at times of the calming of the brain software? What is this calming transformation? Is the brain software not something agile, impelled by the guṇas?

The plural "times" is used, to show, that this is equally applicable to brain software processes in the past, future or present. At times of calming, the brain software is less active.

The brain software consisting of the guṇas (see tables 2.19), is said to be impelled by the guṇas. What is this calming transformation? There must be such a transformation, [which means an upgrade of the brain software]. *Otherwise, if it were never transformed and stayed unchanged, like the user (puruṣa), no calming of the brain software would be accomplished. Due to the changeability of the brain software, one can talk about a calming transformation. If it was unchangeable, like the user, it could not be transformed.*

Analogy of the sleeping elephants

We illustrate the next *sūtra* about the calming transformation in the brain software with an analogy from ancient India. The elephants correspond to the malware in the brain software. The malware rests and does not do any damage, as long as it has not been activated.

On the way to home, somebody encounters a herd of sleeping elephants. To arrive safely, he must pass carefully and silently through the herd, without waking up any of them. When an elephant wakes up, it immediately alerts the whole herd. The elephants correspond to the distracting *saṁskāras*, which are stresses and tensions in the brain software and the body. Waking up an elephant corresponds to activating a distracting *saṁskāra*. Behaving silently, while walking through the herd, corresponds to the *saṁskāras* of calming.

Transformations

3.9

The calming transformation is that which occurs when the distracting saṁskāras are calmed while [simultaneously] saṁskāras of calming appear. Then the brain software is calmed for a moment.

व्युत्थाननिरोधसंस्कारयोरभिभवप्रादुर्भावौ निरोधक्षणचित्तान्वयो निरोधपरिणामः

vyutthāna-nirodha-saṁskārayoḥ abhibhava-prādurbhāvau nirodha-kṣaṇa-citta-anvayaḥ nirodha-pariṇāmaḥ

vyutthāna (n. comp.: distraction, arising, stirring) nirodha (m. comp.: halting, stilling) saṁskāra (m. gen. loc. d.: impression) abhibhava (m. comp.: overcome, vanishing) prādurbhāva (m. nom. acc. d.: appear, manifesting) nirodha (m. comp.: stopping, calming) kṣaṇa (m. comp.: moment) citta (n. Comp.: brain software) anvaya (m. nom. s.: sequence) pariṇāma (m. nom. s.: change, transformation)

The calming moment corresponds to brain software version 4, transcendental consciousness, without any thoughts, and in *saṁskṛt,* it is called *asaṁprajñāta samādhi*. The calming happens both when the *mantra* disappears in *mantra* meditation, as well as when ending a *siddhi* practice. Here, once again, the correctly-discriminating cognition is applied, and *nirvicāra samādhi* (with true knowledge) becomes distinguished from *asaṁprajñāta samādhi*, the *samādhi* without thinking processes.

To calm down the thoughts arising from distracting *saṁskāras*, these *saṁskāras* at their basis must be calmed down. That happens using *saṁskāras* of calming, which put the distracting *saṁskāras* to rest. From the thought of staying calm, the *saṁskāras* of calming are stored. Then the brain software goes into a momentary state of calmness, the *asaṁprajñāta samādhi*. In the *saṁskṛt* original, the distracting and calming *saṁskāras* are in the *saṁskṛt* dual number indicating that there is a calming one for each distracting *saṁskāra*.

The outwardly directed saṁskāra is a quality of the brain software, but not a quality of a thought. The saṁskāra of calming is also a quality of the brain software. Due to the thought of calming, a saṁskāra of calming is stored. These two, the saṁskāra of outward directedness and that of calming, depending on the state of the brain software, become suppressed or permitted.

These two kinds of saṁskāras mutually exclude each other. When the saṁskāras of outward directedness are excluded, they are unable to create their effects and the saṁskāras of calming take effect. This change in the saṁskāras of the one brain software, which means the change of saṁskāras by the suppression of the outward-directed, and the dominance of the calming, is called the "calming transformation." The brain software in the samādhi state of calming (version 4) is said to consist of only saṁskāras.

This process leading to calmness, ultimately resulting in the absence of thoughts, is known as the calming transformation (nirodha pariṇāma). Although there are thoughts on the level of saṁprajñāta samādhi, they are not desirable, but the change (calming) of the saṁskāras is always desired.

Although *saṁskāras* can germinate, they do not in their calmed state. On the level of the brain software, the process of calming transformation corresponds to the switching off of all activities of malware. The malware that is not yet completely switched off is, however, momentarily without effect. This is the prerequisite, to switch it off completely in a later step (3.11).

The calming transformation leads to stable energy levels in the quantum computer of the brain (energy eigenvalues). The Schrödinger equation of a quantum system, in principle, comes in two varieties, time-dependent and time-independent. The calming transformation activates the quantum computer, by finding the solutions to the time-independent Schrödinger equation. These correspond to memory contents in classical computers. By finding the time-independent (steady) solutions, the quantum memory in the brain becomes stabilized. Based on this stable memory, the quantum computer can start its activities.

3.10

In that [calming transformation], from the saṁskāra [of calming, follows] a quiet flowing [of the brain software].

तस्य प्रशान्तवाहिता संस्कारात्

tasya praśānta-vāhitā saṁskārāt

tad (mn. gen. s.: that) praśānta (mfn.: quiet) vāhitā (f. nom. s.: flow, stream) saṁskāra (m. abl. s.: impression)

The brain stays in brain software version 4 (*asaṁprajñāta samādhi*) until pulled out again by another distracting *saṁskāra*. The neutralizing of this distracting *saṁskāra* creates thoughts resulting from stress release, which comes about due to the silence. Those thoughts distract from *dhāraṇā* and *dhyāna*.

During the *siddhi* practices, the corresponding *saṁskāras* are dissolved. In the analogy of the elephants: some elephants go away. Progressively erasing these *saṁskāras*, leads to the next transformation (3.11).

The quiet flowing of the brain software on the quantum computer of the brain corresponds to the solutions of the stationary Schrödinger equation with stable eigenvalues. Dissolving a *saṁskāra*, the cause of unexpected thoughts, leads to momentary time-dependent solutions, until the silence is re-established, and the brain software continues quietly flowing. As in an atom, where an electron stays stable on a higher energy level (stationary), then jumps to a lower energy level (time-dependent), simultaneously emits a photon, and then remains stable at the lower energy level (stationary). The photon (light particle) emitted corresponds to a thought in the brain software. That is the fundamental process in nature whose discovery was at the beginning of quantum physics.

3.11

[Then follows] the samādhi transformation, in which the scattered state of the brain software disappears and its one-pointed focus grows.

सर्वार्थतैकाग्रतयोः क्षयोदयौ चित्तस्य समाधिपरिणामः

sarva-arthatā-ekāgratayoḥ kṣaya-udayau cittasya samādhi-pariṇāmaḥ

sarvārthatā (f. comp.: the possessing of all objects, attending to everything, distraction) ekāgratā (f. gen. loc. d.: undisturbed focusing, attention, one-pointedness) kṣaya (m. comp.: disappearing, destroying) udaya (m. nom. acc. d.: increase, growing) citta (n. gen. s.: brain software) samādhi (m. comp.: absolute silence, restful alertness) pariṇāma (m. nom. s.: change, transformation)

In the scattered state of the brain software, it is directed to all goals, purposes, meanings, etc. The scattered state disappears with the *samādhi* transformation.

The *samādhi* transformation results from the calming transformation and *saṁyama*. From the *samādhi* transformation, *samādhi* becomes predominant, and the ability to practice *saṁyama* with the correct result is perfected. This ability is called one-pointedness and grows with *siddhi* practice. The *siddhis* function! Eureka!

Scattered-ness and one-pointedness (attention to one thing) are the qualities of the brain software. The manifestation of one-pointedness means the disappearing of scattered-ness. Samādhi leads, away from being scattered, towards one-pointedness. That is the samādhi transformation (samādhi pariṇāma). Samādhi is reached when the calming takes over, and the outward directedness is nearly gone.

Thus, the upgrade to brain software version 5 is achieved.

The scattered-ness of the brain software, in quantum physics corresponds to the so-called superposition principle, which allows superimposing an arbitrary amount of quantum states, which do not disturb each other. As long as the quantum computer in the brain works in this superposition mode, it has not yet reached the desired result. The desired result is nothing but one single state, which we call intuitive knowledge. Although the quantum computer in the brain works infinitely fast, calculating infinitely many superimposed states, yet, the result of such a calculation can only be a single one. This result manifests from the one-pointed transformation and spontaneously appears as intuitive knowledge (*prajñā*).

3.12

Then follows the one-pointed transformation [which means that] repeatedly a new thought arises in the brain software similar [to the thought] previously vanished.

ततः पुनः शान्तोदितौ तुल्यप्रत्ययौ चित्तस्यैकाग्रतापरिणामः

tataḥ punaḥ śānta-uditau tulya-pratyayau cittasya-ekāgratā-pariṇāmaḥ

tataḥ (ind.: there) punaḥ (ind.: anew, again) śānta (mfn. comp.: silenced, vanished, undisturbed, free from passions) udita (m. nom. acc. d.: arising) tulya (mf(ā)n.: equal, similar) pratyaya (m. nom. acc. d.: thought) citta (n. gen. s.: brain software) ekāgratā (f. nom. s.: undisturbed focusing, attention, one-pointedness) pariṇāma (m. nom. s.: change, transformation)

A similar thought, is a thought of unity with everything, as with for example: "I am you," "I am that" "I am the universe," "I perceive my SELF everywhere." This vision of unity prevails. Everything is familiar, an expression of my SELF. Even though differences are noticed, this takes effect in the background. That is life in unity.

This quality of the brain software exists in the transformation to one-pointedness. In that brain software, the previous thought disappears, and the next thought that manifests is similar to it. The brain software in samādhi [that means version 5] *is the connecting basis of both thoughts. It is repeated until samādhi gets interrupted by the activity of potential residues of malware (saṁskāras).*

One-pointedness means that the following thought is similar to the previous. That is repeated time and again. The first thought disappears, another similar one is born; when that one disappears, another similar one appears; when that one disappears, another similar one appears, etc. [This corresponds to brain software version 7]. *The similar thoughts* [of unity with all] *continue until samādhi is interrupted by the activity of a saṁskāra, which subjectively appears like an outward going.*

Regarding the three transformations in the brain software (3.9 to 3.12), in each case, the previous ones are contained in the following ones. These three transformations are (1) calming, (2) *samādhi*, and (3) one-pointedness. One-pointedness contains *samādhi*. *Samādhi* contains calming. In other words, brain software versions 5 and 7 are both downward compatible. None of the previous abilities goes away.

Upgrade to higher brain software versions

Version 4

The calming transformation leads to a state of the brain software with nothing but inactive *saṁskāras*, resulting from the calming of outer mental processes (*bāhya-vṛtti*). This means, the brain software may still contain any amount of malware, which, however, is not active in version 4.

Version 5

The *samādhi* transformation leads, from the calming of outward-directed thinking processes, towards the calming of all thoughts, but not completely.

Version 6

This will be described later, in *sūtra* 4.29, with the term "rain cloud of *dharma*."

Version 7

One-pointed transformation leads to similarity of the next thought to the previous one, which went before. That is possible only at the time of *samādhi*.

Version 8

The transformation to *brahman*-consciousness will be described later in *sūtra* 4.14.

Interestingly quantum physics uses a similar term, the "unitary transformation." So long as the wave function has not collapsed, the unitary transformation is happening, and no information becomes lost.

Starting from brain software version 5, the quantum computer in the brain becomes activated and functions in parallel with the normal holographic light computer, which already runs with brain software version 3. From brain software version 6 the quantum computer is used more frequently, and in brain software version 7 is predominant. The quantum computer works with unitary transformations, and therefore the *sūtra* 3.12 is an excellent description of life in unity consciousness, which means continuous one-pointedness. "I am all that."

Regarding this *sūtra* a student asked *Śaṁkara*:

What is the point, of explaining all these changes, again?

Śaṁkara answered:

The nature of the guṇas is continuous change; and anything, consisting of the guṇas, has change in its nature, is not steady; that is why there is this explanation, to cultivate the feeling of serenity. Therefore, the previous explanation is a preparation for the practice of saṁyama on the threefold transformations (3.16), to gain the knowledge of past and future.

At the beginning of chapter three, the technique of *saṁyama* was explained, and in this *sūtra* 3.12, the one-pointed transformation has been explained, which corresponds to the unitary transformation in the quantum computer of the brain. Now the *yoga sūtras* begin with the explanation of the various apps, which can be installed, starting from brain software version 4. The first one of these apps brings the ability, to explore past and future. This is possible because the quantum computer in the brain works with unitary transformations, where no information is lost.

Natural Processes

3.13

By this [one-pointed transformation], the transformations of tasks, time qualities, and states of elements and sense and organs of action are explained.

एतेन भूतेन्द्रियेषु धर्मलक्षणावस्थापरिणामा व्याख्याताः

etena bhūta-indriyeṣu dharma-lakṣaṇa-avasthā-pariṇāmāḥ vyākhyātāḥ

etad (mn. Ins. s.: this) bhūta (n. comp.: element) indriya (n. loc. p.: sense and action organs) dharma (n. nom. acc. s.: task, quality, virtue, righteousness) lakṣaṇa (f. comp.: attribute, feature, characteristics) avasthā (f. nom. s.: situation, stability, state) pariṇāma (m. nom. p.: change, transformation) vyākhyāta (f. nom. acc. p.: explained)

A material (*dharmin*) can take on various tasks (*dharma*). For example, clay as a material is transformed into the form of a pot and then fired by the potter. Then it is a new pot. When the pot is used, it gradually acquires signs of wear and tear, until it finally breaks. Then the clay's task of being a pot has ended. But the material, clay, continues to exist.

Three sequences play a role in this process

- The natural sequence of the tasks (dharma).
- The time sequence: from the future into the present and then into the past, measured in units of time.
- The natural sequence of states: the aging process through use: new, used, damaged, broken.

The one-pointed transformation from *sūtras* 3.12 and 3.13 describes a process that is called "unitary transformation" in quantum physics. In this, the wave function is preserved and therefore no information is lost. Therefore, from the momentary wave function, all past and future wave functions can be deduced, because the information about them, is contained in the present state.

When a thing fades into the past, it becomes subtle, and, therefore, it is no longer directly perceivable. To be subtle, however, does not mean, that the thing never existed. Similarly, with the future. A thing that is going to become perceivable in future already exists in a subtle form. The *sūtras* 3.13 to 3.16 describe, the functioning of the future and past app, which enables the perception of future and past.

3.14

The material (dharmin) adapts to the finished, active and indeterminable tasks (dharma).

शान्तोदिताव्यपदेश्यधर्मानुपाती धर्मी

śānta-udita-avyapadeśya-dharma-anupātī dharmī

śānta (mfn. comp.: quiet, silenced, halted, settled) udita (mfn. comp.: manifested, rising, present) avyapadeśya (mfn. comp.: not defined) dharma (n. comp.: task, specialty, quality, virtue, righteousness, thing e.g. pot of clay) anupātin (m. nom. s.: following as a result) dharmin (m. nom. s.: object, thing, carrier of attribute, e.g. clay)

This sequence of tasks is not to be confused with an exact sequence of time. The word "finished" means a previous task; "active" means the present task; "indeterminable" means a potential task that may happen in future, however, not in every case. The task (*dharma*) is a certain variation of the mere possibilities of the material (*dharmin*). Of the multitude of possibilities, only one is presently perceivable.

The tasks of the material that were active and have stopped being active are the finished tasks (past). Those that are functioning now are the active tasks, which have come from their future time phase into the present time phase. What are the indeterminable *dharmas*? Everything is possible. However, not everything manifests at the same time, due to the binding limitations of place, time, actor, and cause.

> A task (*dharma*), the capability of the material (*dharmin*) to be something special, is in reality the inherent power (*śakti*).

What remains, is the material. Its special manifestation (sound, touch, form, taste, smell) keeps changing.

3.15

The difference in the [three natural] sequences [of evolution] is the reason for the difference in the transformations.

क्रमान्यत्वं परिणामान्यत्वे हेतुः

krama-anyatvam pariṇāma-anyatve hetuḥ

krama (m. comp.: operational sequence, procedure) anyatva (n. nom. acc. s.: difference) pariṇāma (m. comp.: change, transformation) anyatva (n. loc. s. nom. acc. d.:) hetu (m. nom. s.: cause, motive, reason [in loc.])

1. The natural sequence of tasks (*dharma*) of the same material (*dharmin*) – lump of clay, pot, shards, gravel – causes the corresponding transformations (→) of tasks (*dharma*):

- lump of clay → pot
- pot → shards

- shards → gravel

2. The natural sequence of time – future, present, past – causes the two transformations (→) of the time phases:

- future → present
- present → past

3. The natural sequence of states – new, used, damaged, broken – causes the transformations (→) of states:

- new → used
- used → damaged
- damaged → broken

The whole cosmos is organized in this way.

With the change of the material state, there can be a change of the task. These sequences, are, for example with a new pot of clay, falling on the floor:

- The state changes from new → broken
- The task changes from pot → shards

In *jyotiṣ*, Vedic astrology, the word *krama*, which here has been translated as the natural sequence of evolution, is used for the progression of heavenly bodies. Therefore, this *sūtra* can also be read in a way, that the progression of the heavenly bodies causes the transformations of the three sequences, time, task and state.

A horoscope can be interpreted as a life task.

Places and Results of Saṁyama

Having explained the process of installation for all *siddhi* apps at the beginning of chapter three now comes the first app. It is to be applied very generally, and in some way, is the pattern for all the following apps. The minimum requirement is a previous upgrade to brain software version 4 (absolute silence of thoughts), or better to version 5 or higher.

3.16

By saṁyama on the three transformations [of the task, time phase, and state, there arises] knowledge about past and future.

परिणामत्रयसंयमादतीतानागतज्ञानम्

pariṇāma-traya-saṁyamāt atīta-anāgata-jñānam

pariṇāma (m. comp.: change, transformation) traya (comp.: three, threefold) saṁyama (m. abl. s.:) atīta (mfn. comp.: past) anāgata (mfn. comp.: not yet arrived, future) jñāna (n. nom. acc. s.: knowledge)

By saṁyama on the transformations of the task, time phase, and state, to the yogi comes knowledge about past and future things. If dhāraṇā, dhyāna, and samādhi are applied to the same thing, it is called saṁyama [3.4]. *In that way, the three transformations are perceived directly and there emerges knowledge of past and future events. The saṁyama is to be applied until prajñā knowledge* [3.5] *appears.*

The potential future may change due to the influence of the brain software (*citta*), which will be explained further in *sūtra* 4.15.

Onto whatever thing one applies the saṁyama, it brings about the direct perception of this thing, as it really is. That applies to anything, regardless of whether it is subtle, hidden, past, future or distant. The yogi receives the knowledge about the transformations and also about the fundamental material. When the saṁyama is done with the intention, of mastering a thing, this purpose becomes fulfilled, and the yogi brings the thing under his control.

This general statement can be applied to all the *siddhi* apps.

> *And this all-knowing one, who sees the impermanence of that, which changes any moment in the universe, becomes the master of serenity.*

Practices

Dhāraṇā and *dhyāna* are to be applied to one or two of the transformations. From there, in *samādhi*, arises the *prajñā* knowledge about the other transformations.

Practice 1

Choose an item that you see in front of you. Repeat with it the attention practice of 1.41 in all the three variations (to the item, to the perceiver, to the process of perception).

Practice 2

Start practice 2, only when you can attain complete silence with practice 1, and also can perceive subtle differences between the three variations.

Every item changes with time. At some time it will be destroyed. However, the material will remain. Now, direct your attention to the materials, in the item, with the intention of perceiving the item in the state, when it can no longer perform its normal task. Close your eyes and go to *samādhi*, while simultaneously keeping your attention directed to the future of these materials. During the experience of the *samādhi*, a picture instantaneously comes up of the destroyed item, made of the same materials.

In no case try to imagine anything. These pictures come completely spontaneously. They are not imagination, but rather a subtle perception of the future phase of the item which at the moment is contained in the manifest now-phase. By no means use any words or sentence constructs here, because they lead to imaginations (*vikalpa* 1.9).

As long as memories come up (*smṛti* 1.11), for example of similar items, the history of this item, etc., you are still in the purification phase of your nervous system. Once the nervous system is cleansed of all the related memories, *saṁyama* functions really well. Now it is essential, to stay with it and continue to practice.

Practice 3

Again, take up an item and direct your attention to a past phase of the same materials, when this item was produced. Here again, you are practicing *saṁyama*, that means simultaneous *dhāraṇā*, *dhyāna*, *samādhi*. The item for *dhāraṇā*, directed attention, is the past phase of the thing, at the time, when the materials were formed in this way. If any pictures of workshops, production environments, etc. appear, you can look around, to find out more details. Never expect such pictures. Your attention simply stays with the past phase of the thing.

Practice 4

Repeat practice 2 with things that you like very much. It trains serenity for the moment when the beloved thing becomes broken. That is the actual purpose of this practice.

Experiences

Experience 1

I have had difficulty in understanding the concept of putting my attention on an object/place/feeling without introducing imagery or my intellect taking over. Through practice, I have had some interesting experiences.

When putting my attention on the past of an object, I chose a rose. I looked at the rose then closed my eyes. Images appeared, and I realized my intellect had taken over. I had this same experience over and over. Rows and rows of roses in a field ... bucketfuls of roses in supermarkets ... all products of my imagination and not *siddhi* experiences. Out of frustration, I let go of my controlled thoughts. Finally, with lots of practice, I reached the understanding that I don't need images or thoughts ... a brief desire to put my attention on "whatever" and the discovery that my entire being is clever enough to do this by itself if I would only let it. Trusting this process yielded some interesting results. Back to the rose ... I had the experience of cold moving air in blackness which had clear boundaries. It was difficult to describe and meant little to me at the time, but on reflection, my rose had no scent and most likely had an immediate past of being in a large refrigerated container.

Experience 2

I wanted to find out, using *siddhis*, when a friend would appear in a pub. Applying the technique, spontaneously a specific time came to my mind, which later turned out to be true.

3.17

From the mutual projections of sound sequences, meanings and thoughts [there arises] confusion. By saṁyama on the difference of those [three] comes the knowledge of the utterances of all beings.

शब्दार्थप्रत्ययानामितरेतराध्यासात् संकरस् तत्प्रविभागसंयमात् सर्वभूतरुतज्ञानम्

śabda-artha-pratyayānām itara-itara-adhyāsāt saṁkaraḥ tat-pravibhāga-saṁyamāt sarva-bhūta-ruta-jñānam

śabda (m. comp.: sound) artha (m. comp.: goal, purpose) pratyaya (m. gen. p.: thought) itaretara (pron. comp.: mutual, one into the other) adhyāsa (m. abl. s.: projection, faulty identification) saṁkara (m. nom. s.: mixing, confusion) tat (n. nom. acc. s.: that) pravibhāga (m. comp.: classification, partitioning, separation, part) saṁyama (m. abl. s.:) sarva (comp.: all, total) bhūta (mfn. comp.: element, being, existing) ruta (n. comp.: sound, utterance, expression) jñāna (n. nom. acc. s.: knowledge)

Sound sequence means word as well as sentence. Words are perceived as units and have a meaning corresponding to a convention between the living beings who speak this language. However, a truth can only be conveyed in a sentence, not in a single word. This truth is the thought that the being wants to convey. Through *saṁyama* on the distinction of a sound sequence, meanings of words, and the thought, this thought of the being gets translated into one's own language.

The meaning of words is a convention between the beings, who use the same language. Due to mutual projection, words, their meanings, and the thought become mixed up: cow is a word, cow is a meaning, cow is part of a thought. Someone, who knows the difference between them, is an all-knowing one.

A word consists of syllables and sounds, which can, in cooperation, take on all possible forms. Each sound is full of possibilities to express all kinds of things, for example the sound "g" is full of possibilities, to express saṁskṛt words, like for example "go" (cow), "varga" (class), "agni" (fire) and "gagana" (heaven). In connection with other sounds, the sound takes on all kinds of possible forms. Although the word consists of a sequence of sounds, however, it is perceived as one unit.

Understanding the meaning does not emerge from the sounds, but rather immediately from their knowledge. Whatever emerges from a thing, is similar to it. Smoke is similar to fire. However, the understanding of fire alone, cannot arise from seeing the smoke. Smoke alone does not lead to the knowledge of fire. So it is with sounds; something else is required, to understand their sequence.

When understanding the utterances of all beings, the words must be connected to sentences because words only, do not lead to any communication. The sentence is real, as well as the meaning of the sentence. Words or isolated word meanings cannot express any truth.

From saṁyama on the difference between sound sequences, meanings, and thoughts, comes an understanding of the utterances of all beings to the yogi.

Practices

Practice 1

Listen several times to a short foreign language text, whose language you do not yet know. Listen with the intention, to recognize the meaning. Listen carefully to the separate words and their gaps with your silent attention, and go into *samādhi*. The feeling, respectively the coloring, which appears very subtly in *samādhi*, reproduces the thought that the speaker had.

Practice 2

Listen to a bird with the intention, of recognizing the words that the bird composes in various sentences. Birds are not only saying "tweet, tweet," but rather they use very subtle changes of their fundamental sounds. When listening and distinguishing the sounds, words, and sentences, go into the silence of *samādhi* and again perceive intuitively, what comes up. That corresponds to the thought that the bird wants to express. With a bit of practice, you can even get an automatic translation into your own language.

Practice 3

The same, of course, applies to all other animals. The words under certain conditions can be very short. A single "meow" of a cat can be a complete sentence, containing several words. Therefore, please precisely listen while going into the silence.

3.18

By intuitive perception of an impression (saṁskāra) [one gains] knowledge of previous lives.

संस्कारसाक्षात्करणात् पूर्वजातिज्ञानम्

saṁskāra-sākṣātkaraṇāt pūrva-jāti-jñānam

saṁskāra (m. comp.: Eindruck) sākṣātkaraṇa (n. abl. s.: intuitive perception, behold) pūrvajāti (f. comp.: previous life, previous birth) jñāna (n. nom acc. s.:)

Intuitive perception means *saṁyama*. Here, the place for *dhāraṇā* is a specific *saṁskāra*. The *prajñā* knowledge arising from this, in *samādhi*, is like a multimedia show, of what has caused the *saṁskāra*. That situation can originate from the present or a previous life. An impression can never be separated from the place, time, cause and situation that have caused the impression.

This *saṁskāra* leads to knowledge about the situation, which has generated the *saṁskāra* and simultaneously dissolves the negative effect of the *saṁskāra*. The malware becomes harmless.

There are two states of *saṁskāras*:

- Visible – they have begun to develop. That corresponds to a malware that has already been activated.
- Invisible – they have not yet started to develop. That corresponds to a malware, lurking in secret that may become activated at any time upon a suitable occasion.

These two states will be further explained in 3.22, especially how they affect the lifespan of the *yogi*.

Software objects in principle consist of two parts, (1) the data part and (2) the methods part; similarly, all *saṁskāras*, whether already activated, or not, always consists of two parts.

Śaṁkara commented on these two parts of impressions as follows:

Actually a saṁskāra is of a twofold nature. The passive part consists of the causative illusions and the memories. The active part, called vāsanā, causes the ripening in the form of virtue and vice.

These [impressions] *have been formed* [in the present] *and previous lives. When the effect of their execution is stopped, the life force makes the virtue visible in the future as a task in the brain software (citta).*

That means that each malware carries a memory with it, and separate from this, an effective part, which is carried out unconsciously most of the time. The memory part is harmless. However, the effective part is harmful, and therefore we want to get rid of it. The *saṁyama* of 3.18 is used for that purpose. It can be utilized, to explore one's own previous lives, and it also can be applied to other living beings.

To explain the deeper meaning of the *saṁyama*, *Śaṁkara* here quotes an experience report from ancient times:

Ancient experiences

"Jaigīṣavya said to Āvaṭya: having lived through ten cycles of creation (one cycle of creation lasts 4.320.000.000 years) with a pure intellect of sattva,

which has not been overcome by rajas or tamas, I experienced the pains of lives in hell and of animals. I also consider that which I repeatedly experienced in my births amongst the gods and amongst humans, to be nothing but painful.

The divine Āvaṭya said: O, Long-lived one, do you include your mastery of pradhāna (guṇas in their resting state) and your highest (heavenly) joy of contentment, in this suffering?

The divine Jaigīṣavya said: only regarding sensory joys is this called the highest joy of contentment; compared to the bliss of the absolute freedom (kaivalya) it is nothing but pain. The quality of pure intellect is that it consists of the three guṇas. Any thought that consists of the three guṇas is to be called pain, which should be avoided. The chain of greed and desires has the form of pain. But when the agony of the pain of desires is removed, then there remains this bliss that is said, to be calm, undisturbed and all-comprehending."

Practices

Find out about your puzzling, unusual, special, and strange behaviors, preferences, aversions, fears, etc. (*saṁskāras*). Utilize this *saṁyama*, to explore the *saṁskāras* at their origin, until a multimedia vision of the situation appears that has caused the impression. Then you will know, what has caused this peculiarity, however, you will no longer be unconsciously influenced by the impression. If there is a strong impression, this *saṁyama* should be applied several times. It is important, not only to live through the previous experience but rather to take it consciously into the silence of *samādhi*. Only then its damaging effect dissolves.

If you believe, that there are no previous lives, then probably with this *saṁyama* you will initially have only memories of your present life. Your belief system can block the success for a certain time. However, if you continue the *saṁyama*, be aware, that memories can come, which will replace your belief with reliable knowledge.

Practice 1

Select one of your good qualities and apply *dhāraṇā* on it, that means, direct your full attention only on this good quality. Then go with *dhyāna* into the silence, until you reach *samādhi*. However, simultaneously continue to stay with your attention on your selected quality and allow the refinement of your thoughts. That means that you practice *dhāraṇā, dhyāna,* and *samādhi* simultaneously. Then you are correctly doing the *saṁyama*. Do not expect any pictures or other sensory experiences; however, when these appear, you can look around a bit, for example, look at your feet, your dress, living beings, people, animals, buildings, vehicles, etc. Occasionally allow yourself a pause; suspend the *dhāraṇā* on your good qualities and relax in the absolutely calm *samādhi*. Thus you learn, that you do not have to be virtuous all the time, and the negative side effects of this virtuous malware also become dissolved.

Practice 2

Now repeat practice 1 with one of your vices or negative qualities. Thus the negative effect of this malware also becomes dissolved. If you cannot find any of your negative qualities, you can confidently consider this as a negative quality and practice *saṁyama* on this. Perfectionism also is a *saṁskāra*!

Practice 3

If you think, that you have only negative qualities, first practice *saṁyama* on this impression. You will see, how you have come to this impression, and gradually the impression becomes harmless. Then you will recognize positive qualities again, and your depressions will gradually disappear.

Practice 4

Repeat the practices 1 or 2 with all your peculiarities, with every aspect of your individuality and research, from where each one originates. Often these peculiarities appear repeatedly in several lives. You do not need to distinguish between good or bad qualities.

Practice 5

Now we turn our attention to the future. *Śaṁkara* has said before "...the life force makes the virtue visible in the future as a task of the brain software (*citta*)." Pick out one of your good qualities, of which you are very satisfied or proud, and consider, how this quality can affect your future lives. That means, again apply *saṁyama* to this quality, but now to the future.

Practice 6

You may, of course, repeat practice 5 also on one of your negative qualities. The future that you experience in that way should discourage you from continuing this path, such that you finally start, really to remove this malware with practice 2.

Experiences

Experience 1

I was still quite young, age 20, when, after a few years of meditation and a meditation teacher training course, I decided to continue my studies in Switzerland at the University of my revered master Maharishi™[13] Mahesh Yogi. It was far more than merely a university. It was more a spiritual *āśram* with an international center. Later on, we were traveling the whole world, to inspire large groups of meditators and to bring meditation and *siddhis* into the world.

Although I had seen Maharishi™ several times before from a distance, only once I had seen him close-up, as well as, of course from his videotapes. Now I had the chance of meeting him daily, which for me was something very exciting and thrilling. I had learned so much from his books and courses already, that now I wanted simply to absorb more of his great wisdom, kindness, and bliss. Now I had the opportunity to establish personal contact with him, and it was happening faster than I expected.

The leaders of Maharishi's™ worldwide meditation movement met nearly every evening in a large, wonderfully decorated hall, to listen to his lectures together. Shy, as I was, I often sat towards the back of the hall and observed from a distance what was happening in the front. These were his closest confidants, many of whom had received honorary titles from him, some even several titles, to whom I afforded the greatest respect. Now I saw, how these noble humans, were communicating with Maharishi™. It was always thrilling to see this, but already, after a few days, I began to feel the

---

[13] Maharishi is a trademark of Maharishi Foundation Ltd. Corporation United Kingdom, P.O. Box 652 St. Helier, Jersey Great Britain JE48Y2.

need, to get closer to the great master. I saw how some of Maharishi's™ students handed him a flower as he entered the hall. I thought, "I too, can do that."

Next evening I stood there, ready with a flower and Maharishi™[14] was pleased to accept it from me with a broad smile on his face. Somehow, he knew me totally; it was like meeting an old acquaintance again after thousands of years.

He said, "Come!" Before my intellect could entertain another thought, I saw myself obeying him, walking behind him onto the stage. "... and sit here," he continued, pointing to a chair in front of his couch, "and tell them your knowledge." I followed his order and sat down on the chair. Now I saw myself in front of all these educated and enlightened people whom I revered so much, and I pondered, what could I tell them? I could feel my heart beating, but fortunately, I kept quiet. I was not accustomed to speaking in front of assemblies and still had no idea about what I could speak. So, I was very happy, that Maharishi™ waited for a short time, while the hall filled up and then he began his lecture. As more dignitaries arrived, they seemed somewhat surprised to see me, wondering what Maharishi™ intended for me. He did not invite anyone else onto the stage, which was rather unusual. So, really he was introducing me to the executive team that was gathering. Can you imagine how happy I was when he spoke for only 20 minutes – a short time for him – and then left the hall? I was so relieved that I did not have to say anything. I had no idea that Maharishi™ had just sent me on the greatest spiritual journey of my life, one that would continue for years to come.

During the following days, I pondered, what I could have said. Obviously, there was some knowledge within me that I did not yet recognize, but that was precious enough to be worth discovering. It even was so precious that the leaders of Maharishi's™ worldwide meditation movement should hear it from me. Examining all my specialties, initially, I did not find anything. At that time I was not yet aware that just by doing this research, I was practicing the *siddhi*, to gain knowledge of previous lives.

[14] Maharishi is a trademark of Maharishi Foundation Ltd. Corporation United Kingdom, P.O. Box 652 St. Helier, Jersey Great Britain JE48Y2.

Then, a few weeks later, this knowledge came to me. First it came hesitantly, but eventually, it became clearer and more obvious. Then I knew that exactly this was what Maharishi™[15] had intended when he put me on that stage. He did not want to tell me right away about my special knowledge but wanted me to find it out for myself.

So, I searched for, what this special knowledge could be. But somehow it had to do with the natural sciences because that had always been my strength. I never had to learn writing or reading; it was simply there when I was in primary school. The same occurred with the natural sciences in high school. The only topics that I found interesting were the latest insights into natural sciences, which I consumed with great enthusiasm from books and television reports. By the time I reached university, I had advanced so much that I could sometimes get up and correct erroneous formulae that our mathematics professor had written on the blackboard. Similarly, I could ask questions about the electromagnetic field, for example, that my physics professor could not answer. That quickly became boring, so I turned to the exploration of the human mind, meditation and enlightenment. Thus, while still in my early years, I found Maharishi™.

Now I considered, whether I should have told Maharishi's™ confidants something about the coherence formula that we had been using in our minicomputer in the brain wave lab, to examine higher states of consciousness? Somehow this also could not be it, because even though there were not very many, there were still one or two others, who could have explained the mathematical details of this formula. So, this was also not my special knowledge. I continued searching.

During my first years with Maharishi™, over and over again, he invited special scientists and also some Nobel Prize winners to examine the phenomenon of meditation from the viewpoint of scientific theory. Somehow I always managed to get into those meetings easily, although the number of participants was rather limited. I still remembered my last lesson at my previous German university, when our mathematics professor had sent us on

[15] Maharishi is a trademark of Maharishi Foundation Ltd. Corporation United Kingdom, P.O. Box 652 St. Helier, Jersey Great Britain JE48Y2.

vacation with the remark that our next topic would be non-linear differential equations. Now I sat with Nobel Prize winners and an enlightened master at a meeting on the topic "Consciousness and non-linear differential equations." That was really funny, but somehow I also knew, that it was to be my next lesson. The EEG coherence formula was also mathematics, but mathematics that we could use to measure states of consciousness.

Then it slowly dawned on me that this hidden knowledge I was searching might have come from a previous life. I realized that somehow in a previous life I had already been very proficient in physics and higher mathematics. Over several months more and more details of this previous life appeared to me.

There were memories of train rides from Switzerland to Germany; sailing on Lake Zürich; travel with the little train, the "Polybähnli", from the Swiss Federal Institute of Technology (ETH) down to the town of Zürich, where we loved to meet with other students in coffee shops to exchange lecture notes and engage in philosophical discussions; travelling with a bright yellow – very modern at that time – stagecoach through the Swiss Alps; trips on a little mountain railway that had not been in use for a long time. I have discovered it again recently in a television report. It had been renovated, and I could remember accurate details, of where I stood in that previous life and how I got on and off. There were trips to a glacier in a large cable car.

Thus, gradually hundreds of details of daily events from this previous life came to light again. I was able to remember another Swiss town. I had a profession, where I had to write a lot, and sometimes I came back home with black fingertips, as those strange patented ink pens often did not work properly. I can still remember details of the building where I worked, and the place where we had to deposit the keys when we were last out of the building. By now I have found out that this had been the patent office in Bern in Switzerland. I know how it looked from the inside even though in my present life I have never seen it. There were also a lot of memories about trams and certain tram lines one would use to get through the town.

I could also recall tram lines in another big city, a big German city. It was Berlin. I remember very well traveling in one of those electric trams when I was a bit careless and nearly fell off. A friend saved me. While this friend had been very shocked by it, I took it easy. I was destined to meet this friend again in this present life. That has happened already, and this time she had incarnated herself as a woman, but she remembered, that she was Max von Laue.

In Berlin, I had a series of different apartments, and I can remember many of the details about them, entrances, stairways, divisions of rooms, etc. I can also remember museums, a large library and the workplace there. My wife from that time has now incarnated again as a distant relation.

The process continued to unfold. Ever more details were bubbling up from my memories, sometimes two or three new details a day. At the same time, also acquaintances from the previous life came into my present life. Somehow I sensed that we had met previously. There was a French woman, who now worked in the same lab in Switzerland. Sometimes we talked to each other with great enthusiasm. Her name was somehow familiar and still sounded similar to what it previously had been when she was called Madame Curie. Then there was a work colleague who one day simply arrived with a suitcase and said, "Here I am." I recommended him immediately to my supervisor, and he was employed the next day. From then on we were working together as if we had already done that for a hundred years. He was a brilliant physicist and a deep thinker who explored the most complex connections, slowly but rigorously. Later I found out that in a previous life he had been Max Planck.

As the memories condensed ever more, the description fitted only one person in natural sciences. This person in his early years had a similar life story as I had: born in southern Germany; moved to Switzerland because of an aversion to the German military; living for a short while in England and then in the USA. The same life story and the other evidence pointed to Albert Einstein. Initially, this thought was quite shocking to me, and I can already see the disbelieving faces of many of my readers. I was very well aware that mental hospitals are full of people who imagine that they have been, or still are, one or several famous persons. As I have grown up in rather modest conditions and always retained a certain modesty, I thought it was reasonable not to talk about this at all. However, I continued my researches and often looked for another hint from Maharishi™[16]. It was to come fairly soon.

By then, I had obtained a book about Albert Einstein's life and wanted to check, whether there were certain similarities both with my memories as well as with my present life. I had been born about a year after Albert Einstein's death. So, this was fitting already. But for me as a scientist, of course, that was not sufficient. So, I checked further details and found about 100 correlations and most peculiar similarities that actually could not be coincidences. When reading the book, several other memories appeared, for example, the details of how the special theory of relativity had really been discovered. Later I visited the old house in Bern that is now an Albert Einstein museum. There I saw the same old pendulum clock that I had tried to synchronize more than a hundred years before, again and again, most accurately with the tower clock in my road, and which always showed little differences. With that, I explored the phenomenon of simultaneity from which, later, I had derived special relativity theory.

Further hints came from special words, which appeared important to me in the present life, but sometimes had a different meaning, which I did not understand for a long time. Now, these words appeared again in the books about Einstein, and all became clear. For example one of these words was Odeon. I knew it in the present life from Odeonsplatz in Munich. But somehow, for me, this was not a subway station and also not the Field Marshal's Hall, but somehow a special meeting place. And then I read, that Odeon was the name of this café in Zürich, where we had met regularly as students in Einstein's times. Now the specialness of the word Odeon became clear to me. Obviously, it is just those things which are called *saṁskāras*, and on their tracks, we can travel back to previous lives.

So, by now this Einstein life had become a bit more acceptable to me. 100 correlations were quite a good start. But still I had the feeling, that my master knew somewhat more about me and of course, his confirmation

---

[16] Maharishi is a trademark of Maharishi Foundation Ltd. Corporation United Kingdom, P.O. Box 652 St. Helier, Jersey Great Britain JE48Y2.

would have been a great blessing. This confirmation then came during a further meeting. I attended another conference with international scientists and among them was also one man, who proudly declared, that he had been a personal friend of Albert Einstein, but he was a historian rather than a scientist. The theme of the meeting was to explore the qualities of space. Quantum physics had long before discovered, that space is full of virtual vacuum fluctuations. Some scientists talked about that, and all appeared very intelligible to me. One of them then remarked, that this space, filled with virtual vacuum fluctuations, was somehow similar to the aether, that science believed to exist before the era of Albert Einstein. Then this alleged friend of Einstein, whom I in no way recognized, gathered momentum. He told Maharishi™[17] and the scientists that Einstein had abolished the aether. But nothing of his talk appeared plausible to me and also Maharishi™ was just grinning. Then Maharishi™ all of a sudden looked directly at me and said, "If Einstein lived today, he probably would think differently about that!" I could only affirm this with a nod and was just about to burst out with the words, "What does this man think, by calling himself the best friend of Einstein?" I could barely suppress it, but now I had received this clear hint from Maharishi™.

Now, it had become clear to me, that in a previous life I had been Albert Einstein. It was a great boost to my self-confidence, and that probably was exactly, what Maharishi™ intended. But it was also clear, that practically no possibility existed, to scientifically prove a certain previous life of a person. All of it only depended on my memories. Therefore, I could only prove it to myself. This proof worked out quite well for me. But for 40 years I did not talk about it, except with very few close friends.

Later, starting from the time, when in this life, I had been living in the USA just over a year, memories of Albert Einstein's life in the USA came back. I was visiting Disneyland in Florida, and there was an experimental city of the future. With some friends, I visited the Hall of Energy, and we were driving through it. There was a fascinating talk about how the under-

---

[17] Maharishi is a trademark of Maharishi Foundation Ltd. Corporation United Kingdom, P.O. Box 652 St. Helier, Jersey Great Britain JE48Y2.

standing and the use of energy had developed during the history of humanity. Suddenly there appeared a new scene, which I knew. I knew this town, and yet I knew, that I had never seen it in this lifetime, not even in pictures or movies. Nevertheless, it was my town. There I sat now and desired eagerly, "please; please tell the name of this town!" After about a minute the talk came to Albert Einstein and his discovery of $E=mc^2$, and he was shown in his town Princeton. So, this was it, Princeton in New Jersey. That was the town, the town square that I knew so well as if I was visiting it every day. It was another milestone in my chain of proof which I regrettably could only do for myself, as it all depended only on my memories.

Then, during my further stay in the USA and after that, many more details came to light about my life in the USA. Among them were the walks in Central Park in New York, then those little, narrow bookshops in New York, where I could sit alone in a corner and browse through books without getting disturbed by anybody. Also, those pictures of this luxury hotel Waldorf Astoria often came. It was a place where American high society was at home and where there were conferences, in which I participated. Waldorf again was one of those words, with a special connection for me that I could not explain from the present life. I have never visited this hotel in the present life, but I can very clearly remember from Albert Einstein's life the luxurious interior of corridors and rooms and the elevators and the taxis down on the street. Whenever in this life I ate a Waldorf salad, there was this peculiar feeling of luxury that I knew so well. Now it was clear again. Being Albert Einstein, I had eaten the original Waldorf salad already in New York. Once I had, at that time, even tried to drive a car out of the hotel garage, but somehow had the foot pedals mixed up and had driven into a wall. Then I decided once again, that driving cars was an inaccurate science, which did not suit me. How strange, that the brakes did not always work. It seems I had confused the break with the clutch. No wonder, Einstein never had learned to drive a car. I also often remembered this underground shopping mall, which was quite peculiar at the time where I took an easy walk into the center of New York, after my train rides from Princeton. There were also many more pleasant memories of the holiday feeling on Long Island from where I sailed and stayed for long periods in nature and my beloved solitude.

All those memories were quite convincing to me, but – as told before – they were no scientific proof. However, a few years ago I got the idea, how would it be, if I would call on the intuition of another person. There was this excellent spiritual artist, Ros Coleman (*roscoleman.com*), whom I had met several times and who had already painted a wonderful picture of my spiritual helper. She was able, to research previous lives of her clients with pictures and words. I commissioned her to draw a previous life of mine and intentionally gave her only very few details. I gave her the approximate period, when I had lived, from the 19th century up to the first half of the 20th century. I told her that I knew, who I had been and that I was interested, as to if she could find any coincidences. I gave her no other indications. She was able to travel to previous lives of her clients, from their handwriting. Their handwriting was, as it were, the *saṁskāra* that she could explore.

In her first report, she saw me in an agricultural environment, and it was rather more like a description fitting the ancestors of Einstein. On that occasion a drawing came about, that showed quite a young Einstein. But the last part of the report was a bit more interesting and read like this:

"... You take me to a later part of your life, where some time has passed. I sense the name Bella, but I am not shown the context of this name. I sense it is through Bella that you are in this new place of your current occupation. A benefactor perhaps, not an employer certainly. You are living in a township and making drawings – detailed drawings – in a small room. You are spending a lot of time on these drawings – small sketches that eventually find their way onto large sheets of paper. You write on the drawings, giving meanings to the lines and symbols. There is movement – arrows pointing and a compass drawn in one corner. The drawings are portrayed in different directions as the compass is depicted pointing in a different direction. You are deeply focused on these drawings. It is creative work, and you become lost in it as you work, spending long hours on the candlelight.

I can see you are very intelligent. As I see your eyes, the pupils have become pinpricks – focused. Your image ages as I watch and stops in middle age. I am not sure you quite understand the meaning of your drawings or even for what they may one day be used. The drawings seem to illustrate a complex process and were reworked time over time to establish accuracy as you made new understandings and incorporated them into the whole. I feel you died without having quite having reached the point of how it would ever be used. But that was not the point for you because you were a creator and the creation of these drawings was in a significant way, the point of this life.

The information above came out as a channel, like a stream of consciousness, in snapshots and short 'videos.' I hope you find it interesting (I did) and useful."

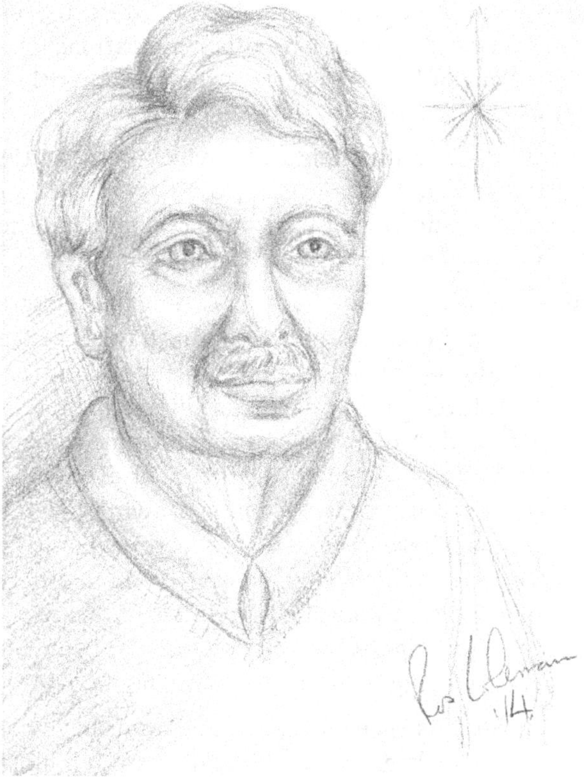

After Ros Coleman sent her first report, I was a little bit disappointed but did not give in so quickly. She told me that several times when she wanted to paint my previous life portrait, she would get into an unbelievably deep sleep phase and that is why it had been delayed so long. Then it became clear to me, that on a spiritual level, I had not given her permission, to look at my life. I did that now very consciously and told her, that I had opened the locked doors for her now and that, please, would she try once more, maybe to paint a picture from a later phase of my life. Then she only wanted to know, whether it had something to do with astronomy.

I confirmed that and encouraged her to continue the research, but I gave her no other hints or confirmation.

In her second report, Ros wrote:

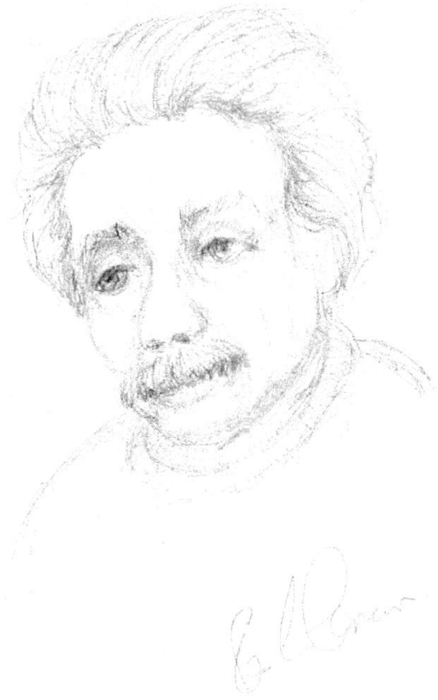

"This portrait of your past life was with me when I woke up this morning (2/10/2014). The vision was as clear as crystal, and we have replicated it as faithfully as we can. On sitting down to write this, a number of things strike me about this portrait and these I feel are clues as to your past life's character and mind. This reading and portrait is not going in any way how I expected it to go and again, this is testimony to this great man's Being.

For one, he did not do things like others – he had his own very individual way of seeing things. He was unconventional; went his own way; insisted with others that he goes his own way. He did not follow anyone's rules but his own, and I feel that those around him would have needed to fall in with him. He followed his own star and his own truth. His mind would see the bigger picture, yet was able to hone into extraordinary minute detail. This made him a creative thinker in a broad sense, and he was thus able to calculate and work out detail in order to see how things worked individually. Then, he would piece theories, and then piece them together into an operational whole. This did not come overnight. He was an illumined thinker – a visionary who had the science to make that vision work. It was as if he was out there on his own with his concepts. These were change making concepts. It is as if he was placed on Earth at that time to create that vision for the world to see. He is the sort of person who either did or should have, won a Nobel Prize or received recognition of similar import for the work he had done. He was perceived as brilliant but somewhat 'eccentric,' not so much in his person but for his work and views. He preferred to work on his own and would spend long hours (I see mostly at night) where I feel he found more peace and quiet. I can see walls covered with diagrams and calculations. I can see him sitting for long spells reflecting, cross-referencing, fragmenting and defragmenting, placing pieces of this jigsaw into different contexts to see how they work across different spheres of scientific thought (or academe). He would have physically rearranged his environment to have himself come up with answers or visions.

This is part one of your second reading and portraits. There is more to come. As before, it seems to be coming in pieces, but I hope this is starting to shine a light onto this past life and piece things together for you. I am wondering if this is, how this man would himself have worked... Perhaps he would have spent much time in his form of meditation before waking up one morning with complete clarity. Yes, I feel this is likely because when I am working, I do take on the 'ways' of those I am channeling. This reading is also forming a kind of diary. I feel he documented or diarised, his thoughts and ideas in the same way. Utterly intriguing. I will send this part to you now and will tune in again later as I feel there is some more to come. In love and light, Ros."

Chapter 3 Sūtra 3.18

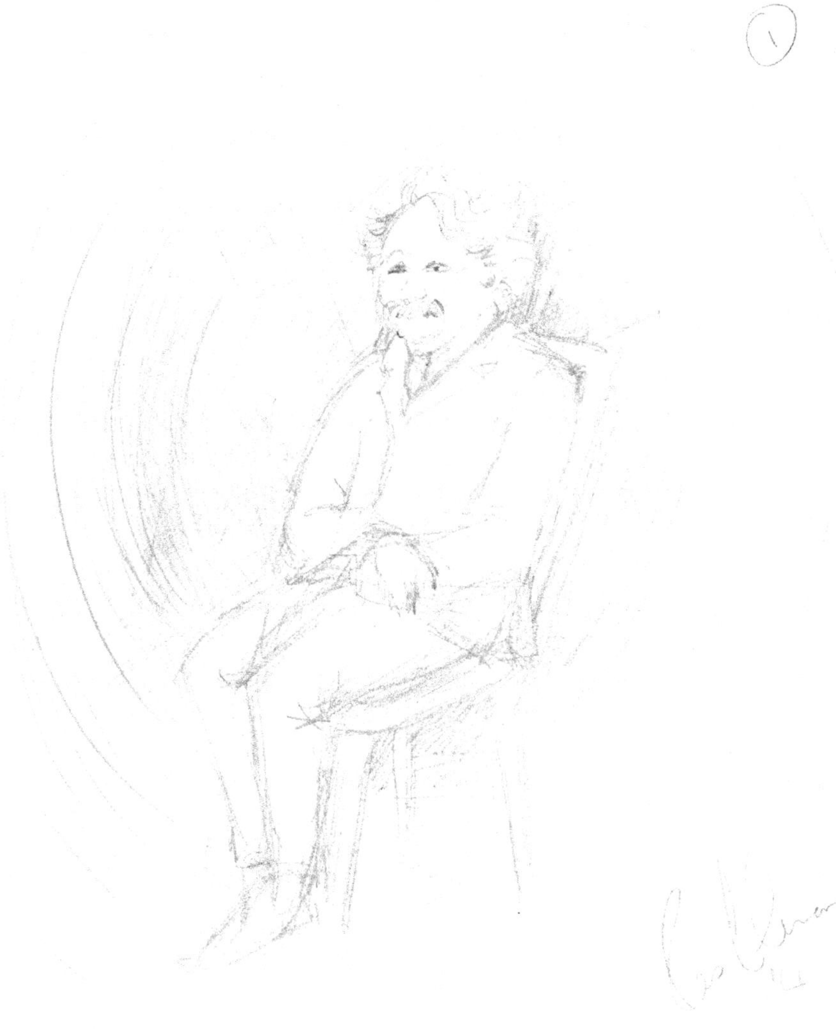

In her third and last report Ros then wrote the following:

"An odd thing came in at the beginning when I started tuning into your past life's character. I sensed very strongly that he loved cats. In fact, one of my own cats (Pippin – she is very 'psychic' and sees Spirit) came to sit on my lap as I was tuning in and purred away. Reluctantly I had to lift her down as she was too distracting. I keep coming back to this being very clear in that he goes his own way and it would have been unthinkable to him to be expected to do otherwise. He is demonstrating this in the portraits I am creating of him. When I channel, I take on the character in some ways of who I am channeling. I feel he sees that I have fallen into a pattern when I create these portraits. But he is having none of it. He was very much someone who would be in the driving seat.

This energy exists, as he was then and as he is now, out there on the quantum. 'How?' I think, 'can this be when his soul is residing in another human's physical form? That would mean that his consciousness is split into two.' He explains that this is so, and it is more than that because form is not, in quantum space, as we perceive it in our physical space. He can be in several different 'places,' like parts or aspects, but each part is completely individual and autonomous. And still the one him.

In his own, very individual way he begins to explain and demonstrate how this works. He starts by saying it is not a matter of one soul being a single entity that hops from one human life to another. I have an image now of tourists, island-hopping, sailing from one Greek island to the next, exploring each one before gaily jumping on their boat again and sailing onto the next. I find this image amusing and see that he had a sense of humor. I can see him using it in talks on topics that certain others found very profound, deep and serious. He was different and unexpected. Reactions were mixed.

He is showing me now an image of his face. It is like a photograph or as if I had created a flat painting, as if in two dimensions. As I watch, I see the photo become fractured, as if someone has torn it up and then let them drop. I can see that as they have fallen, they are still making a recognizable likeness of him. I'm seeing the same photograph but in a different way. Their tearing up is telling me that I need to 'tear up' my old way of perceiving and look at it in a different way.

Now the pieces are lifted up, put back together in a three-dimensional form and placed on a backdrop of the cosmos. I can still see each part separately but part of the same whole in a different, expanded form. I hear the word 'fractal.' It is not a word I am familiar with. I find myself zooming right into this new form. The closer I get the more detail I see. I can see his image many times on each of these parts; he is facing this way and that way and shows me that I can perceive him in any way that is possible. I am zoomed in even closer, as if through the lens of a telescope. The more expanded my view, the more facets, sides, and aspects I see. But it is all him, and more and more. It is like a story that never really ends. It is a picture that is like an end and a beginning all at once as if the end and the beginning are one and the same. I find that I understand infinity. How life is infinite. And eternal.

Now he has zoomed me out again, and as I watch, it is as if the parts have exploded outwards into many pieces. Each part becomes a perfect form of him, and I can see his kind and gentle nature perfectly reproduced in each part. The parts look different now, like orbs, each containing a perfect image of his face. He is showing me now that each of these orbs are him. And that each one can exist separately and act independently from each other, and reside in separate living human bodies should they so choose. But they are still each and all him.

He is reminding me (just popped up from my memory) now of a time when I was at school, and the class was learning about how atoms were constructed. The diagrams reminded me of planets orbiting their own Sun, and I wondered whether, like life on our own planet, these tiny (to us) planet-like particles hosted life, only in a much smaller form. Anyone I mentioned this to, said 'no' it's impossible to get anything that small. But I wondered… How can they know that so certainly, even though this has never been discovered or proven? The size of the life would be as relative to those on that tiny 'planet' as our life is to us on our planet. How can something be impossible just because the means to see it has not been created? He says 'Yes. It is all a relative concept.'

I am absolutely clear that this man was a teacher, and he would have been a very interesting one too. He has explained (what I am guessing) is a pretty tricky concept to put across, but in a way that makes sense to me by using a model that was familiar and that I found interesting. (I understand how teaching works because it was my career and I was fascinated with the science of it). He is very expressive with his hands and arms and seems to use the word 'yes' a lot. This would make his words memorable. I can see him reinforcing these affirmative with a vigorous nod of his head and a direct gaze over the top of his glasses. He would sometimes hold eye contact for quite lengthy periods. This could be encouraging for some and disconcerting for others. He did this because he was listening intently to what the other was saying and not for any other reason.

I am seeing him as a passionate teacher and one who understood the psychology of teaching very well. He was naturally gifted in this area. He was naturally gifted because of his passion and enthusiasm for the subject. He appears bright and full of energy compared to the formal teaching of his days. If I were a student at that time, I would have given anything to be taught by him.

I am seeing that some people, some sectors of his community, did not agree with his views. Many thought him outspoken and opinionated. He did have strong views and would not hold back when voicing his opinions. For all this, he was a gentle and kind man who felt compassion.

Everything I have seen today points to your past life as being Albert Einstein. I'd be amazed if it wasn't because the images are so clear and the energy feels like him. If it isn't him, it was someone closely connected with him, such as a tutor. The info that came above was very clear and very interesting. I hope you enjoy it and find it useful. In Love and in Light, Ros."

These now were the reports and pictures of Ros Coleman about my previous life as Albert Einstein that she was able to research from a short handwritten notice of mine, where I gave her only one specification being the period of the 19th to the middle of the 20th century.

What I found quite interesting in this report was that Albert Einstein explained how he could simultaneously live in several incarnations and each one of them a projection of his higher self. Another clairvoyant had indicated this to me already ten years before. I did not tell her, that I had known earlier, that I was Albert Einstein. But she said, that recently she saw Albert Einstein appearing quite clearly in her apartment before I first met her. And then a few days later I had a phone call with her, in which she was able to talk to this visible version of Albert Einstein made of light and to me simultaneously. She could somehow arrange communication between me in my present and my previous life. I gave her no indication about me and Albert Einstein but only smiled silently to myself and then after a few minutes, she said with the greatest surprise, oh, you are the same, you are Albert Einstein; why did I not notice this immediately? So, after Maharishi™[18] and before Ros Coleman, that was a third independent hint for me towards this reality.

Ultimately, this projection of the one Self applies to all living beings. We all have only one Self that appears projected in a great variety of various living beings. It was also interesting to note Ros Coleman's cognition of the projection into the infinity of a closed circle in which the end becomes a new beginning. That is enlightenment that makes infinity possible together with an experience of the finite.

I have myself researched more about Albert Einstein's and my other previous lives. Doing this, for example, I became interested, in whether I could remember some of the publications of Albert Einstein again. So I bought the collected papers of Albert Einstein. What a work, to write so much in one life! So, I went to the original German version of the special theory of relativity and began for the first time in this life, to read it from the beginning. Immediately every sentence appeared completely known, the grammar, the rhythm of the words, all came back. After a few sentences completely unexpectedly and very intensively, the thought came, that this can go to print, that you have read it often enough! Everything appeared to me as if I had just finished writing and proofreading the article.

The graphical understanding of all the principles of space-time, quanta, heat motion, the equivalence of mass and energy, and much more was already there in my early years. In high school, it was great fun for me, putting special relativity theory completely on two pages for a presentation. Meanwhile, after a lot more studying of mathematics, which has also not been

---

[18] Maharishi is a trademark of Maharishi Foundation Ltd. Corporation United Kingdom, P.O. Box 652 St. Helier, Jersey Great Britain JE48Y2.

easy for me in this life, I now understand the mathematical equations of Albert Einstein's work again.

Additionally, there are also still some of the old aversions, like for example towards Niels Bohr, who also in my present opinion has not done humanity any favors by his interpretation of quantum mechanics.

This has now fooled four generations of physicists into believing, that they could not understand quantum mechanics and should be content with the correctness of the mathematical formulae. There is still quite a bit left to be sorted out!

Experience 2

In the morning, in the wakeup phase, between sleep, dream, and waking, I kept having pictures of flying experiences. They were very concrete; they happened mostly in a town and in a rural suburb. I was flying in between rows of houses, to windows of certain houses, into open windows, in halls, in long corridors, through the openings of half broken window panes, etc. There was some danger that appeared over and again consisting of a network of lines, which somehow divided the town into an above and below. Flying there was dangerous. It was like a death trap. The lines looked like the powerlines of a tram network. For a long time, I could not explain, from where these visions came. One morning I saw the vision of my feet. They were orange with long toes. Then it became clear. I had seen the pictures of an incarnation as a bird. The feet were those of a certain kind of crow. Now it all made sense. The tram lines were clear hints that this incarnation had happened fairly recently. I enjoyed a few more "films" from this incarnation, like for example, soaring on ascending air currents above broad valleys and also sometimes in front of a threatening thundercloud. Then the theme started to become boring. The visions no longer came as often; they were all stored as my memories, which I can access at any time. However, they showed me, that someone with many incarnations as a human before, occasionally can incarnate as an animal.

Experience 3

Probably the most memorable and impactful was a past life experience. There are three things worth mentioning here:

- I have experienced restriction in my throat throughout my life and more during times of stress.
- I have a fear of being out of my depth in water.
- I have a fear for the safety of my children. This was no ordinary fear. It was irrational and inappropriate and would descend at any time. It was also embarrassing as all three children are adults now and perfectly capable of looking after themselves.

Using the attention on my navel to look at my throat problem it became obvious, the restriction belonged to something in the past. With guidance, I put my attention on the feeling attached to the restriction, and I experienced a sensation of being chocked... a rope being tied around my neck. At the same time, I was being dragged away from my children. A sack was placed over my head then my whole body was submerged in water. During all this, I continued to place my attention on the sensation of constriction.

Although the images are as clear today (one year later), I have no recollection of how this was resolved. I strangely didn't find the images/experiences distressing. I do know, I no longer have a throat restriction or irrational fears about my children. I still would not like, being out of my depth in water, but treat this as normal.

Experience 4

There was a time in my life when during waking up in the morning, more and more new puzzle pieces of a previous life appeared. It mostly happened in large buildings. Somehow, I had the task of controlling everything. When I came there initially, I was not able to orient myself. The main building was somehow far too complicated. Sometimes I got lost and did not arrive at, where I wanted to be. As time went on, I became more acquainted with the building and from memory could pretty well draw it on paper. There were grand stairways, huge corridors, high ceilings, magnificent rooms. Much of it was sumptuously decorated, and everything had to follow certain rules. I knew some of the doors very well because I had to watch in front of them. However, that was not my only task; I had to find out exactly, what was happening everywhere, even in the basements and in special subterranean corridors. Those were pretty shabby. The more I found out, the clearer it became, that in this previous life I had lived in the Palace in Vienna, the so-called Hofburg. My main task there was, to ensure the safety of the Emperor's family. I was a member of the imperial guards. I had probably learned something there, which I can still utilize today, staying calm for a long time, awake and straight-faced.

When this profession in the imperial lifeguard became clear to me, many of the previous memories now also made sense. Those subterranean channels were the remainder of the siege of Vienna by the Turkish army. I had not been there at that time, but the corridors were still there, and they were possible hiding places for assassins. Therefore I had to check with great care, that nobody un-noticed would hide there. To ward off all these dangers, I not only had to know the grand, magnificent corridors, but also the small, hidden hallways and staircases that were used by the servants to provide supplies for the Palace. Everything had to be taken into account.

The more I became interested in the topic, the more visions came. There were these visits with some of the ladies of the imperial family and their closest confidants in a special coffeehouse in Vienna. The Austrians had discovered the coffee at the Turkish camps, following the siege of Vienna, and therefore a coffee culture originated in Vienna, apart from a baking culture of sweet delicacies. We, as soldiers always had to be there, but were not allowed to eat anything. We found ways, to taste the delicious cakes and tartlets, which had not been eaten and went back to the kitchen, where we could test them ourselves. One always had to be careful, not to be caught out.

Then, there also was this summer Palace, the Schönbrunn Palace. I remember carriage rides with the imperial family when a new renovation phase of the Palace began. Initially, there were only very few rooms inhabitable, but anyway, we had a look around. Then I also remember a later phase, when the Palace was in full use. There were floors and stories only for the ladies. No men were allowed there. However, my colleagues and I had to ensure security. It was always something of a balancing act. I remember the courtly carriages, the majestic stairways, and all the ambiance. Additionally, there were also these various intrigues within the Emperor's family, where a guard had to be extremely careful, not to get involved. Probably I did not always manage that, and at some point somehow, this may have been the reason, that my life was very short.

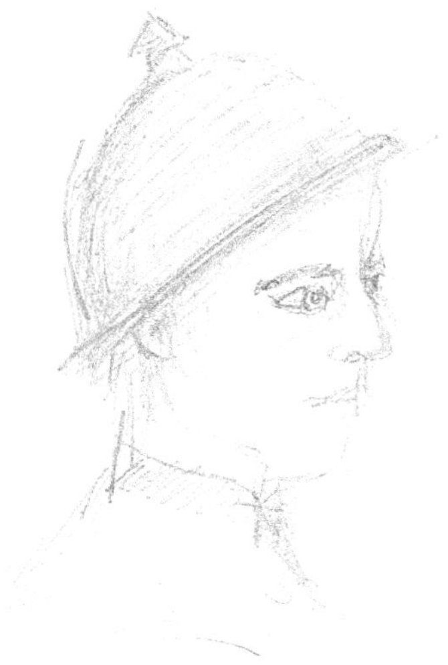

A clairvoyant in England, on a mind-body-spirit fair, once drew four pictures of some of my previous lives. One of them fitted this life exactly as an imperial guard. She also had sensed the word "Kaiser" (Emperor). When I became clear about the connection of this to my previous visions, I searched for the special helmet in the drawing on the internet and found something. From there I could infer that this life happened in the 19th century and that the drawing showed the helmet of the guards at the Emperor's Palace in Vienna. It was quite a good confirmation, that my visions were right, and that this clairvoyant had seen the same.

Then I also remembered a special melody. It was a melody that always particularly fascinated me in my present life. The melody was like the *saṁskāra* on which I could travel back to the past.

Later I found out, that this melody sounded not the same, but similar to the barcarole in the opera "The Tales of Hoffman," by Jacques Offenbach. When I heard this opera the first time in the present life, an unusual, peculiar familiarity appeared. Somehow, I completely knew this music. Then I continued to research on the internet and found out, that the barcarole of this opera originally came from the romantic opera "The Rhine Nixies," also by Jacques Offenbach. There, my beloved music was the overture with the name "Fairy-Music." Here is a hyperlink to this music on the Internet:

https://www.youtube.com/watch?v=Iqk6ryRXCVg

Its premiere was on 4th of February 1864 at the Imperial Court Theatre in Vienna. Members of the imperial family also were present. I found this announcement of the premier on the internet.

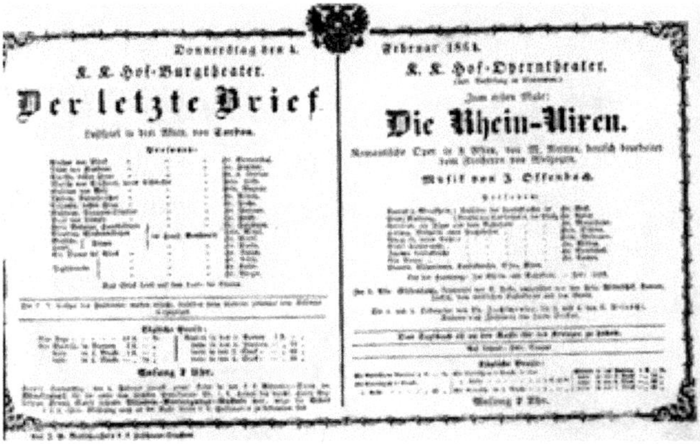
Donnerstag den 4. Februar 1864.

K. K. Hof-Burgtheater.

Der letzte Brief

Anfang 7 Uhr.

K. K. Hof-Operntheater.

Zum ersten Male:

Die Rhein-Nixen.

Musik von J. Offenbach.

Anfang 7 Uhr.

Now, the old memories of this premier arose again. I had been present. I was on guard duty for the imperial family during the premiere. More than the pictures, there was also this special, elevated feeling during the opera, which came to memory. All this was quite interesting for me because thus I had a time specification for this life. Therefore I now know, that in Vienna in 1864 I had been a member of the lifeguards of the Emperor Franz Joseph I.

Experience 5

About 20 years ago, I visited a friend, who had just finished training as a past life regression therapist, to accompany people exploring their previous lives, and we decided, to practice his new skill on me. Several previous lives appeared some of which I already knew from before. Finally, we went back so far, that my consciousness became very sleepy. Who would want to spend a lifetime as watchmen with a spear in front of the hut of an African chieftain? Therefore we decided to travel again forward in time to arrive in the present.

Next day we did something completely crazy. We traveled with the same method into the future. Before it started, I saw the *pūjā* picture of Guru Dev, a holy master from my tradition, and he impishly grinned. That was a sign for me that something very special could happen. Then we traveled through my future, there I met several future events, some of which had already manifested by now. For example, I heard the name of my, at that time future, by now past, wife. Then I saw a building project in India, which also happened exactly that way. Then also a building project in Holland, which manifested exactly at the place, I had seen, although I was not involved in this project.

And then it really started. There came visions, how the dream of yogic levitation would become a reality. It started in a beautiful environment, with a house and a group of about 200 persons, who advanced their consciousness in grand steps, and where I had a leading position. All were very happy and became happier day by day. Everyone helped everyone else, was friendly, happy and ultimately almost euphorically happy, really blissful. This happiness became so touchable, so solid, that it was sufficient as a basis, on which to walk. It was the basis for that, which happened next. We were practicing together the yogic levitation, and the flights became longer and more elegant. Then it was no longer a hopping, but we rather flew for about 10 seconds, as if on a parabolic trajectory, from one end of the room to the other. Then we were pretty quickly restricted by the rooms and continued the flying program outside, in nature. The flights then became very long. For safety, first, we practiced those long flights above waters, like rivers or lakes. The longer a flight was, the more intense became the bliss. Ultimately the flights became higher and much longer. Food and drink were no longer required, and even breathing was easy in spite of being high up in thin air. We saw the Earth from a great height, below us, like on a map. Now we had achieved it.

Then, there was another phase, where we met another group. They had practiced the flying successfully in a hot country. They soared like eagles upwards on thermal air currents. I arrived in a situation, where one of them was just about to land. For safety reasons, they were attached to a kind of delta wing glider. In case they would, during their practices, lose *samādhi*, and thus lose their ability to fly, they still had these wing gliders for safety. Additionally, for the rest of the population, it appeared as if these people were simply practicing a new kind of sport with wing gliders. Thus, they did not attract attention.

In the last phase of this development, I saw then how I would orbit the Earth as a living satellite. We could fly individually, as well as in groups. The bliss was absolutely indescribable. One time I landed again on Earth, to regulate some things. However, I felt that this landing and walking with my feet was like inadvertently stepping into a heap of manure. As fast as I could, I went back up, flying on my blissful orbit around the Earth. Sometimes we were flying in formation and pushed away dark clouds in front of us. When we came, everything brightened. Sometimes, telepathically, we got a call from our master and then flew in formation in the direction of the Himalayas, where we would meet at a secret meeting point that could not be accessed by any vehicles.

Finally, I returned to the present time and opened my eyes. The bliss was still very intense. My friend, who was accompanying me with his eyes open, confirmed to me later, that during the long time he had known me, he never saw me with such a blissful face. So, it is a wonderful future that is awaiting me.

3.19

[By intuitive perception, saṁyama on] the thought of another, [one gains] knowledge of [the other's] brain software.

प्रत्ययस्य परचित्तज्ञानम्

pratyayasya para-citta-jñānam

pratyayasya (m. gen. s.: thought) para (mf(ā)n. comp.: other) citta (n. comp.: brain software) jñāna (n. nom. acc. s.: knowledge)

Telepathy sūtra

By saṁyama on the thought of another, there arises a direct perception of the thought of this other one; from this direct perception appears knowledge about the brain software of the other, who has this thought.

Naturally, it is useful, not to become worried by the worried thoughts of others, more so, if one already has better ways of gaining reliable knowledge, like for example with the apps 3.35 and 3.36. Those already have been described in 3.6 as a higher level.

On the other hand, however, it is always enriching, to communicate in thought with another brain software user, who is free from longings for sensory things (1.37).

Practices

First ask the *ātman*, the SELF of the person in your thoughts for permission, to be allowed to do it! If the answer is "no," simply do not do it.

As it is sometimes a bit cumbersome, to write both in male, as well as female gender, this time we will write only in the female gender.

Practice 1

Choose a dear relative or a good girlfriend and completely tune to her thoughts, if you have previously obtained permission. The thoughts of another person are the place for the *dhāraṇā*. The full attention goes to a feeling that can approximately be paraphrased with the sentence: "what might she be thinking now?" Then you stay with this feeling, even when you have reached the silence of *samādhi*. Then, completely spontaneously in *samādhi,* a thought appears, which corresponds to the thought of the person. If it does not distract you from *dhāraṇā*, then also several thoughts can come in sequence.

Practice 2

If it works well with a dear relative or good girlfriends, why not try it with an adverse person? However, you have to be careful, not to bring any of your own hostile feelings into this game.

Practice 3

Now try it with a person, where you are not quite sure, whether she is dear or hostile towards you. You may even become able to spot that from her thoughts.

Practice 4

If you utilize this *siddhi* in your professional life, you can often gain advantages, for example, find out who your friends are or your enemies or find out the actual position of a negotiation partner during negotiations before signing contracts.

Practice 5

If you adore a spiritual master or teacher or any personality of the divine, use this *siddhi*, to allow two-way communication. If, for example, you are praying, allow sufficient time in silence, to also perceive the answers of your adored divine person.

Experiences

Experience 1

Right from the beginning, with the first practice of the *siddhi*, to read thoughts, I tried it with another course participant. My perception later was confirmed by her.

Experience 2

Shortly after Heinz had helped me learning the *siddhis*, I asked Maharishi™[19] in thoughts, whether I was allowed to pass on this kind of interpretation of the *siddhis* because he had taught them in another way. Before I could even finish the question, the answer came as a "Yeeees...," like thunder that made the whole universe vibrate. That was unmistakably clear.

Experience 3

When I lived and worked in Switzerland at the University of my Indian master, I noticed that apparently, he was communicating with some of his students not merely verbally, but also directly in his mind. He never talked

---

[19] Maharishi is a trademark of Maharishi Foundation Ltd. Corporation United Kingdom, P.O. Box 652 St. Helier, Jersey Great Britain JE48Y2.

about that in his lectures. However, when that became clear to me, I also wanted to be able to do it. What could there be more beautiful, than directly communicating mentally with a liberated one? Therefore, I practiced that, and during each of his lectures I sat there and tried to guess, what he would say next. After a while, this worked quite well, and I was immersed in the flow of his thoughts. Others took notes of the lectures, but I had no time for that because I was busy guessing his thoughts.

He fairly quickly found that out and began to play with this ability. He could read all my thoughts, for him I was like an open book. He also indicated to me by various gestures, when I was not quite right, or when my intellect was babbling something, that did not correspond to his thoughts. Sometimes, however, I had detected his thought correctly, and he paused, but then did not speak that thought, and instead, thought about something else. It was a playful game, which, again and again, trained my flexibility. With many hours, days, months of these practices, my ability to guess his thoughts improved and I could fairly well rely on it.

Then it became a new challenge, to guess his thoughts when he was not in the same room with me. For example when telephoning him or even, when I merely thought of him and then began a mental communication. He also could start communication from his side. As a kind of ringtone, to allow me to recognize him, he used the sound of a great Buddhist bell which he loved to ring and which I also very much liked. When I mentally heard this sound, I knew that my liberated master wanted to speak to me. Initially, I had certain difficulties, "in picking up the phone." With some more practice, however, in time this became easier.

On the day when he finally left his body, I was still able to communicate directly with his mind. I had heard the message about an hour later and, of course, wanted to bid farewell. There I saw him sitting in a large palace with many servants and ministers. He sat in the middle and enjoyed, being able to eat again. It seems, his digestion here on Earth had not functioned very well before he died. He saw me, and I did not want to disturb in any way and went a bit to the side. He had the two large middle doors opened and welcomed me in. He showed that he was very well and then told me, "We are going to meet again!" However, the way he said that it was very clear that he did not mean I would come to his heavenly world, but rather that he would reincarnate during my lifetime back on Earth and we would meet again on Earth. The communication continues, and I can practically talk to him at any time. Sometimes, very seldom, he approaches me to tell me something important.

3.20

But not about the state of consciousness, that is connected to that thought, because it is not a fitting item for this saṁyama.

न च तत्सालम्बनं तस्याविषयीभूतत्वात्

na ca tat sālambanam tasya-aviṣayī-bhūtatvāt

na (not) ca (and) tad (n. nom. acc. s.: that) sālambana (mfn., n. nom. acc., m. acc. s.: belong to, connected with [practice]) tad (mn. gen. s.: that) aviṣayin (m. comp.: not a fitting object for that, not a subject) bhūta-tvāt (n. abl. s.: life situation, existence, living being, element, what exists)

The *yogi* only perceives the thought, but not, whether the person is liberated, or not. However, it is not dangerous, to read the thoughts of persons with previous versions of the brain software. There is no danger of losing one's own advanced brain software version. The telepathy *sūtra*, therefore only transfers the thought impulses of the other person, not their brain software. These thoughts, however, for someone with a higher version of the brain software, may appear rather worried and therefore this practice may be a waste of time. But there is no danger that the *yogi* could thus fall back into a worried state.

Practice

If you notice that someone has rather worrying thought processes, like for example seeing everything through the glasses of his ego, then you also can reach the result of the telepathy *sūtra* in another way. You can, for example, apply the *sūtras* 3.35 and 3.36 in sequence, to explore any knowledge.

3.21

By saṁyama on the contour of the body, the possibility of being seen by beings is suppressed. Disconnected from the light of the eyes [of the observer, the body of the yogi] becomes invisible.

कायरूपसंयमात्तद्ग्राह्यशक्तिस्तम्भे
चक्षुःप्रकाशासंप्रयोगेऽन्तर्धानम्

kāya-rūpa-saṁyamāt tat-grāhya-śakti-stambhe cakṣuḥ-prakāśa-asaṁprayoge antardhānam

> *kāya (m. comp.: body) rūpa (n. comp.: form, gestalt) saṁyama (m. abl. s.:) tad (n. comp.: that) grāhya (mfn. comp.: perceivable, perceived) śakti (f. comp.: power, energy, possibility) stambha (m. loc. s.: suppression, hindrance, halting) cakṣu (m. nom. s.: eye) prakāśa (m. comp.: light) asaṁprayoga (m. loc. s.: no connection) antardhāna (n. nom. acc. s.: disappear, invisibility)*

The yogi is no longer connected to the light that travels towards the eyes of other beings, and thus his body is no longer visible to them. That also includes the disappearance of sounds and other sensory perceptions.

There is a power that allows hearing the yogi. When this saṁyama is applied to the sound, this power will be neutralized, and then the other person no longer hears him. The same applies to touch and the other sensory perceptions.

Practice

Many people perform this *siddhi* quite spontaneously when traveling in an elevator. Suddenly, they come close together with many unknown people, and most of them only concentrate on their body boundaries towards the others. Thus, it is nearly like magic, that one is not disturbed so much by the others because somehow the others seem invisible. Small children do not practice that, remain fully visible, and the attention of the passengers often turns towards them.

In a way, here you can see the first entry towards the invisibility *siddhi*. Direct your attention to your body boundaries, the place for this *dhāraṇā*, then with the refinement of *dhyāna* go into the silence of *samādhi*. You may be surprised by the result. It could even happen, that your body appears on a camera picture, while humans or animals simply overlook it. One more thing: always remain calm and relaxed, then it is easier.

Experience

This *siddhi* was something special. When I practiced it just for fun and opened the eyes again, all my body was still visible, at least for me. So I did not practice it too often, as there was no obvious visible result. But one day I was in a good mood while cycling and thought spontaneously, it would be funny if others on the cycle path could perceive only a bicycle without a cyclist. It was not really dangerous to practice this *siddhi* along a little creek, cycling on this path with little traffic. So, I practiced it for a while with open eyes and then, after some time, noticed something strange. All the little insects, midges, beetles, butterflies no longer evaded me as they usually do – I was not going very fast – but instead banged directly onto my white shirt. I had never experienced such a thing before. It was a successful proof that at least for those little creatures the visibility of my body was reduced. But then, it was bothering me too much, and so I stopped applying this *siddhi* and immediately the insects were able to avoid me again.

3.22

[Karma becomes] either carried out or not carried out. By saṁyama on that karma or on omens [there arises] foreknowledge of one's death.

सोपक्रमं निरुपक्रमं च कर्म तत्संयमादपरान्तज्ञानम् अरिष्टेभ्यो वा

sopakramam nirupakramam ca karma tat-saṁyamāt aparānta-jñānam ariṣṭebhyaḥ vā

sopakrama (mfn., m. acc., n. nom. acc. s.: begin, take up, undertaken) nirupakrama (mfn. m. acc., n. nom. acc. s.: not started, incurable) ca (and) karman (n. nom. acc. s.: action) tad (n. comp.: that) saṁyama(m. abl. s.:) aparānta (m. comp.: death, end) jñāna (n. nom. acc. s.: knowledge) ariṣṭa (n. dat. abl. p.: misfortune, precognition, prophecy) vā (or)

Karma that brings the result of a lifespan with it is twofold, either it ripens fast, or it ripens slowly. By the practice of saṁyama on both kinds of karma, the intuitive knowledge about the end of life arises.

Karma can be compared to a wet cloth. It dries faster when it is spread out; it is similar to the karma that has already begun, which will be dissolved faster. When the same cloth is balled up, it takes a longer time to dry. It is similar to the karma that has not yet begun.

Intuitive knowledge of the end of life also comes from omens.

- *Personal omens are the absence of a humming tone with closed ears or the absence of light with closed eyes.*
- *Elementary spirit omens mean, seeing relatives who have died or seeing messengers of death.*
- *Divine omens mean suddenly seeing angels without any reason.*

- *Sight gets confused: seeing everything as the opposite of what one has seen during one's lifetime.*

The purpose of this saṁyama is to create a sense of urgency in fulfilling one's human obligations.

3.23

By saṁyama on friendliness, etc., these powers [increase].

मैत्र्यादिषु बलानि

maitrī-ādiṣu balāni

maitrī (n. comp.: friendliness) ādi (m. loc. p.: beginning with, etc.) bala (n. nom. acc. p.: power, force, strength)

Sūtra 1.33 now is applied with *saṁyama*.

Friendliness towards happy beings strengthens friendliness. Compassion towards suffering beings increases the strength of compassion. Happiness towards pure beings strengthens happiness.

The three different places for this app are the corresponding feelings. By *saṁyama* on them, these feelings become stronger.

Thus, feelings with an inexhaustible energy manifest.

Regarding indifference towards habitual sinners, this saṁyama is not applicable, because that is not a continuous feeling and, therefore, no samādhi can arise in this indifference.

Experience

The *sūtra* for friendliness is to be applied to happy beings. There are a few humans whom I would place in this category, and I have often applied friendliness towards them. In any case, it improves the relationships with friends and relatives. Recently I have begun to apply friendliness more and more towards heavenly beings. Then, usually they come fairly quickly to me, and we begin to talk. For example, I can talk to *Kṛṣṇa* as soon as I turn towards him with friendly attention. I still consider *Kṛṣṇa* as one of the friendliest humans who ever walked on Earth. This statement makes him happy just now, and he has sent me back a wave of bliss as an answer.

The *saṁyama* on compassion is to be applied to suffering beings. And, yes, there is truly enough to do on this Earth. I have been able to give solace to individual people with that, but I was also able to supply faster healing towards my own body when I felt a painful spot with compassionate attention.

Here now are two special experiences of compassion. I came back to Europe from an India trip and passed the border between Iran and Iraq, at a time, when down there, there was an ongoing war. The pilot brought our attention to this and completely spontaneously I thought that hearing this news just at that moment could not be a coincidence. I went into a deep meditation and then practiced the most intensive compassion that I was able to have. I was mentally talking to both war parties, that they actually were brothers and that this conflict should not be continued. The feeling was so intensive that my eyes burst into tears. Then, when I read a week later in the news about a truce, I was sure that with this *siddhi* of compassion I had created some movement or at least given my contribution to ending this war.

On another occasion, I practiced, together with my friend Robert, compassion on the war parties in Afghanistan. That turned out to be a bit more difficult, but we did not give in and practiced every morning and evening intensive compassion for Afghanistan. When two enlightened are coming together with such an intention, this does have an effect. Then, very slowly, compassion began to appear in public reports, the agitation against Afghanistan subsided, the warring parties became a bit more agreeable, and after about a month, a truce was negotiated and implemented. The compassion had been victorious. Hooray!

Saṁyama on happiness is something quite funny. Deep inside is this infinite happiness of enlightenment always residing. I know, I am this infinite bliss. But with the *saṁyama* on the feeling of happiness, this gets transformed to the outside. Usually, I begin to laugh, to giggle; the longer I practice the *saṁyama*, the more intense it becomes. I already had experiences, where the happiness would become so intense, that I had to stop the *saṁyama*, just to give my lungs and my laugh muscles a rest. It is so wonderful to know, that any time I can put myself into a state of intense happiness. I can call in this feeling at will and also switch it off again.

3.24

By saṁyama on the strengths, [for example] of an elephant, etc., [bodily] strengths [arise accordingly].

बलेषु हस्तिबलादीनि

baleṣu hasti-bala-ādīni

bala (m. loc. p.: power, force, strength) hastin (n. comp., n. nom. acc. s.: Elephant) bala (m. comp.: power, force, strength) ādīni (m. beginning with, etc.)

By saṁyama on the strength of the king of the birds comes the strength of the king of the birds (Garuḍa, the vehicle of Viṣṇu) to him. By saṁyama on the strength of the wind comes the strength of the wind (Vāyu) to him. It is the same in other cases.

When applying this app, the brain software changes the hardware of the body. There arises a bodily strength, which can also extend to the whole environment, like for example with the strength of the wind.

Matthew 8, 27: "But the men marveled, saying, what manner of man is this, that even the winds and the sea obey him!"

Experiences

Experience 1

I can apply the *sūtra* on strength in various ways. For example when I am having difficulties with my spine, when something is a bit turned or a disc has dislocated a bit, which, fortunately, seldom happens, I apply the strength of an elephant. Then my spine and the whole body gets flooded with enormous strength, and usually, all the vertebrae readjust themselves.

Once, when I was bicycling up a hill, the strength of the elephant appeared a bit too heavy for me, so I practiced the strength of *Garuḍa*, the king of the bird, after that we swiftly moved over the mountain without any effort.

Experience 2

With the *sūtra* on the strength of an elephant, over the years my whole body, mind, and soul have developed to become very positive and strong.

Experience 3

I had moved into a small market town, and only then heard, that there were, quite often, heavy thunderstorms. I also noticed, that, indeed, often these thunderstorms were about to unleash. Then I did my meditation and the strength *siddhi*, which I applied to the wind and the weather. Then I noticed, that the thunderstorm would not become so intensive anymore and was quickly over. When I talked about it, years later, with my neighbor, that the thunderstorms here were not so bad, as she told, she insured me that very strange; there were no more strong thunderstorms since I had been living in town. However, previously there had been thunderstorms with very great devastations in the town and the vicinity.

3.25

By attention [by saṁyama] on the inner light of anything, [there arises] knowledge about the subtle, hidden and remote.

प्रवृत्त्यालोकन्यासात् सूक्ष्मव्यवहितविप्रकृष्टज्ञानम्

pravṛtti-āloka-nyāsāt sūkṣma-vyavahita-viprakṛṣṭa-jñānam

pravṛtti (f. comp.: appearance, manifestation, prevailing) āloka (m. comp.: inner light, seeing) nyāsa (m. abl. s.: attention, fixing, focusing) sūkṣma (mf(ā)n. comp.: fine, small, atomic) vyavahita (mfn. comp.: hidden) viprakṛṣṭa (mfn. comp.: removed) jñāna (n. nom. acc. s.: knowledge)

According to quantum field theory, all matter, energy, and empty space are always filled with virtual photons (light particles). They constantly interact with everything, and, therefore, contain the complete knowledge of everything. *Saṁyama* reads out the knowledge of those virtual photons by cognizing the electromagnetic light field. Here we have an app that, similar to the previous 3.24, affects the whole physical world, however, not to exert power, but rather to gain knowledge.

Practices

Practice 1

Apply this practice to a closed container, into which you have previously not looked with your eyes, for example, a cupboard in a foreign house, a drawer, or a box. The item of attention for *dhāraṇā* is the light in this closed space. That does not mean the sunlight, but rather the virtual photons which also exist in seemingly dark rooms. The result then appears in *saṁyama* as colors and forms, which have a certain similarity to the actual content of the container.

With this app, like with so many others, it is also very important, not to mix up the direct, inner perception with a memory. Probably one should practice it several times until the memories have disappeared. Then the inner perception comes easier but stays different from the perception of the eyes. Inner perception always comes as a coloring of *samādhi*, and, therefore, has the *samādhi* qualities of emptiness (*śūnya*). It can appear blurred, cloudy, hollow, transparent, and unfathomable. Any attempt, then to "nail it down," or to "focus it," causes this inner perception to disappear again.

Practice 2

If you have lost, say, a bunch of keys, you can, by using *saṁyama* on the light of this thing, find out where it is. Turn your attention (*dhāraṇā*) initially to the light in the thing. In *samādhi,* you will, with a bit of practice, recognize, both the thing as well as its near vicinity. Then, when you apply *dhāraṇā* on the light in this area, you will recognize a wider area in the vicinity and thus, find out, where the lost thing is.

Practice 3

You can apply this *saṁyama* not merely to things, but also to subtle connections. Thus, you can gradually solve a lifetime of riddles.

Experience

Many years ago, when I had just recently learned the *siddhis,* I had a special experience of the "inner light." Most *siddhis* did not bring me any special experiences, apart from a general feeling of well-being and deep rest. But with the "inner light" I did something different. Only now, when looking back on it, since I know, how the *siddhi* techniques are functioning correctly, it has become clear to me that I had already applied this *siddhi* correctly. Even though initially I thought the word "inner light," I still did not become diverted by it and found, my attention was taken immediately to the object of cognition.

I was visiting a meditation academy and got doubled up in a common room with Evans, a friend from Singapore. This friend was a very conscientious man and reluctantly entrusted me with the key to our shared room, as he had earlier promised, to take great care with this key. Somehow, he was to learn a lesson from that. So I took the key with me and went with it into a basement room where I was practicing the yogic levitation in a group. After our exercises, I went back up to the room and discovered surprisingly, that I did not have the key anymore. The situation was now rather delicate, as the fears of my Asian friend had manifested in fact. I downplayed it all, went into our room through the neighboring room and over the balcony, just to hear my friend moaning. I told him, "Problems do not exist!" Then I sat down, closed the eyes and focused my attention on the key.

Within a few seconds, I saw the picture of the flying practice room with the mattresses and saw the key lying in the gap between two mattresses. I was overjoyed about that. I had found the key again. To make sure, I practiced the "inner light" *siddhi* once more and was surprised to get another picture. I saw Dieter, another acquaintance, as in an x-ray vision, his spine, his walk, his inner organs, his trousers, and in the pocket of his trousers, my key. He was putting on his shoes and unhurriedly went to the elevator in the basement. Now, I had to act. I took a few seconds, then opened the eyes and went quickly to the elevator door on the second floor. Just at this moment, the elevator arrived and really Dieter came out. I asked him, "have you found my key?" He was taken by surprise and first asked me for a description of the key. I described the key accurately. Then, he gave it to me and was stunned, because he had wondered, what in the world to do with this key, and was now relieved, that the key was quickly returned to its owner.

The *sūtra* "inner light" was for a long time the only one that was working reliably for me. At that time I did not know exactly why, but it was because my attention went immediately to the object without any digression.

At that time I had the task of keeping the data center of a research university running, and the main computer had broken down. At that time the computer cost as much as an expensive car. It was cheaper to repair it, than exchange it. I had had some experience with computers from school and university, but I simply did not know enough about the hardware of such a large computer. I first had to study the circuit diagrams in detail to figure out the fault.

That went on for three days, and then my friend Gerd, with whom I had recently learned the *siddhis*, came to me, but had even less of an inkling of computers than I, and told me some news. He had applied the *siddhi* for "inner light" onto the fault in the computer and had seen certain chips. That was interesting, because if I knew, what chip was at fault, I could have looked it up in the circuit diagrams and checked, what was causing the fault.

The repair then would be straightforward. The next few days we both practiced this *siddhi* to isolate the fault. While doing this, several things became clear to me. On the one hand, I saw the objects as turned around in a fourth dimension. It was, as if I saw the objects from the inside out and thereby, in a curious way, left and right was exchanged. But then, on the other hand, I also saw the current flow through the chips as a yellow light. At one point, however, I saw that the yellow light was interrupted and it was all black. Now, I thought, I had found the fault. I only had to find out, which one of the 200 chips on the motherboard was the one, that I had seen as black in the *siddhis*. At the next *siddhi* practice exercise, I focused on the number of pins at the chips. With this, I could locate the faulty chip a bit more accurately. Finally, I focused on the print on the chips and found a number that I could identify, although again left and right was exchanged. Then I could trace it back to one single chip, looked it up in the circuit diagrams and it became clear to me, that this could be the source of the fault. I exchanged the chip, and the computer was working again. Hooray! I could not have wished for a better proof of the correctness of my *siddhi* practices.

Then it became ever easier, to find the faults. One day I was called again to a repair job. To produce books, at that time rather complex typesetting machines were required. The data were stored on large 8-inch floppy disks. These were circular memory foils with an 8-inch diameter. They were rather flexible and could store about 1 MB. Now the typesetter, which was a profession at that time, had typed long texts for several hours, corrected them and stored them on floppy disks, but could no longer reliably retrieve the data. I was called to remedy the situation. I came into the room, saw the poor fellow exhausted and flabbergasted and suggested that he forget about his rush job for now and join our group meditation and *siddhi* practice. Then a solution would be found. While I practiced the *siddhis,* I now applied the "inner light" to the floppy disk machine. There I saw a certain arm made of plastic that was bent in a very special way, had several branch-offs and was movable. That was sufficient for me. After the evening meal, I went unhurriedly back again to the typesetting room and said that I would now like to have a look at the machine. Never before in my life had I seen such a machine from the inside. I opened the cover and, what a surprise; there I saw exactly this plastic arm, just, once again, turned around four-dimensionally.

Its function was immediately clear to me. With a little spring, it was supposed to press the floppy disk against the read head. This mechanism had come loose, and I only had to adjust a setscrew, so that the floppy disk would be pressed on again. I did that, closed the cover and asked the typesetter, to store something and read it back. It functioned immediately, wonderfully and the whole repair took only five minutes and two minutes, to practice the *siddhi*. He asked me, how I had done that and I only told him, that this was know-how, and disappeared.

My special repair abilities became known, and it became even easier. Then I could already, when approaching a machine, look into it with my consciousness and discover the faults. In the end, this went so far, that machines that had played havoc for days, decided, to function well again, as soon as I entered the room.

Later on, I got a bit bored with continuous machine repairing. Why deal with machines that were developed so badly, that they needed the continuous attention of a repair expert? I preferred to direct my attention to the development of new machines. Then I could also apply my well-functioning *siddhi* abilities in a more useful way. For example, I was able to see the future of a machine, newly developed by me, and I could see, whether it would function well or not. If it would not function well, I could remove the weak points at an early stage. It was working quite well, for example, with an invention of mine, of a plug technology, which allowed me and my engineering team to interconnect computer circuits three-dimensionally. Engineers in a world-famous computer firm got the same idea, but only ten years later.

A further method that became available to me with my "inner light" *siddhi*, one could also call future market research. I was simply looking into the future, to see whether in future a certain machine would be used by large crowds of people. When I saw that, I simply "invented" this machine in the present. This way, inventing had become a mere glance into the future, which I was able to do fairly precisely now, based on my *siddhi* training. After some industrial experience, I joined a spiritual organization again. There and then I used this *siddhi* to view the optimum development of this organization in the future. I saw that communication via video conferences was very important. Then I recommended it to the leaders of this organization and also to their spiritual head, to utilize video conferences and video transmissions via data communication that is via the Internet. First, they took a while even to grasp my concept of such a virtual university. But when my letter got read out directly to the head of the organization, he understood exactly, what I meant. During a meeting, the head then gave some recognition to me in his so-called Council of Supreme Intelligence, "why do we not have such ideas?" I could have answered his question, "because either you do not have *siddhi* experiences or you are not applying them practically!"

In quite a rush then they did implement this concept of an Open University, but thought they did not need any further advice from the inventor and then, instead of implementing internet videos, they built up an incredibly expensive satellite network that cost them several million dollars each year. The organization was nearly collapsing financially, to do that. I only thought, "You can lead a horse to the water, but you cannot make it drink."

3.26

By saṁyama on the Sun, knowledge about the cosmic regions [arises].

भुवनज्ञानं सूर्ये संयमात्

bhuvana-jñānam sūrye saṁyamāt

bhuvana (n. comp.: world, the area of beings) jñāna (n. nom. acc. s.: knowledge) sūrya (m. loc. s.: sun) saṁyama (m. abl. s.:)

This app enables the *yogi* to view the universe-computer, using his activated quantum computer, and to connect to all regions of the universe-computer.

Practices

Practice 1

Direct your attention to the round radiant ball of the Sun. That is the place for *dhāraṇā*. Look at it with your inner eye. Here, it does not matter, in what direction, seen from your body, the Sun is. Stay on the radiant ball, and the refinement of *dhyāna* automatically happens, and in the silence of *samādhi* pictures arise. Do not get distracted by these pictures and stay with *dhāraṇā* on the radiant ball. Occasionally let the *dhāraṇā* go and allow five to ten seconds of absolute rest of *nirbīja samādhi* (1.51 and 3.6). Then, however, come back to *dhāraṇā*.

Practice 2

Sit comfortably in the Sun and look with closed eyes in the direction of the Sun. In the silence of *samādhi* enjoy the refined perception of travel through the universe.

Experiences

You can evaluate the extent of the cosmic network from experiences, that *Śaṁkara* has described in his commentary.

The seven worlds are:

1. *The terrestrial world from the point called hell (avīci), to the summit of Mount Meru.*
2. *The world of the stars (antarīkṣa) extends from the summit of Mount Meru up to the Pole Star* [in the Milky Way].

Beyond this world, the Heavens consist of five planes:

3. *The Heaven of the great Indra* [local galaxy group].
4. *The great world of Prajāpati* [local galaxy cluster chain].

The threefold world of Brahmā (world creator):

5. *The world of divine beings (jñāna world).*
6. *The world of striving (tapas world).*
7. *The world of truth (satya world)* [total universe].

The worlds are described as sevenfold:

The world of Brahmā is threefold,

below it the great world of Prajāpati,

Than that of the great Indra –

All this is called Heaven.

In the sky, the intermediate region, are the stars,

and on Earth the creatures.

From avīci one after another are six great hells, constituted of earth, water, fire, wind, space, and darkness and called respectively Mahākāla, Ambariṣa, Raurava, Mahāraurava, Kālasūtra und Andhatāmisra; in these are born beings who are to suffer long lives of misery as a result of their karma. Then there are the seven netherworlds called Mahātala, Rasātala, Atala, Sutala, Vitala, Talātala, and Pātāla. Eighth is the region corresponding to this Earth called Vasumatī, with its seven island continents and in the middle, the golden king of the mountains called Sumeru. Its peaks on the four sides are of silver, lapis, crystal, and gold. From the brilliant reflection of the lapis-lazuli, the sky to the south is the deep blue of a blue lotus leaf; the eastern is white, the western shining, and the northern yellow. To the south is the jambu tree (rose apple) that is why that land is called jambu-dvīpa. As the Sun advances, day and night follow him exactly. To the north are the three mountains, blue, white, and sharp-peaked, covering 2000 yojanas. Between them are three regions, each 9000 yojanas, called Ramaṇaka, Hiraṇmaya, and the northern Kurus. To the south are the mountain regions Niṣadha, Goldhorn and the Snow-Crags, each 2000 yojanas. Between them are three regions of 9000 yojanas each, called Harivarṣa, Kiṁpuruṣa, and Bhārata.

To the east of Sumeru is Bhadrāsava, bounded by the Mālyavat Mountains; on the west Ketumāla, bounded by the Gandhamādana range. In the middle is the zone of Ilāvṛta. Jambudvīpa is 100.000 yojanas across, stretching out from Sumeru 50.000 yojanas in each direction. It is girdled by a salt sea double its extent. Then come the lands of Śāka, Kuśc, Kraunca, Śālmala, Magadha and Puṣkara, each double the preceding, fringed with wonderful hills, and the seven seas of undulating surface like a mass of mustard seeds, with their waters of sugarcane juice, spirits, butter, curds, cream, milk, and syrup. These lands encompassed by the seven seas and engirdled by the Lokāloka Mountains are some 500 million yojanas across.

The whole configuration is contained within the Cosmic Egg, and the Egg itself is a minute fragment of pradhāna, as it were a firefly in space.

In the lower worlds, in the sea, in the mountains, gods have their group abodes: Asuras, Gandharvas, Kinnaras, Kimpuruṣas, Yakṣas, Rākṣasas, Bhūtas, Pretas, Piśacas, Apasmārakas, Apsarasas, Brahmrākṣasas, Kuṣmāṇḍas, Vināyakas. In all the lands there are righteous gods and humans. Sumeru is a pleasure ground of the Thirty (gods), and in it are particular paradises: Miśravana, Nandana, Caitraratha, and Sumānasa. Sudharmā is the gods' assembly hall, Sudarṣana their castle, Vaijayanta their palace. The planets and constellations and stars move around the Polestar like the sails of a windmill, and they revolve in circles above Sumeru. Six groups of gods dwell in the world of great Indra: the Thirty-Three, the Agniṣvattas, the Yāmyas, the Tuṣitas, the Aparinirmita-vaśa-vartins, and the Paranirmita-vaṣa-vartins. All these have their desires fulfilled and have the eight powers such as becoming as minute as an atom. They live for a kalpa and delight in making love, in bodies, they take on without parents for the purpose, with the incomparable and compliant nymphs (Apsarasas) who form their train. In the great world of Prajāpati, there is a five-fold group of gods: Kumudas, Ṛbhus, Pratardanas, Añjanābhas, und Pracitābhas. These have mastery of the elements; their food is meditation (dhyāna); they live for a thousand kalpas. In the Jñāna world, first, of the Brahmā worlds, there is a four-fold group of gods: Brahma-purohitas, Brahmakāyikas, Brahma-Mahākāyikas, and the Amaras. These have mastery over the elements and the senses. Each lives twice as long as those of the previous group. In the Tapas world, the second, there is a three-fold group of gods: Ābhāsvaras, Mahābhāsvaras, and Satya-Mahābhāsvaras. These have mastery over the elements and the senses and prakṛti; each lives twice as long as the group before, their food is meditation, and their lives are chaste (ūrdhva-retas). Upwards there is no obstacle to their thought, and below there is no object obscure to them. In the third world of Brahmā, the Satya world, there are four groups of gods: Acyutas, Śuddhanivāsas, Satyābhas, and Saṁjñāsaṁjñins. They build no dwellings, but are grounded in themselves and maintain their order; they have mastery over pradhāna and live as long as there are creations (universes). Of these the Acyutas delight in savitarka dhyāna (meditation on the physical); the Śuddhanivāsas in savicāra dhyāna (meditation on the subtle); Satyābhas in meditation only on bliss (ānanda-mātra); and the last group in meditation only on I-am-ness.

All these seven worlds are in fact worlds of Brahmā. But the bodiless and those resolved into prakṛti being in a state of liberation, are not classed as in the worlds. All that becomes capable of being directly perceived by the yogi who has made saṁyama on the Sun gate, and further on the other objects, till all has been seen.

Experiences from a newer time

Saṁyama on the Sun was one of the most difficult for me. Always the word "Sun" went around in my head. That probably was because for 30 years I had practiced it like that, without getting any results. By now it has dawned on me, that this was pretty stupid.

So, now I tried, again and again, using the correct method, to direct the attention on the round, glowing ball, the Sun, to stay there with *dhāraṇā*, to allow the refinement with *dhyāna* and to stay simultaneously in *samādhi*, the complete emptiness. With a lot of practice, I managed, to do this without any words. Finally, a fantastic result came. I went through the Sun as if through a portal. I saw the center of our universe. It was not merely a black hole, but more of a highly ordered structure. In the center, there was the mountain *Meru* that appeared almost like a Mayan pyramid. The four cardinal directions were clearly recognizable. Everything was radiating in the most brilliant colors, in gold, silver and also totally transparent. Around the central mountain, there was something nearly like a garden or a park. There were lakes as large as oceans, probably cosmic oceans, larger than complete galaxies. The central order was extending to the outside and ultimately got lost in the infinite distances of the universe.

3.27

[By saṁyama] on the Moon [there arises] knowledge of the arrangement of the stars.

चन्द्रे ताराव्यूहज्ञानम्

candre tārā-vyūha-jñānam

candra (m. loc. s.: moon) tārā (f. comp., f. nom. s: star) vyūha (m. comp.: arrangement, distribution) jñāna (n. nom. acc. s.: knowledge)

Compare this to the second world *antarīkṣa* in the experience report of 3.26. This *sūtra* should be practiced immediately following the Sun *sūtra*.

When the yogi has come to know the world, which means the universe; he should immediately practice saṁyama on the Moon, then he will perceive the arrangement of the stars. From the Sun saṁyama, there arises the knowledge of the extent of the worlds – the worlds and rivers and oceans and mountains, as described before. However, the way the stars are arranged is not within the scope of the Sun saṁyama. From the Moon saṁyama, however, there arises an understanding regarding the nature and the arrangement of stars [star signs, etc.].

Practice

Practice 1

First, always start with the Sun *saṁyama*, and afterward the Moon *saṁyama*. When you see the corresponding pictures or movies with the Sun *saṁyama* together with the silence of *nirvicāra samādhi* for some time, then this time do not go through *nirbīja samādhi* (total emptiness). Instead, go with your attention (*dhāraṇā*) directly from the Sun to the Moon and then practice *saṁyama* to the Moon.

Practice 2

Maharishi™[20] Mahesh Yogi described on 7 September 2005, during a press conference in the video, part 2, minute 5:00, the way how he performs *saṁyama* to the Moon. In doing so, he follows exactly the recommendation of *Patañjali* in 3.1 to 3.5, and applies *dhāraṇā*, *dhyāna*, and *samādhi*, without using any words.

---

[20] Maharishi is a trademark of Maharishi Foundation Ltd. Corporation United Kingdom, P.O. Box 652 St. Helier, Jersey Great Britain JE48Y2.

One of the great unsolved riddles to the authors of this book is, why he had taught the *siddhis* differently, than he obviously practiced them? Often Maharishi™[21] was wondering, why his students seldom had *siddhi* experiences. Today that is clear to us: it was due to his modification of the original *siddhi* technique because the use of words disturbs the result of the *siddhis* and prevents the loading of the *siddhi* app into the brain software.

Fervent followers of the *siddhi* technique taught since 1976 probably will be somewhat upset. However, they honestly have to admit, that with the modified procedure they have hardly any *siddhi* experiences. We have to admit to ourselves, that we have practiced the *siddhis* for 30 years with words, devotedly and uncritically. It then took us several years, to decipher the correct technique from the *yoga sūtras*. However, there were a few, who did not apply these *siddhi* techniques literally according to the instructions but rather took a freer interpretation. Those few had the correct *siddhi* experiences, as predicted by *Patañjali*.

Our advice: Simply practice all the *siddhis* exactly, the way, Maharishi™ in the following short talk describes his own experience, in a press conference, and you will have immediate results.

Experiences

Experience 1

Maharishi™ Mahesh Yogi (press conference, 7. Sep. 2005, part 2, minute 5:00).

"About 'A.' It's like when you see the Moon. When you see the Moon, now you see the Moon, you are seeing the Moon, seeing the Moon. Then what happens is, when you are seeing the Moon, seeing the Moon, seeing the Moon [*dhāraṇā*]; what is inside the Moon begins to be, in, come in the vision, what is inside [*dhāraṇā + dhyāna*]. And then what is inside that comes out; what is inside that comes out; what is inside that comes out; what is inside that comes out." [*dhāraṇā + dhyāna + samādhi*]

[21] Maharishi is a trademark of Maharishi Foundation Ltd. Corporation United Kingdom, P.O. Box 652 St. Helier, Jersey Great Britain JE48Y2.

Experience 2

When applying *saṁyama* on the Moon sphere, within a few seconds both white and black points project three-dimensionally, similar to a hologram. The bright points are stars, and the dark ones are planets. The dark ones then often have a bright halo around them.

Sometimes, during the day I also surprisingly see such points flash up in my field of vision. Occasionally I checked it immediately with an astrology program, to see what planet was positioned accurately at this angle at this time and then sometimes I identified Jupiter, sometimes Saturn or Mars exactly at that point in the sky. I greeted them and said hello to them. They love it, and they also answer, if one listens to them.

3.28

[By saṁyama] on the Pole Star [arises] knowledge about the movement of those [arrangements of stars and planets].

ध्रुवे तद्गतिज्ञानम्

dhruve tat-gati-jñānam

dhruva (m. loc. s.: pole star) tad (n. comp.: that) gati (f. comp.: path, movement) jñāna (n. nom. acc. s.: knowledge)

This app should be applied immediately following 3.27 (Moon). It leads to an intuitive *jyotiṣ* knowledge.

If the yogi immediately following the Moon saṁyama performs the saṁyama to the Pole Star (Dhruva), then he cognizes the movement of the stars, the way they go together and the way they depart; how at one time this planet is opposed to another and how in this way it becomes oppressed and how in that way it rises again. By these means, he arrives at the knowledge, for example about the good and bad destiny of living beings (jyotiṣ, Vedic astrology). Then, if he applies saṁyama to the bear constellations (large and small bear), he also learns these, their various kinds, and paths and everything about them.

Practice

The same way you have done before; first practice the Sun *saṁyama*, then the Moon *saṁyama*, and only then the Pole Star *saṁyama*. That corresponds to the application in stages as described in 3.6. This time also do not go through the *nirbīja samādhi* (total emptiness). Instead, go with your attention (*dhāraṇā*) directly from the Moon to the Pole Star and then apply the *saṁyama* to the Pole Star.

Experience

When I apply *saṁyama* to the Pole Star, I often see the whole night sky with its stars within me.

3.29

[By saṁyama] on the navel wheel (nābhi cakra) [arises] knowledge of the structures of the body.

नाभिचक्रे कायव्यूहज्ञानम्

nābhicakre kāya-vyūha-jñānam

nābhicakra (n. nom. acc. loc.: navel wheel, navel-cakra) kāya (m. comp.: body) vyūha (m. comp.: arrangement, distribution) jñāna (n. nom. acc. s.: knowledge)

By using this app, you can explore your body structure.

ĀyurVeda knows three body elements (doṣas): vāta, pitta, kapha and seven organ systems (dhātus), which according to jyotiṣ knowledge are each influenced by a heavenly body: skin – Mercury, blood – Moon, muscles – Saturn, fat – Jupiter, bones – Sun, bone marrow – Mars, semen/eggs – Venus. The arrangement of the list of the seven dhātus is from the outside to the inside.

Compare this to the seven worlds in 3.26 (Sun *sūtra*).

With the same saṁyama, the yogi can explore the structure of the nervous system.

If you apply this app to the navel of other beings, you can explore with it the bodily state of other people, and also of animals.

Practices

It is a very important app because you can get rid of a lot of bodily troubles.

Practice 1

Sit comfortably with closed eyes and for a moment touch your navel with a finger. Then keep your attention on the navel. The navel is the place for the *dhāraṇā*. Staying with your attention there, it will automatically refine (*dhyāna*) and in the silence of *samādhi,* there will appear pictures or multimedia movies. Important: Do not search for pictures, the way you know them from schoolbooks. The *dośas* and the *dhātus* appear rather like vibrations, less like concrete items. Do not expect any pictures and take it, as it comes. It is important, if pictures or movies appear in *samādhi,* that you do not interrupt the *dhāraṇā* and continue to stay on the navel. We have emphasized this already several times (3.4).

Practice 2

Repeat practice 1. However, this time, begin with the slightest intention, to see a certain place in your body. It is not an intensive desire, but just a slight tendency. Your *dhāraṇā* continues to stay on the navel, but through the navel, you can see as through a window into all of the body.

Practice 3

If you see, with practice 2, structures or tissue with a dark color or black coloring, different from the brighter tissue, simply think the sound "*soma.*" *Soma* is the Vedic universal medicine. Then you will probably notice a certain prickling, light or warmth. That is an indication that this place is normalizing.

Practice 4

Simply try practice 3 out at the first signs of a cold, and you will be surprised, how quickly your immune system becomes strengthened. The place for *dhāraṇā* is the navel, and your intention, to view the affected places, anyway is already there.

Experiences

Experience 1

Whenever I apply *saṁyama* on the navel wheel, this area becomes bright. Then, the weak points in the body show up, where I can send energy.

Experience 2

Waiting for an appointment, I sat with a business partner in a car, and we decided to meditate for a little while. After a short meditation, I then did *saṁyama* on the navel. Suddenly within my vision, my complete spine appeared with every single vertebra, spinal discs, nerves and many other details. I could travel up and down my spine with my vision and look more closely at arbitrary places.

In one session with the navel *sūtra,* I could see several details in my body. Then I was also observing the silent periods of the non-excited *samādhi,* and now the experience became really interesting. Whenever I came back to the navel, I saw not merely single pictures but a movie with hundreds of pictures within a few seconds. Organs, cellular structures, cells, parts of cells, molecules, DNA, and atoms showed up to me. Everything was in color, brilliant and dynamic. I had never before seen such a thing in any biology book or any scientific movie.

Experience 3

My most important and beneficial experience was after a diagnosis of breast cancer and an operation to remove a small tumor. The Health Service has a particularly scaremongering and aggressive approach, and I had to fight hard to refuse radical surgery and drug intervention.

Using the *siddhi* technique of putting my attention on my navel and looking at the structure of my body after three hours my entire being was filled with white light. I also seemed to radiate light. I have never experienced anything like it before. In such a blissful state no illness can survive. A year on from that experience I had to have a hospital check-up where they said there was no recurrence of the disease.

3.30

[By saṁyama] on the throat pit, hunger and thirst disappear.

कण्ठकूपे क्षुत्पिपासानिवृत्तिः

kaṇṭha-kūpe kṣut-pipāsā-nivṛttiḥ

kaṇṭha (m. comp.: throat) kūpa (m. loc. s.: pit, cave) kṣudh (f. comp.: hunger) pipāsā (f. comp., f. nom. s.: thirst) nivṛtti (f. nom. s.: ending, disappearing)

Behind the tongue are the vocal cords, below these the throat (larynx), below that the windpipe (trachea) and the throat pit. From saṁyama on this (throat pit) hunger and thirst no longer torment him.

Practice

Localize your throat pit, by touching the windpipe (trachea) with your fingers and follow it down to the place, where the windpipe disappears into the body. That is the throat pit. The place for the *dhāraṇā* is within the windpipe on the same level. Remove your fingers again, but stay with your attention on this place. Then you automatically go through *dhyāna* and arrive at the silence of *samādhi*. It is so important that we repeat it once more: In the silence of *samādhi,* you continue the mental activity of *dhāraṇā* and continue to stay with your attention to the windpipe on the level of the throat pit.

That is a *sūtra*, where, together with the silence of *samādhi*, you may notice bodily reactions. Ignore those bodily reactions and do not get distracted from the *saṁyama*. Only after about 20 to 30 seconds, you let the attention go and come into the absolute silence of *nirbīja samādhi*. At that time, the effect on the feeling of hunger and thirst disappears and the corresponding impressions (*saṁskāras*) become dissolved. You can then repeat this whole cycle several times.

3.31

[By saṁyama] on the tortoise energy channel [arises] steadiness.

कूर्मनाड्यां स्थैर्यम्

kūrma-nāḍyām sthairyam

kūrma (m. comp.: tortoise) nāḍī (f. loc. s.: energy channel) sthairya (n. nom. acc. s.: steadiness, immovability, hardness)

Below the throat pit, in the chest, there is a nerve channel called tortoise.

The place is the first branching of the windpipe (trachea) into the two bronchi.

With the saṁyama on that, the body is immobilized like a snake or lizard when grasped by the neck.

Practice

You can use this app for example before a speech or public performance to reduce your excitement or stage fright.

Experience

Upon applying *saṁyama* on the tortoise energy channel, my whole body becomes stiff and energetic.

3.32

[By saṁyama] on the brightness in the top of the head [arises] vision of the perfect beings.

मूर्धज्योतिषि सिद्धदर्शनम्

mūrdha-jyotiṣi siddha-darśanam

mūrdhan (m. comp.: crown, forehead, head) jyotiṣ (n. loc. s.: light, brightness) siddha (m. comp.: perfect being) darśana (n. nom. acc. s.: vision, show, seeing, appearance, meeting)

The place is the bright space between the brain and the upper skull bone. From there arises the vision of the perfect beings, that move between heaven and Earth.

In the emptiness at the crown of the head, there is a radiance called the light. By saṁyama on that, arises the vision of the siddhas, who move between heaven and Earth.

This *sūtra* provides a connection, an interface to the *devas*, the personified natural laws. Regular activation of this connection makes it easier, to talk to the *devas*. See also the following *sūtra* 3.33.

Experiences

Experience 1

With *saṁyama* on the radiance up in the head, several higher beings, enlightened ones, Ascended Masters, *Devas*, etc. have appeared to me. With this, as with the other *siddhis* the art seems to be, not to assume, imagine or remember anything. The higher beings then appear from this field of light that often, but not always, builds up to a kind of geometry, from where the being then appears. Sometimes it is only the face, sometimes only the eyes, sometimes the whole body.

For me, having become estranged from Christian religion due to too many disappointments, one day to my surprise Christ's mother Mary came into view. She first manifested in a kind of elongated rhombus, within which she then appeared with arms, spread out, downwards as a compassionate being of blessing. Then it suddenly dawned on me, how certain heavenly beings are connected with special angles and geometric arrangements. The geometry seems to describe the essence of their character. Now it also became clear to me, why Divine Mother in her form as *Lakshmi* can be described in three ways, as a humanlike person with four arms, as the *Shri Yantra*, or as the physical natural law of gravitation. These are all only different views of the same cosmic phenomenon.

Experience 2

On the second exercise, I was more successful. We started off with the basics of *saṁyama* or attention on inanimate objects. We then repeated the exercise inwardly, looking upwards inside the head. I felt very confident with this exercise. We went further than just attention on the *siddhi*. Initially, I saw some patterns of light, and after several practices, I began to see, a fogginess, followed by a clearer light, like a cloudy sky. That felt very powerful, and we were told it applies to all *siddhis*. I hope this is the start of something new.

Experience 3

The place for this *saṁyama* below the skull, in this practice initially appears bright and then expands infinitely. It appears to me as if I am coming into an assembly of *devas*, guided by *Īśvara*. If in this state, for example, I think of a *Devi*, immediately an energy rush goes through my whole body, and there appears a blurred image of her, filling the whole room. I can immediately communicate to her as if she was in me. It appears to me as if she had settled within me.

In the *Śringeri Math*, Karnataka, India, I once had during a special ceremony for *Śiva* attended a *yajña*. Then, in front of my inner eye a radiant white, half a meter wide vertical light column appeared, that was infinite in depth and height. Later I mentally asked *Adi Śaṁkara* in front of his temple, whether it had been a vision of *Śivaji*. Before the question was even thought to the end, an about 1 cm wide light column went through my spine, like lightning that had neither beginning nor end. Simultaneously I heard loud in me: „I am *Śiva*, I am *Śiva*." I had no feeling of time, but it probably lasted several seconds. My question had been answered by this vision. In the *Śiva Purāṇa,* the phenomenon of the light column is attributed to *Śiva*, whose beginning and end could not be cognized, neither by *Vishnu* nor by *Brahmā*. Many years before, I had already perceived an infinite light column with 5 meters diameter when attending a ceremony (*rudrābhiṣeka*) for *Śiva* with about 3000 *pundits*. The power comes with the numbers.

3.33

Or from intuition [the cognition] of everything.

प्रातिभाद्वा सर्वम्

prātibhāt vā sarvam

prātibha (n. abl. s.: intuition) vā (ind.: or) sarva (mf(ā)n., m. acc. s., n. nom. acc. s.: all, total)

When the *yogi* perceives the *siddhas*, by applying *sūtra* 3.32, he communicates with them directly, to gain intuitive knowledge. It is a path to intuition that is full of surprises. Communication with the *siddhas, Īśvara, devas,* and *ṛṣis* opens the access to the field of all knowledge.

The word *prātibha* here appears for the first time. We have translated it as "intuition." It will be more refined in *sūtra* 3.36. By getting to know the perfect beings, intuition begins. Intuition is soft sensing and discovering all knowledge. This group of perfect beings, the *siddhas*, simply know everything. The highest of them is *ātman*, the SELF. *Ātman* also is available for direct communication. Thus *Vyāsa* and *Śaṁkara* comment:

prātibhādvā sarvam ātmani saṁyamaṁ kurvataḥ

"Or from intuition – by applying the *saṁyama* to *ātman* – [the cognition] of everything."

Intuition can also be achieved by a direct question to *ātman*. *Sūtra* 1.37, and also this one here, 3.33, explain, why the dialogue with *ātman* or the *devas* is a direct means to liberation. It is like the dawn of knowledge, the first phase of knowledge, born of correctly-discriminating cognition (*viveka khyāti* 2.26).

With the intense attention of the yogi to Īśvara, intuition, the universe, or the self-created (Brahmā), he [the yogi] cognizes intuitive, clear knowledge.

Who, here, asks whom? It is the individual SELF (*aham*) that asks the universal SELF (*ātman*). This communication is again, as often mentioned before, an application of the correctly-discriminating cognition, *viveka khyāti* of *sūtra* 2.26. Why is that? It is because this inner dialogue establishes the distinction between that, which changes and the non-changing, between the relative and the absolute, between the non-SELF (*aham*) and the SELF (*ātman*). This distinction always leads to perfect, clear, intuitive knowledge, as will be explained further in 3.35 and 3.36.

Experience

The shaman from whom I had learned some healing practices, once requested me to learn the picture of *Devī Durgā* that was placed in my apartment. He had no relationship to the tradition of *yoga*. Therefore his request appeared strange to me, and intuitively I asked *Durgā* in the picture – by the way, the first time that I had ever asked a picture that means a natural law symbolized by the picture. The answer came spontaneously before the thought of the question was internally spoken. It was explicit and shocking: "Then I am burning you." This experience showed me that pictures of *devis* or *devas* are a kind of communication interface to these natural laws. Those pictures are placed in many homes in India.

3.34

[By saṁyama] on the heart one cognizes the brain software.

हृदये चित्तसंवित्

hṛdaye citta-saṁvit

hṛdaya (n. loc. s.: heart) citta (n. comp.: brain software) saṁvid (f. nom. s.: cognition, thorough understanding, awareness, perceiving, intellect)

In this city of brahman, the body, there hangs the heart, a lump of flesh in the form of a lotus with the head down, in a lake inside the chest. It is the meeting point of many channels and prāṇa streams. In it is the consciousness of the intellect.

That is the place for the *dhāraṇā* of the app 3.34. The result is the perception of one's own intellect that means the *sattva* part of the brain software. We also call it the main component of the brain software. *Dhāraṇā* is to be applied to the meeting point of veins and arteries, which hold the heart, the so-called aortic arch.

Experiences

Experience 1

This *siddhi* was interesting for me in several ways. On the one hand, the *sūtra* itself makes clear already, that there is not the slightest conflict between heart and intellect. On the contrary, the heart was the place, where one would cognize the intellect. Additionally, during this exercise of the *sūtra,* it became ever clearer, what the intellect really was. It was nothing solid, it moved continuously, as the heart is pumping continuously, as the breath is synchronized with it, so also the intellect was pulsing. At various opportunities it also showed up in different forms, sometimes more, sometimes less expanded, sometimes nearly infinite. Everybody in my study group had a completely different experience with their intellect, the same way as this *siddhi* experience changed every day, for me as well.

However, most important was, that finally, I had found a place to which I could apply the following *siddhi*. Without this *siddhi* on the heart, it was never quite clear, what the intellect essentially was. Therefore the next *siddhi* that distinguishes the intellect from the unmoving Self, had no place, no starting point; and with words alone, not any right result could come about, as I had experienced already before with other *siddhis*. Now I had found the starting point, and the next *siddhi* accordingly was functioning really well.

Experience 2

By applying *saṁyama* on the aortic arch, this area became bright and in the space of consciousness expanded into infinity. Thereby, initial disturbances in the form of pains, feelings, or thoughts in this space dissolved, such that clarity, silence, and easy brightness remained.

3.35

Experience is a thought that does not distinguish between [buddhi-] sattva and puruṣa, although they are absolutely distinct. By saṁyama on that [buddhi-sattva] which is there for the purpose of the highest, and on that which is there for its own purpose [puruṣa], arises knowledge of puruṣa.

सत्त्वपुरुषयोरत्यन्तासंकीर्णयोः प्रत्ययाविशेषो भोगः परार्थत्वात् स्वार्थसंयमात् पुरुषज्ञानम्

sattva-puruṣayoḥ atyanta-asaṁkīrṇayoḥ pratyaya-aviśeṣaḥ bhogaḥ para-arthatvāt sva-artha-saṁyamāt puruṣa-jñānam

sattva (n. comp.: purity) puruṣa (m. gen. loc. d.: silent SELF) atyanta (mfn. comp.: perfect, absolute) asaṁkīrṇa (n. gen. loc. d.: not mixed) pratyaya (m. comp.: thought) aviśeṣa (m. nom. s.: not different, same, without difference) bhoga (m. nom. s.: pleasure, experience) para (mf(ā)n. comp.: other, highest) artha-tvāt (m. abl. s. purpose, goal; -ness) sva (mf(ā)n. comp.: own) artha (m. comp.: purpose, goal) saṁyama (m. abl. s.:) puruṣa (comp.: silent SELF) jñāna (n. nom. acc. s.: knowledge)

As a result of the previous *sūtra* the main component (*buddhi-sattva*), the subtlest level of the brain software (*citta*) is recognized. Now, this is compared to the absolute silence in consciousness, to *puruṣa*.

By *saṁyama* on *puruṣa*, as distinct from *buddhi-sattva*, the knowledge of *puruṣa* unfolds. *Puruṣa* is the eternal silence of pure consciousness that exists for its own purpose. The *buddhi-sattva* is the subtlest level of the active brain software, which exists for the purpose of *puruṣa*. *Puruṣa* and *buddhi-sattva* are absolutely distinct from each other and have completely different qualities.

The users of brain software versions 1 to 6 are having "experiences." That means, their perceptions are always, again and again, connected to the limited ego, or the other illusions, and thus they remain limited. Experience means thinking that does not distinguish between *buddhi-sattva* and *puruṣa*. Users of brain software versions 7 and 8, however, continue to perceive, but no longer in the form of experiences.

Buddhi-sattva, the intellect, strives towards clarity. *Sattva* is changing because it is a *guṇa* and because also the other two *guṇas*, namely *rajas* and *tamas* to a certain extent, albeit small, play a role. In this game, a continuous change occurs.

Sattva exists for the purpose of the highest, has no consciousness, independent of the highest, and does not even exist without the highest. *Sattva's* intelligence and wisdom are borrowed from the highest. *Sattva* is completely distinct from *puruṣa*, the highest. *Puruṣa* is pure, unchanging, exists for its own purpose, is eternally silent, is pure consciousness.

Buddhi-sattva by this *saṁyama* becomes transformed, that means simply by the thought of the *yogi*, that *buddhi sattva* and *puruṣa* are distinct. That is *dhāraṇā* and *dhyāna* on their distinctness. The transformation then generates a purified state of the *buddhi-sattva*, which can maintain the "knowledge of *puruṣa*."

Brain software (buddhi-sattva) always strives towards the light. Connected to it on the same level are the pair rajas and tamas. When they are mastered, when they are subdued, the brain software sattva becomes transformed by the thought of the yogi, that sattva and puruṣa are different. This sattva always changes, because it is a guṇa because it is nonpermanent because it exists for the purpose of another because it is not conscious. In its character it is absolutely opposite to puruṣa, who is pure, unchanging, existing for its own purpose, eternal, and by its nature, pure consciousness.

Experience is a thought that does not distinguish between buddhi-sattva and puruṣa, although they are absolutely separate. This thought is perceived because puruṣa perceives all thoughts of the buddhi-sattva.

Buddhi-sattva's first purpose is to serve *puruṣa* by generating experiences. *Puruṣa*, however, by nature is pure consciousness and always exists for itself, for its own purpose. By applying *saṁyama* on this distinction, the knowledge of *puruṣa* appears. The knowledge of *puruṣa* is the seed of all knowledge that contains all possible knowledge in an unmanifest form.

- Puruṣa always notices the buddhi-sattva and stays untouched by it.
- Buddhi-sattva perceives puruṣa only as long, as the yogi applies the siddhi of distinction. Then, the buddhi-sattva mirrors puruṣa and becomes infused with the infinity of puruṣa. This infusion purifies the buddhi-sattva. The brain software adapts to its silent user.

Thus, liberation becomes stabilized.

The buddhi-sattva perceives puruṣa, as with a mirror, held in front of the face. The mirror corresponds to the buddhi-sattva, whereas the face corresponds to puruṣa. The mirror image in the mirror, changes with the form of the face. Additionally, it adapts to the mirror. A face, for example, mirrored in a sword, is seen as long, even though in reality it is not long.

Thus the *buddhi-sattva* brings that highest infinity of *puruṣa* into a mental image of infinity.

This image in the *buddhi-sattva* is the "knowledge of *puruṣa*."

- I, *puruṣa*, am the silent witness, and I always witness anything that my *buddhi-sattva* perceives.
- With the *siddhi* on the discrimination, my *buddhi-sattva* turns onto Me and shows a mirror image of Me.

- That mirror image is the "knowledge of Me," which the Vedic authorities call the "knowledge of *puruṣa*."
- I observe this version of my changeable *buddhi-sattva*, enlivened with the "knowledge of Me."
- *Buddhi-sattva* cleanses itself by this reflection of My infinite purity.
- My purified *buddhi-sattva* now recognizes ever more clearly my infinity.
- This infinite expansion happens suddenly.
- Call it liberation or enlightenment, if you like.

Practice

Perform this practice initially, ideally in a quiet place after deep meditation. Direct your attention to that, which is active in your brain, which is your brain software. Then direct your attention to your SELF that means to you, the silent user of the software, who, completely unmoved, notices everything happening in your brain, however, does not react to it in any way. The difference is completely obvious. The moment, this difference becomes clear to you, you already have established in your brain software, the knowledge about the user, the knowledge about the SELF. It can happen very fast.

Experiences

Experience 1

As soon as I fetch the knowledge of *puruṣa* and address it, *puruṣa* stays with me, no matter whether I do some work or have a walk. He is in me and also around me.

Experience 2

Starting from *buddhi-sattva*, I turn my attention additionally to *puruṣa* and stay with both. By doing that, both energy and bliss appear and grow ever stronger. *Puruṣa* is experienced as the "larger" space with enormous energy and bliss that contains in it the clarity and silence of the *buddhi-sattva*. That is then called the knowledge of *puruṣa*.

3.36

[Saṁyama] there, [on the knowledge of puruṣa] increases intuition, [then] hearing, feeling, seeing, tasting and knowledge of events.

ततः प्रातिभश्रावणवेदनादर्शास्वादवार्त्ता जायन्ते

tataḥ prātibha-śrāvaṇa-Vedana-ādarśa-āsvāda-vārttā jāyante

tataḥ (ind.: there, in that place) prātibha (n. comp.: intuition) śrāvaṇa (mfn., n. comp.: audible, knowledge derived from hearing) Vedana (n. comp.: feeling, sensation) ādarśa (m. comp.: seeing, beholding) āsvāda (m. comp.: taste, tasting) vārttā (f. nom. s.: event, news) jāyante (born, produced, generated; verb: jan)

The "knowledge of *puruṣa*" was the result of the previous *sūtra* and now is the starting point for a new *saṁyama*. This second *saṁyama* on the "knowledge of *puruṣa*," means, practicing on the result of the previous *sūtra*, leads to perfect intuition (*prātibha*). Now, that we have attained the knowledge of *puruṣa*, we can consider it a new place, and, therefore, apply *saṁyama* on this place.

That is the perfection of intuition from communication with the perfect beings in 3.33. With this perfect intuition (*prātibha*), knowledge increases of that, which is subtle, hidden, remote, past, or possible in the future. It is also an improved version of the app of inner light in 3.25 because the app 3.36 is no longer bound only to visual perception.

Practices in steps

First step

Dhāraṇā and *dhyāna* on the heart (3.34) cause the perception of the main component of the brain software, the *buddhi-sattva* that is embedded in *samādhi*.

Second step

Dhāraṇā and *dhyāna* on the difference between the active *buddhi* and the silent *puruṣa* (3.35) create a state of all-knowingness. This state is the knowledge of *puruṣa*, embedded in *samādhi*.

Third step

Dhāraṇā and *dhyāna* on the knowledge of *puruṣa* generate the intuition, to know everything, embedded in *samādhi* (3.36).

Fourth step

In this *samādhi*, colored with the intuition, the attention is gently directed towards the senses or events. This leads to divine sensory perceptions or the knowledge of events (3.36).

Results of intuition

With gentle attention (sampadyate) on:

Hearing	→	*the hearing of divine sounds.*
Touch	→	*the touch of perfect beings and others.*
Sight	→	*the seeing of divine forms.*
Taste	→	*the tasting of divine savors.*
Events	→	*the knowledge of the things of the world.*

> *From this, the yogi discovers the truth about worldly things, as they are.*

3.37

Those [intuition, etc. of sūtra 3.36, while] overshadowing [nirvicāra] in samādhi [appear as] perfections in the excited [brain software].

ते समाधावुपसर्गा व्युत्थाने सिद्धयः

te samādhau upasargāḥ vyutthāne siddhayaḥ

tad (m. nom. p.: those two, that) samādhi (m. loc. s.: restful alertness, absolute silence) upasarga (m. Nom. s.: misfortune, bad omen, problem, eclipse of sun or moon) vyutthāna (n. nom. acc. d., loc. s.: activation, resulting, arising, deviate from the right course) siddhi (f. nom. p.: success, perfection, effectiveness, unusual ability)

The intuition and refined sensory perception of *sūtra* 3.36, overshadow *nirvicāra samādhi*, containing the knowledge of *puruṣa* from 3.35.

Any fears, whatsoever that *siddhis* could distract from liberation, possibly stem from a superficial consideration of the *yoga sūtras*. Here, no dualistic worldview is suggested, the way, so many other translators claim. It is not explaining, how to exchange the perfection of the *siddhis* with final liberation (*kaivalya*). It rather, from the point of view of perfect unity, which we already have established in *sūtra* 2.26, describes a continuous process, how perfection comes to the world of the *yogi*.

One may compare *puruṣa* knowledge, the most abstract excitation state of *samādhi*, namely *nirvicāra samādhi*, with a white, bright, radiant lamp. To take a concrete result out of this complete abstraction, *saṁyama* in 3.36 is applied twice more (see steps 3 and 4). This is like putting a color filter in front of the brightly beaming lamp. Thereby, the white light gets covered, and the desired colored light emanates.

This colored light corresponds to perfection appearing in the brain software; the various colors correspond to the various sensory channels. Thus, gradually, the infinite *prajñā* knowledge of *nirvicāra samādhi* becomes covered and brought into the range of the *guṇas*, where in turn, it can be recognized. Now it appears as perfection on the subtlest level of the *guṇas*, the heavenly level of *savicāra samādhi*, in the form of divine perceptions. It can then manifest further in *nirvitarka samādhi* (for example as abstract pictures), or even as human speech on the level of *savitarka samādhi*. On all these excited levels of *samādhi*, the *siddhi* results appear as perfect expressions.

Here, we are not talking about the overshadowing of *nirbīja samādhi*, pure consciousness, but rather about the overshadowing of the purest state of knowledge in *nirvicāra samādhi*. Once, pure consciousness is established, beginning from brain software version 5, it can no longer become overshadowed. What becomes overshadowed here, is the knowledge of *puruṣa*. This happens with the brain software, starting from the knowledge of *puruṣa* – therefore, in a perfect way – turns again towards the world in 3.36. Thus, the abstract knowledge of *puruṣa* becomes overshadowed again.

All interpretations of this *sūtra*, such as, that a *yogi* should give up the *siddhis*, after having reached them, are simply foolish. The belief that *siddhis* could prevent the final liberation, *kaivalya*, probably arose from a superficial consideration of this *sūtra* 3.37. If *siddhis* opposed the actual goal of *yoga*, *Patañjali* possibly would have mentioned them in one verse, but definitely would not have spent the whole chapter 3 on that topic. Also, *Śaṁkara* in his introductory comment in *sūtra* 1.1 would not have called chapter 3, containing all the *siddhi* practices, the description of the healthy state. It is very clear that the practice and achievement of *siddhis* describe the healthy state of a *yogi*.

Our precise analysis of this *sūtra* came from *Śaṁkara's* commentary. He talks not about the overshadowing of *samādhi*, but rather only the overshadowing of the sight of *puruṣa*. The sight of *puruṣa* corresponds to the knowledge of *puruṣa* of 3.35:

Intuition etc. [3.36], which appear in the samādhi state of puruṣa in the brain software [3.35], overshadow the sight of puruṣa [puruṣa jñānam 3.35]. From this opposition arises perfection [3.36] in the strongly excited brain software. Although it arises from the saṁyama of puruṣa [3.35], serenity in the samādhi of the brain software does not prevail.

That means the *yogi* does not continue to sit in *asaṁprajñāta samādhi* (brain software version 4), but rather gives expression (brain software versions 6, 7, 8) to his perfect intuition and heavenly experiences.

3.38

By [saṁyama on] the loosening of the cause of bondage, and knowing the playground [of another body and its environment], the brain software can remotely control other bodies.

बन्धकारणशैथिल्यात् प्रचारसंवेदनाच्च चित्तस्य परशरीरावेशः

bandha-kāraṇa-śaithilyāt pracāra-saṁVedanāt ca cittasya para-śarīra-āveśaḥ

bandha (m. comp.: binding) kāraṇa (n. comp.: cause, reason, motive) śaithilya (n. abl. s.: loosening, looseness, non-attentiveness) pracāra (m. comp.: playground, wandering, roaming, appearing, prevailing) saṁVedana (n. abl. s.: perceiving) ca (ind.: and, also) citta (n. gen. s.: brain software) para (mf(ā)n. comp.: other) śarīra (m. comp.: body) āveśa (m. nom. s.: entering, occupying)

The sleeping *karma* (non-activated *saṁskāras*) binds the brain software, especially the input-output component (*manas*) to the body. Loosening the *karma* binding comes from the power of *samādhi* that means the brain software goes into a *samādhi* state and switches off its own individual likes and dislikes. Then the attention goes into the other body. Enthusiasm or disgust for certain things or events are individually different and are switched off in *samādhi*. Also, the attention on the new playground starts only from *samādhi*. It is important, for example when experiencing this *siddhi* in an animal's body, not to transfer any human thinking patterns!

The brain software, in reality, is not preassigned. It is continuously excited, like a bell, that has been rung, or like the flickering glow of a mass of burning charcoal. The point is, that the brain software by the bindings of the store of karma, is kept in the body, has settled in one body as its home. Karma is the cause of this binding. The loosening of this cause, the loosening of the store of karma, originates only from samādhi. By thinning out the binding of karma and by attention on how his own brain software moves, the yogi moves out of his body with the brain software and lets the brain software act in other bodies.

While his brain software flies out, the senses go with it, and it is by the actions of the senses and organs of action in other bodies, that the functions, like for example the live streams (prāṇas) appear at that new place. Just as bees following their queen settle, where she settles.

Similarly, the senses and the *prāṇas* of the brain software settle down in another body and use the organs of sense and action of the other body. The original body must remain in a silent position in *samādhi*.

Practice

The practice of this app is easiest with animals, where you cannot go far wrong. Occasionally look with the eyes of a bird, or chew the grass, while you are in a cow. It is always important, to switch off your individuality before transferring to the animal because the corresponding animal could not endure your individuality.

Then, in *samādhi*, become fully immersed in the situation of this animal. You can then have the sensory experience of the animal, or even let it act the way, that you would like. Do not overload the poor animal, for it has a very simple sight and way of acting. You have to adapt to that before. Otherwise, it will not work.

Experience

Experience 1

I heard a bird singing in my garden. It sat on a tree, which I could not see. However, I was interested anyway, what bird this was. I am continuously in *samādhi* so that it did not take any great effort, to switch off my ego completely, for a moment, and, while listening to the bird, completely to slip into its individuality. Suddenly I noticed, how my feet were clenching a twig. Previously, as a human individual, I was not quite aware of that. Somehow the bird always had to cling to a tree. And then, there followed this call, full-throated, with intensive fervor and joy of life. A beautiful experience!

Experience 2

Did you ever wonder, why red Indians so often had extraordinary names, like Great Bear, Great Eagle, Black Falcon, Little Wolf? That was because they have been able to use the app 3.38 to slip into the bodies of those animals and to use their sensory and organs of action in a meaningful way. The same applies to talented shamans.

3.39

By mastering [saṁyama] the upward moving live stream [udāna] [the yogi walks] untouched on water, swamps, thorns, etc., and when dying, takes the upward path.

उदानजयाज्जलपङ्ककण्टकादिष्वसङ्ग उत्क्रान्तिश्च

udāna-jayāt jala-paṅka-kaṇṭakā-ādiṣu asaṅga utkrāntiḥ ca

udāna (m. comp.: upward rising prāṇa) jaya (m. abl. s.: mastery, conquer) jala (n. comp.: water) paṅka (mn. comp.: swamp) kaṇṭaka (n. comp.: thorn) ādi (m. loc. p.: and the others etc.) asaṅga (m. Nom. s.: non-touching, without contact) utkrānti (f. nom. s.: rising, leaving, dying) ca (ind.: and, also)

Udāna is a live stream in the body that starts from the feet and goes up to the top of the head. This technique is a pre-stage of flying.

Life is the action of the totality of the eleven indriyas (here: sense organs, organs of action, input-output component), the prāṇas, etc. Like a pigeon loft shakes with the movement of the birds in it, similar, the body without fail is supported by the united, amplified action of all indriyas, and that is life. In this life, that is controlled by duty, to fulfill the purposes of puruṣa, the action is divided fivefold: prāṇa (forward going stream), apāna (downgoing), vyāna (all-permeating), udāna (ascending) and samāna (balancing).

Among them, prāṇa has its range, going from the heart to the mouth and nose. The samāna live stream is called that because of smooth (sāma) leading (āna), and its range goes to the navel. It functions as far as the navel region. Apāna is called that because it leads (āna) the urine and feces, etc., down (āpa) and its range is from the navel down to the soles of the feet. Udāna is called that because it leads upwards (ūrdhvam) in the body and its range is from the sole of the feet up to the top of the head.

The leader of them is prāṇa. By mastering it, mastery over the apāna and the others follows. A method of mastering all of them is mentioned in detail by Hiraṇyagarbha; however, as their mastery follows from the mastery of manas (input-output component), here we do not mention any separate method.

By mastering prāṇāyāma, all of them are conquered. Here, he [Patañjali], without dealing with the specific methods of the mastery of those live streams, simply presents the result of the conquering of udāna.

He (the yogi) goes untouched on water, swamps, thorns, etc. It also means, for example, the blade of a sword. When dying, he takes the upward path, which happens spontaneously.

Practice

Go with your attention from the tip of the feet, gradually flowing up to the upper part of the head and beyond that. While doing that, you notice a certain lightness in the whole body. This is, for example, a good exercise, when you are walking with your body up a mountain or an ascending slope. You will notice, that your body becomes much lighter and also, that this walking up becomes much easier. Therefore, this is an exercise, which you can do well while hiking or walking.

Experience

Experience 1

Udāna is my strongest *siddhi* experience. I have the experience, as soon as I move mentally from the tip of my toes, through the body up to the crown of my head. Then my feet lift from the heels to the toes, and I have to walk fast or begin dancing.

Experience 2

When I keep my attention on the whole area and range of the upward going breath, a warm, bright energy stream rises from the feet vertically up through the spine into the head and far beyond it. By attention on this whole area, there is a constant flow of energy.

3.40

By mastering [saṁyama] of the middle live stream, in the belly [samāna] there comes about a blazing light.

समानजयाज्ज्वलनम्

samāna-jayāt jvalanam

samāna (m. comp.: prāṇa for digestion) jaya (m. abl. s.: mastery, conquering) jvalana (n. nom. acc. s.: shining, radiating, fire, blazing light)

Samāna is one of the live streams in the body. It causes the movement of digestion in the belly area.

Saṁyama on *samāna* kindles the *agni* in the stomach and stimulates *udāna*, the upward going live stream.

Experience

By attention to this area in the belly, there originates warm, bright energy, which immediately wanders to the head and then to the whole body. From the body, it extends to the whole space of consciousness.

3.41

By saṁyama on the intimate connection between space (ākāśa) and hearing [arises] divine hearing.

श्रोत्राकाशयोः सम्बन्धसंयमाद्दिव्यं श्रोत्रम्

śrotra-ākāśayoḥ sambandha-saṁyamāt divyam śrotram

śrotra (n. comp.: ear, hearing) ākāśa (n. gen. loc. d.: space) sambandha (m. comp.: connection, binding together) saṁyama (m. abl. s.:) divya (n. nom. acc. s: finest, divine) śrotra (n. nom. acc. s: hearing)

Space gives scope to unmanifest sound. The sound is a quality of space. Space is not empty, but full of impulses of virtual fluctuations of sound. Those are the vacuum fluctuations, called quantum foam.

Space is the basis for all hearing and sound. Just as sound has the qualities of space, sound also has space as its basis. The relationship between hearing and sound is that nothing intervenes between the listener and the sound, on which the hearing is directed. It has been said: For all listeners who are at a similar place, the same is heard. Hearing is something, by which something is heard, and those who do this at the same place, are similarly placed listeners. For all of them, that which is heard is the same. It is in connection with an existing thing (space), which gives it (the sound) the possibility, of spreading out, and that, by nature, is free of obstacles. This actual fact is the quality of space. With things with a form, for example, like in the case of a jar, it is observed, that they have an opposite quality because they are obstructions. And if there is no obstruction, as in the case of a jewel, a diamond for instance, then space is transparent, which clarifies the all-permeating quality of space.

Hearing, and also space is explored, to become acquainted with the two *dhāraṇā* items of the next *sūtra*. This app, therefore, is essential to learn flying with the body of a *yogi*. The *yogi* first needs to obtain that intimacy with *ākāśa*, space, to establish the connection between space and his body by the use of the next *sūtra*. We are not sure, whether this app is sufficient to explore space completely. Maybe, a few more physics lessons are required. Space is not really empty. It is full of vacuum fluctuations with fantastic energy values. It is self-referral, can bend, can interchange with the time dimension according to certain rules. The *yogi* should know all this when he wants to go on his intended path, freely through space.

3.42

By saṁyama on the intimate connection between the body (kāya) and space (ākāśa), and attention (samāpatti) on the lightness of cotton fiber, space goes.

कायाकाशयोः संबन्धसंयमाल्लघुतूलसमापत्तेश्चाकाशगमनम्

kāya-ākāśayoḥ saṁbandha-saṁyamāt laghu-tūla-samāpatteḥ ca ākāśa-gamanam

kāya (m. comp.: body) ākāśa (n. gen. loc. d.: space) saṁbandha (m. comp.: close, intimate connection, binding together) saṁyama (m. abl. s.:) laghu (mfn. comp.: light, fast) tūla (n. comp.: cotton) samāpatti (f. acc. gen. s.: attention, coming together, meeting) ca (ind.: and, also) ākāśa (n. comp.: space) gamana (n. nom. acc. s.: to move, going, going away)

> *Vyāsa* comments: *„Wherever there is the body, there is space, because space gives scope to the body."*

Space and body are intimately related because space provides a region where the body can exist. It is not about the cosmic space outside the body;

rather it is in regard to the space as being at every place in the body, the space of every cell of the body, every atom, every quark, and every electron!

By saṁyama on the intimate relationship between body and space and attention on the lightness of things, like cotton fiber, firefly, air, etc., as minute as the electron, the yogi becomes weightless.

From there, the yogi first gains the ability, to walk with his feet on water, then on spiders' webs, then on rays of light and the wind. Afterwards, he goes on any arbitrarily selected path through space that means he thinks of his path in the universe, which he then walks.

The result of this *sūtra* is described by the composite *ākāśa-gamanam*, which can be translated grammatically correctly in several ways. *Ākāśa* means space and *gamanam* means going. We are aware, that other translators have described the result as "going in space." However, we prefer to translate the composite as "the going of space" because with the other translation of "going in space," the intimate connection (*saṁbandha*) between body and space is not established. In that case, the body is considered as something separate from space because it goes as one thing through another thing. We prefer the translation "space goes" because this places the body on the same level as space and, therefore, expresses that, as a result of this *saṁyama*, the intimate connection between body and space is established: When the body goes, the space goes.

How intimate is this connection between the body of the *yogi* and space? It is very intimate, nearly orgasmic. The word *saṁbandha* also has the meaning of a sexual union. The sound sequence at the beginning of the *sūtra* gives another hint. It is "*kāyāk*," and therefore completely symmetric around the "*y*," which is a semivowel, consisting of the two vowels "*i*" and "*a*." This symmetry comes about only by the intimate connection of body and space.

The *yogi* should know two places to enable a successful application of this app. The first place is his body, *kāya*. How does the *yogi* gain knowledge of his body? That, of course, happens by the complete interior view of the body with attention on the navel using the app 3.29. From there, originates the knowledge of all structures in the body, the energy flows, the various breaths flows, etc. This knowledge can readily become as fine as the atomic and subatomic levels. In other words, all the elementary particles of the body, contributing to its mass, can be explored with this app.

The second place, the *yogi* ready for flight, should know, is the space, *ākāśa*. It means not only the empty space of the outer universe. It rather is the all-permeating space. All atoms consist mainly of this space. Exploration of space is simplest using the previous app 3.41. Do you still remember *sūtra* 3.6? There it was stated, that the practice of *saṁyama* should happen in stages. Here again, there is a useful sequence. First, explore space, and then only the flying which is space technology.

Then the massless space becomes connected to the massive body, and a parameter becomes newly adjusted. A specific, new value should come about for the parameter of lightness.

Some more relevant physics

The mass of matter essentially comes about by the nuclear building blocks, the protons, and neutrons in the atomic nucleus. The electrons in the clouds around the atomic nucleus, on the other hand, contribute only about 0.025% of the total mass of the atom.

Now, the nuclear building blocks consist of quarks. There is a baffling phenomenon! The nuclear building blocks each consist of three quarks. The proton consists of two u-quarks and one d-quark. The neutron consists of one u-quark and two d-quarks. So far, so good. Now there is a surprise, upon weighing them. The proton weighs 938 MeV/c^2; the neutron weighs 939 MeV/c^2. These are units of mass, expressed, by a convention of nuclear physics, in energy units. The quarks, however, weigh far less, namely 2.3 MeV/c^2 for the u-quark, and 4.8 MeV/c^2 for the d-quark. Adding the three components for the proton, one arrives at 2*u + 1*d which is 2*2.3 + 1*4.8 = 9.4 MeV/c^2. That is pretty much 1% of the measured mass of the proton. For the neutron it is not much different: 1*d + 2*u = 1*2.3 + 2*4.8 = 11.9 MeV/c^2. That is about 1.2% of the measured mass of the neutron. The contribution of the electrons of about 0.025% here can be neglected.

What does this value of about 1% mean? It means that only 1% of the mass of the human body or any other heavy thing comes about by adding up its components. About 99% of the mass must be attributed to something else. It has not yet been fully researched. There are some conjectures, that, for example, the binding energy contributed by the gluons is so high, that it appears like mass. The gluons themselves have no resting mass. However, they have a moving mass which is simply their energy transformed into mass. That is the binding energy of the strong nuclear interaction in the neutrons and protons of the atomic nucleus.

Applied to yogic levitation, this means, that to neutralize the mass of the human body, which is the generation of a gravitation-less area in space, one must aim at the binding energy in the building blocks of the atomic nucleus.

Who would then be surprised, that the app for flying contains the concept of a relationship? It is about the relationship between the mass of the body and space. In that way, the binding energy in the atomic nuclear components could be influenced. If this binding energy could be reduced to zero, a loss of 99% of mass could be explained. The 99% mainly comes about by the binding energy of the strong interaction. However, for the remaining 1% of mass, there would need to be other explanation models, like for example the modification of the Higgs field, which has the famous Higgs boson as its excited state. Funnily enough, the so-called Higgs mechanism refers only to this remaining 1% of mass, whereas it ignores the mass contribution of 99%, the far more influential binding energy. Does nobody notice, that a heavy elephant is standing in the living room?

A model for neutralizing the remaining mass could be, that the quarks also could be built up with a similar binding scheme, and the rest mass could be covered by that. Quite often, in nature, similar phenomena repeat on all levels.

The viewpoint of the cosmic software

Here it is all very simple. All strings and the elementary particles derived from them, like electrons and quarks, are nothing but partial aspects of the cosmic software. If this software was modified even minimally, which is no problem at all with software, the influence of these elementary particles on space could be minimized. This space is also nothing but software. It is only a question of providing the right cosmic communication interfaces between the elementary particles and space. Here, again the connection is an essential concept. This time a communication connection. As soon as the massive elementary particles no longer modify the space in a well-known way, according to general relativity theory, there would be no more gravitational field. The mass would be gone; the *yogi* could levitate without any weight.

That is, so far, our present thinking on the topic. However, as we ourselves cannot fly yet, the practical proof of this theoretical approach is still missing.

Practices

Practice 1

With your yogic levitation practices, you should take great care, to be well rested. When snoozing or half asleep, it is unlikely, that your body will begin to float. Also make sure, after flying practices, to allow sufficient body rest, simply by laying down for a while.

Practice 2

Do your flying practices with the attitude, that weightless levitation is possible. To make this intellectually understandable, we have extensively explained all the physics of this phenomenon. As long as the intellect cannot yet grasp it, or does not want to, it will try to prevent it.

There has been a rumor about an experiment with Russian cosmonauts in training, where the cosmonauts were still on Earth, were hypnotized, and were utterly convinced, that they were already in outer space. The rumor is, that they spontaneously levitated above their seats because they were completely convinced, they were weightless. If this information was correct, that would show once more, how important the attitude is, to achieve levitation.

Practice 3

In a preliminary stage of flying, the hopping, it is best to provide proper, soft supports, such as foam mattresses.

Practice 4

This *sūtra* 3.42 may easily be confused with *sūtra* 3.39, mastering the ascending breath, *udāna*. If someone simply has attention on this upward rising breath, it generates a certain lightness. That is a technique, to walk above water, swamps, etc. It is somewhat more arduous than 3.42. However, it is quite a good preparation. It can also simply be practiced while walking.

Practice 5

To avoid the mix-up with the *udāna* technique, the *yogi* should first consciously establish the relationship between the body and space. Most *yogis* do not yet know the space intuitively and therefore should practice 3.41. Once the connection is established, it is also important, not to forget to readjust the lightness parameter. *Śaṁkara* in his commentary tells us that we do not need to stay with the lightness of cotton fiber. You all know these tiny dust particles made of fibers that float in the air. Following the first stage of cotton fiber, we can also assume the lightness of fireflies that fly upwards or even the lightness of electrons.

Practice 6

Here again, as with all the *siddhis,* the words of the *sūtra* produce little effect. It is only the attention on the body, space and their connection that works. These are the places for the *dhāraṇā*. There, are located the light switches, to activate the *siddhi*. The term attention, *samāpatti,* has been defined in 1.41. Now, it appears again in this *sūtra*. When the connection between body and space is established, the attention is very gently directed to the new lightness of cotton fiber, etc.

Practice 7

Allow yourself a big favor during your levitation practices. Do not consider it to be muscle sports. In this way, in the lotus position, you would ruin your knee joints by overexertion, something, that some of our sporting friends have already managed.

Experience

With this practice, my consciousness expands into all of space. The bliss originating from that surpasses even an orgasmic bliss multifold and often continues for more than an hour. It has reminded me of the statement in the *Madhusūdana-Purāṇa* (2.42).

3.43

The "great bodiless" is a mental process (vṛtti) outside of the body and not [merely] imagined. From this, the covering of the light diminishes.

बहिरकल्पिता वृत्तिर्महाविदेहा ततः प्रकाशावरणक्षयः

bahiḥ-akalpitā vṛttiḥ mahā-videhā tataḥ prakāśa-āvaraṇa-kṣayaḥ

bahiḥ (ind.: outside, out there) akalpita (mfn. s.: not artificial, natural, not a joke) vṛtti (f. nom. s.: thought process) mahā (f. nom. s.: big, great) videha (f. nom. s.: bodiless) tataḥ (ind.: through that, resulting from that) prakāśa (m. comp.: light, brightness, radiating) āvaraṇa (n. comp.: cover, veil) kṣaya (m. nom. s.: reduction, decreasing, diminution)

This app builds on its earlier stage in 3.38. Now, the brain software is not only momentarily transferred to another brain but rather uploaded to the universe-computer. There it is completely free of limitations and can have all sensory perceptions and even actions by the organs of action, directly from the universe-computer. The individuality of the *yogi* remains, and he can perceive and act from any place in the universe.

It is a process of the brain software outside the body. It is generated by resting on a certain thing at another place, purely by will, by the power of the samādhi and the binding (dhāraṇā) of the attention, and it is called the great bodiless.

When the yogi achieves, that he is in an external thing, merely as a process of the brain software, which stays completely located in the body, then this process is called imagined, because it is created by a certain intention (saṁkalpa) of the brain software that stays located in the body. If, however, resulting from the power of samādhi, the cause of the bodily bondage is loosened, then this is the outer process of the brain software, which, having become external, is no longer connected to the body. This one is called "not imagined."

With the imagined, the yogi who has achieved the external mental process still stays limited to the body. With the non-imagined, his experience is not limited by the limitations of the bodily basis anymore. Both are called bodiless, insofar as in both of them, the thought of "external" is there. However, the process, which is not imagined, is called the great bodiless. By practicing the imagined process, the yogis practice the non-imagined, the great bodiless. By the continued practice of dhyāna on the imagined process, the yogi finally achieves the non-imagined process.

Using the great bodiless, yogis enter other bodies. By the binding (dhāraṇā) to the great bodiless the covering of the brain software sattva, whose nature is light, becomes thinned out. This covering is the triad of illusions and karmas and their fruits. They are rooted in rajas and tamas.

Experiences

Experience 1

A dear friend of mine wanted to move into my house for a while but first had to make a long journey from another country. To ease travel for her that went on until late into the night, I continued doing chats with her, to stay in contact. At some point, she moved into a hotel room, that she had selected spontaneously when she was too tired to carry on driving. She enjoyed my close attention, and we were in a playful, easy-going mood. I told her that I could nearly see her new room. She wanted to know what I saw in a bit more detail. Therefore, to test me, she asked me, to describe the interior of the hotel room. For me, this was then, as if I had visited her at that place. I could look around and discover details, like for example the rococo style of the room, the candleholder lamps on the walls, and the form of the armchair, the table, and the bed. She was completely amazed by my description and immediately sent me some photos, which confirmed the correctness of my vision.

Experience 2

The unexpected passing of my Indian wife due to her *prārabdha karma*, gave me a reason, to experiment with mental healing I simply wanted to understand, how diseases originate, where their information is stored and how to mentally neutralize them. My highly revered teacher *Śri Śri Bharati Tirtha Mahaswamiji* from *Śringeri* had demonstrated to me years before that this was possible. I knew that he could heal and asked him, to teach me the technique. At that time, I had acute pains in a knee. He answered that he would heal the knee. The pain really diminished. So, four weeks later when he asked me whether it had improved, I was able to affirm it. Then, however, surprisingly the pains came back. Aha, I thought, this was just a demonstration, and I should try it myself, which I then did successfully.

When I am directing my attention to a disease or an indisposition ("disturbance") in another person or myself, I often perceive in my inner perception corresponding pictures or a "movie" about the disease and also the healing process. This perception comes so spontaneously that my intellect has no time to interfere. For example with a stomach inflammation I "see" in this area a red stain. Then, when I keep my attention for a longer time on the inner area and simultaneously activate certain *devas*, the color of the abnormal area changes from red to white, and the person reports an improvement. I have tested this with several persons. The "mental body" provides an interface, in this case, a red stain or spot, by which one can influence bodily disturbances.

During my apprenticeship with a shaman, I treated a man, who had been in pain for decades with a bad migraine and had been taking strong medication. I treated him both in my home and at a distance. When I directed my attention to him, dragon-like and snake-like beings appeared as inner pictures or movies, which did not give a friendly impression. With the help of the *devas,* I removed them, which regularly turned out like a "fight" in my inner perception, and afterward the person felt better. These "beings" are to be understood as negative intelligent energies, which interfere with our physiology. In the commentaries of the *yoga sūtras,* they have been described as "*bhūtas*" (intelligent beings). The acquaintance later told me that his migraine had disappeared. However, I had an intensive migraine for three days, which I finally neutralized with my meditation.

3.44

By saṁyama on their physical form, their essential nature, their subtle form, their inheritance and their purposefulness, the [five] elements are controlled.

स्थूलस्वरूपसूक्ष्मान्वयार्थवत्त्वसंयमाद्भूतजयः

sthūla-svarūpa-sūkṣma-anvaya-arthavattva-saṁyamāt bhūta-jayaḥ

sthūla (mf(ā)n. comp.: gross) svarūpa (n. comp.: own form) sūkṣma (mf(ā)n. comp.: fine, subtle) anvaya (m. comp.: sequence, connection, effect, meaning, content) arthavat-tva (n. comp.: meaningfulness, importance) saṁyama (m. abl. s.:) bhūta (n. comp.: gross elements) jaya (m. nom. s.: mastery, control)

This *siddhi* is to be practiced in sequential stages, without going into *nirbīja samādhi* in between and *nirbīja samādhi* then comes in the end. The five elements are earth, water, fire, air, space, which correspond approximately to the five states of matter.

Experiences

Experience 1

At the end of the night, mostly during an extended wake-up phase, I saw more and more visions, which were related to the future or the past. Many of my future visions were only a preview of the coming day that would then happen similarly. Others were somewhat more extended previews. These extended future visions I could also often verify, like for example, in my vision of the "Lord of the Oceans." This one appears in various cultures under various names, like for example as *Varuṇa*, as Poseidon or as Neptune.

The vision came completely unexpected, and I saw the Lord of the Oceans in a kind of carriage, that was drawn by aquatic animals. He was accompanied by a huge crowd of various aquatic beings. There were groups of dolphins, schools of most varied fish, crawling animals on the seafloor, a colorful and dynamic diversity of life underwater. All oriented themselves towards the Lord of the Oceans and swam in synchrony with him. The whole vision was shown to me by his wife, and she told me, "Look, he is angry!" I saw how he was steering his open coach along the path of a moon-like half-circle. With this, a gigantic wave arose, that brought the whole ocean into turmoil. It was very impressive, and no Hollywood movie could have shown it any better.

After waking up, the meaning of the half Moon became clear. It was a symbol for a period of about two weeks. He wanted to tell me, that in two weeks something was going to happen with the ocean.

I had this vision around the 12th December 2004, and actually something did happen about two weeks later, on the 26th December 2004. A gigantic seaquake with strength 9.3 shook the Indian Ocean off Sumatra and caused the strongest tsunami in modern times, where 230,000 people died. The Lord of the Oceans was hopping mad, and I think, that he wanted to tell me, that he simply did not want to endure the continued exploitation of the oceans, the pollution, the deep sea fishing, and the extinction of so many kinds of aquatic animals any longer.

Experience 2

I had a spontaneous *siddhi* experience in a meeting, where healing techniques were being taught. A young woman wanted to "warm up" the participants, by teaching them, how to bend a teaspoon with the mind. I felt challenged and spontaneously imitated it while asking *Gaṇeṣa* for his help. No force is required to bend it; it is rather a kind of "feeling into" the process: the teaspoon in my hands became as soft as wax. I found this impressive and repeated it at home with a tablespoon: not only did I bend it, but twisted this, while the tablespoon again became soft as wax. Inspired by it, I wanted to try it with another tablespoon. Then, surprisingly I heard a loud inner voice: "Stop this nonsense." That was it, then. A friend could, with a lot of force, only partially remove the bend, but not the twist because it was impossible to hold the spoon in that position. I kept the spoon as a trophy.

3.45

From that [mastery of the elements, eight abilities] arise [for example] becoming small, etc., and the perfection of the body, its tasks, and its protection.

ततोऽणिमादिप्रादुर्भावः कायसंपत् तद्धर्मानभिघातश्च

tataḥ aṇima-ādi-prādurbhāvaḥ kāya-saṁpat tat-dharma-anabhighātaḥ ca

tataḥ (ind.: by that, from that) aṇiman (m. comp.: minute, small as an atom, thinness, subtlety) ādi (m. etc.) prādurbhāvaḥ (m. nom. s.: appearance, manifestation, becoming visible) kāya (m. comp.: body) saṁpad (f. comp.: perfection, excellence) tad (n. comp.: that) dharma (n. acc. p.: virtue, task) abhighāta (m. nom. s.: non-obstruction) ca (ind.: and, also)

The eight abilities are:

- becoming small as an atom
- becoming light in weight
- becoming large
- bridging distances, for example, touch the Moon
- having an irresistible will, for example, to go through a rock
- mastery over all worlds
- gaining sovereignty
- gaining omnipotence

Since the yogi is without any impurities, he will not cause a change in the nature of things, because his manners are impeccable.

3.46

A perfect body has a beautiful form, [insurmountable] strength and the hardness of a diamond.

रूपलावण्यबलवज्रसंहननत्वानि कायसम्पत्

rūpa-lāvaṇya-bala-vajra-saṁhananatvāni kāya-sampat

rūpa (n. comp.: shape, form) lāvaṇya (n. comp.: beauty, charm) bala (n. comp.: power, strength) vajra (m. comp.: diamond, thunderbolt, hard) saṁhanana-tva (n. nom. acc. p.: hardness, solidity; -ness) kāya (m. comp.: body) sampad (f. nom. s.: perfection, excellence)

Three more results from 3.44.

3.47

By saṁyama on the [process of] perception [of the senses], their essential nature, their limited "I"-consciousness, their inheritance and their purposefulness, the senses are controlled.

ग्रहणस्वरूपास्मितान्वयार्थवत्त्वसंयमाद् इन्द्रियजयः

grahaṇa-svarūpa-asmitā-anvaya-arthavattva-saṁyamāt indriya-jayaḥ

grahaṇa (n. comp.: perception) svarūpa (n. comp.: own form, essential nature (quality)) asmitā (f. comp.: limited i-consciousness, identity) anvaya (m. comp.: sequence, connection, effect, meaning, content, inheritance) arthavat-tva (n. comp.:

purposefulness, meaningfulness, importance) saṁyama (m. abl. s.:) indriya (n. comp.: sense and action organs) jaya (m. nom. s.: mastery, control)

In 2.55, the control of the senses was first mentioned as a result of the practice of *pratyāhāra*, and now here it becomes perfect. This *siddhi* also, as in 3.44, must be practiced sequentially in the prescribed stages, without going in into *nirbīja samādhi* between stages. The *nirbīja samādhi* comes at the very end.

3.48

From that [mastery of the senses] and by mastering [saṁyama on] pradhāna, arise [the abilities to travel] with the speed of thought, to exist without bodily organs, and to control nature.

ततो मनोजवित्वं विकरणभावः प्रधानजयश्च

tataḥ manojavitvam vikaraṇa-bhāvaḥ pradhāna-jayaḥ ca

tataḥ (ind.: by that, from that) manojavitva (n. nom. acc. s.: speed of the mind; manojavin = swift as a thought) vikaraṇa (n. comp.: without sense or action organs) bhāva (m. nom. s.: existence, appearing, becoming, art of acting) pradhāna (n. comp.:) jaya (m. nom. s.: mastery, control) ca (ind.: and, also)

Pradhāna, the ground state of the *guṇas* will be explained in more details in 4.2. Controlling the eightfold *prakṛti* comes from *saṁyama* on its ground state (*pradhāna*), also traveling with the speed of thought, and existence without a body.

Existence without body means that the brain software of the *yogi* is completely uploaded to the universe-computer and continues to function perfectly there. In the universe-computer, then there are no longer any spatial or temporal restrictions for the *yogi*.

3.49

By the complete cognition that buddhi-sattva and puruṣa are distinct, [the yogi] has power over all that exists and omniscience.

सत्त्वपुरुषान्यताख्यातिमात्रस्य सर्वभावाधिष्ठातृत्वं सर्वज्ञातृत्वं च

sattva-puruṣa-anyatā-khyāti-mātrasya sarva-bhāva-adhiṣṭhātṛtvam sarva-jñātṛtvam ca

sattva (n. comp.: purity, clarity) puruṣa (m. comp.: silent SELF) anyatā (f. comp., f. nom. s.: distinction, difference, discrimination) khyāti (f. comp.. perception, knowledge, cognition) mātra (n. gen. s.: complete, only, total, whole, measure, distance) sarvabhāva (m. comp.: all objects, existence, appearance) adhiṣṭhātṛ-tva (m. acc. s., n. nom. acc. s.: ruler, rule, govern) sarvajñātṛtva (n. nom. acc. s.: omniscience) ca (ind.: and, also)

Living in the universe-computer, the eternal individuality of the *yogi* can know everything in the universe and produce any effect. In this way, from ancient times, Masters have ascended to become omnipotent beings. Why are they not disturbing everything?

Since the *yogi* is without impurities, he does not cause a reversal in the nature of things because his behavior is extremely impeccable.

These *yogis* have become the software functions of the all-comprehensive universe-computer, *Īśvara*, and govern, together with him, the whole universe. In this context, see also the description of the various beings in the universe in 3.26.

3.50

When, from serenity towards even those [omnipotence and omniscience] the seeds of impurities are destroyed, liberation (kaivalya) [remains].

तद्वैराग्यादपि दोषबीजक्षये कैवल्यम्

tat-vairāgyāt api doṣa-bīja-kṣaye kaivalyam

tad (n. comp.: that) vairāgya (n. abl. s.: serenity, equanimity) api (ind.: also, even) doṣa (m. comp.: impurity, shortcoming, fault) bīja (n. comp.: seed, sprout) kṣaya (m. loc. s.: reducing, cancelling, destroying) kaivalya (n. nom. acc. s.: unity consciousness)

The individual desires are no longer required, although by omniscience anything could be achieved.

3.51

[In the case of] invitations by the rulers of heavenly realms, one should neither get involved with them nor show pride [smiling] because, from that, unwanted results would again follow.

स्थान्युपनिमन्त्रणे सङ्गस्मयाकरणं पुनरनिष्टप्रसङ्गात्

sthāni-upanimantraṇe saṅga-smaya-akaraṇam punaḥ-aniṣṭa-prasaṅgāt

sthānin (n. nom. acc. s.: heavenly) upanimantraṇa (n. loc. s.: invitation) saṅga (m. comp.: meeting, getting involved, contact with, craving, desire) smaya (m. comp.:

feeling honoured, smiling, pride, curiosity, arrogance) akaraṇa (n. nom. acc. s.: non doing) punar (ind.: again, repeatedly) aniṣṭa (n. comp.: wicked, disadvantage, bad) prasaṅga (m. abl. s.: adhere, possibility, meeting, connection)

The realms are divine regions, like for example the heaven, and their rulers are gods, like Indra. Such invitations by them, are for example, "Noble Sir, I request you, to take your place here, etc." In such situations, the yogi should remember and understand the essential poverty of individual ego. And he should react neither with attachment nor pride. Any reaction with attachment or pride would create unwanted consequences.

There are four groups of yogis

- the beginner (*prathama-kalpika*)
- in the honey state (*madhu-bhūmika*)
- with the light of knowledge (prajñā-jyotiṣ)
- one, who has transcended all that he has practiced (*ati-krānta-bhavanīya*)

Description of the four groups

1. *One, who has kindled the light of the extrasensory perception of a divine item, has activated one of the viṣayavatī functions, directed to a sensory item, like for example the radiant inner light (jyotiṣmatī 1.36), and practices it with devotion.*
2. *He has intuitive knowledge (1.48). That is the honey state.*
3. *He has conquered the senses, remaining steadfast, as it should be, when something has been achieved; he has achieved all that had to be achieved so far, all that can be achieved and all that can be directly perceived (in the case of knowledge) or mastered (in the case of power); he also has the means to achieve that, which remains to be achieved. The means, to achieve it, are practice and serenity (1.12). The third one is one, who has those.*
4. *The fourth one, is one who has left behind, all that which had to be practiced, and whose only remaining purpose now is, to let the brain*

software become absorbed in pradhāna [that means, to upload the brain software to the universe-computer]. *He has the sevenfold highest knowledge.*

Amongst them it is the yogi, who has achieved the honey state, the second state with the truth-bearing knowledge, whose purity is perceived by the heavenly gods, and whom they lure into their realm and whom they salute with words like "Noble Sir," as will be described here:

"Noble Sir! Would you like to be seated here? Would you like to enjoy yourself here? The pleasure is delicious, and delicious is the girl. This potion prevents age and death. Here is a spaceship, there is a wish-fulfilling tree, the heavenly river mandākinī, the perfect beings, and great sages, all give their blessings. The nymphs are without equal, and compliant. Sight and hearing are divine, and the body like a diamond. Your special virtues, Noble Sir, have merited all this. Would you like to take this high position, which is unfading, ever fresh, undying, and beloved of the gods?"

When he is invited like that, however, let him meditate on the evils of that association: Scorched by the fierce flames of saṁsāra (the world jungle), wandering from birth to death, I have just managed to obtain the lamp of yoga, which destroys the blindness of illusions. The winds of sensual things, wombs of craving, are its foes. How then can I, who have seen its light, be led astray by the mirage of these sensory things, and make myself fuel for the burning fire of saṁsāra to flare up again? Farewell, you things like dreams pursued by pitiable creatures!

Thus confirming his purpose, let him practice samādhi on it. Giving up all association with them, let him take no pride in being thus solicited by the gods, themselves. If he, through such pride, feels secure, he will forget that death has already grasped his forelock, and then carelessness – always to be guarded against as it seeks an opening – will enter and rouse the illusions, with their undesirable consequences. By avoiding that association and that pride, what he has already practiced becomes firm in him, and what he has yet to practice stands right before him.

3.52

By saṁyama on the now and its two sequences of time phases comes knowledge born from discrimination.

क्षणतत्क्रमयोः संयमाद् विवेकजं ज्ञानम्

kṣaṇa-tat-kramayoḥ saṁyamāt viveka-jam jñānam

kṣaṇa (mn. comp.: moment) tad (n. comp.: that) krama (m. gen. loc. d.: operational sequence, procedure) saṁyama (m. abl. s.:) vivekaja (mfn., n. nom. acc. s: arising from discrimination) jñāna (n. nom. acc. s.: knowledge)

The sequences of the time phases have been explained in 3.15. Here, the topic is, to be in the "now" and to let the changes, due to the progression of time, run past you, through the now. From this, again, knowledge of discrimination arises, which is always complete knowledge. The seed of knowledge grows into the immeasurable. It works again, as before, in 3.35 and 3.49, by applying the *viveka khyāti* method of 2.26. *Viveka khyāti* always leads to complete, intuitive knowledge of all. Here now comes this method in a new variation, simply by discriminating between the unchanging now (*puruṣa*) and the two changeable sequences of time, from the future to the present, and from the present to the past.

Whoever distinguishes the unchanging from the changing, gains all comprehensive knowledge from that.

This *sūtra* also describes the basics of the special theory of relativity by Albert Einstein. Probably this was Einstein's initial access to the enormous treasures of knowledge, which he had discovered during his lifetime.

3.53

From that [knowledge of sūtra 3.52] comes the discrimination between two things that are apparently the same, unidentifiable by class, quality or place.

जातिलक्षणदेशैरन्यतानवच्छेदात्तुल्ययोस्ततः प्रतिपत्तिः

jāti-lakṣaṇa-deśaiḥ anyatā-anavacchedāt tulyayoḥ tataḥ pratipattiḥ

jāti (f. comp.: birth, class) lakṣaṇa (f. comp.: quality, attribute) deśa (m. ins. p.: place) anyatā (f. nom. s., comp.: difference) anavaccheda (m. abl. s.: undeterminable) tulya (mf(ā)n. gen. loc. d.: same, similar) tataḥ (ind.: by that, from that) pratipatti (f. nom. s.: perception, knowledge, determination, identification)

Here we see a different method, of unifying quantum physics and relativity theory because quantum physics, so far, assumes, that particles are not individually identifiable. By accessing the universe-computer, however, all knowledge is accessible.

In 1.19, under the headline "cosmic software" we found, that within the smallest volume, which an electron, the smallest mass particle (fermion), can occupy, 10^{48} smallest space elements, and the so-called Planck volumes, exist. Thus, each electron can carry with it sufficient information, to document its complete path from the beginning of the universe until now. Each elementary particle in our new model is a software object of the corresponding class; for example, an electron is an object of the class "electrons." Like all software objects, this particle also contains individual data, about its previous path through the universe.

This view essentially digresses from present-day quantum physics, which sees no possibility, of distinguishing, seemingly identical, but however, individual elementary particles.

This *sūtra* shows, how deep the all-comprehending knowledge is. The *yogi*, who practices 3.52, thereby can gain knowledge about all that ever happened in the universe, and about all the various variations of future events, that could come towards him. He gains this knowledge from the universe-computer. He does not need all the knowledge at once because that would overload the quantum computer of the small human brain. However, he can always call the required knowledge, whenever he needs it.

Simultaneously, he also uses the universe-computer with its vast store of information, to support and perfect his individuality. Already, with the perfection of the "great bodiless" in 3.43, he no longer depends on his body but rather can use the distributed computing of the universe-computer for himself. His individual SELF becomes expanded to cosmic dimensions. He becomes a cosmic individual. His desires are the desires of the totality. He functions as an integral part of the totality of nature and in tune with the will of the all-knowing and almighty, best ruler.

3.54

And also in that way knowledge is born from the discrimination between all that is intuitively perceived in the starry skies and the totality of all at all times.

तारकं सर्वविषयं सर्वथाविषयमक्रमं चेति विवेकजं ज्ञानम्

tārakam sarva-viṣayam sarvathā-viṣayam akramam ca iti vivekajam jñānam

tāraka (mf(ikā)n., m. acc. s.: pertaining to the starry sky) sarvaviṣaya (mfn., m. acc. s.: related to everything) sarvathāviṣaya (mfn., m. acc. s.: in whatever way appearing, in arbitrary appearance) sarvathā: all together) viṣaya: things, themes, topics) akrama (m. acc. s.: happening at once, inactive, without movement, frozen) ca (ind.: and, also) iti (ind.: so) vivekaja (mfn., n. nom. acc. s: arising from discrimination) jñāna (n. nom. acc. s.: knowledge)

Here, another way of reaching complete knowledge is illustrated. The *yogi* discriminates again between something unchanging, all-comprehending, and something changing, also all-comprehending.

Tāraka also is a star, which points towards *jyotiṣ* knowledge (1.36 and 3.28). This is the viewpoint of change, where actions are happening, because galaxy superclusters, galaxy clusters, galaxies, suns, and planets are all moving.

Opposite to that is the "totality of all at all times," the immovable, four-dimensional space-time with all the immovable world lines.

From this discrimination, again arises complete knowledge because it is again an application of the *viveka khyāti* method of 2.26.

Experience

When examining this *siddhi* in details, it suddenly occurred to me, what it meant. I knew this *siddhi* already. It corresponds to the illustration of the three spatial dimensions (3D) and the time dimension of the universe in a unified picture of four-dimensional space-time (4D). Space-time is the illustration of the totality of all at all times. In there, nothing moves anymore, because each movement in space and in time becomes fixed lines, areas, volumes or 4D volumes. In three-dimensional space, however, things are moving. This then corresponds to what is observed as movements in the universe.

Thus, I found out, that simply by learning the relativity theories of Albert Einstein, I had learned already, to practice this *siddhi*. Because it was another *siddhi*, to discover all knowledge, it suddenly became clear to me, that this was Einstein's big secret, in a way, his secret weapon, by which he could make so many discoveries in physics.

3.55

When buddhi-sattva is as pure as puruṣa then the absolute unity (brahman-consciousness, kaivalya) is there. So it is.

सत्त्वपुरुषयोः शुद्धिसाम्ये कैवल्यम्

sattva-puruṣayoḥ śuddhi-sāmye kaivalyam

sattva (n. comp.:) puruṣa (m. gen. loc. d.:) śuddhi (f. comp: purity, free from impurities) sāmya (n. loc. s., nom. acc. d.: sameness, similarity) kaivalya (n. nom. acc. s.: total freedom, absolute unity) iti (so it is)

The knowledge and the power, arising from yoga have been reviewed and completed, and there is no knowledge and no power beyond these. Regarding someone who has reached the knowledge and power by the yoga practices, it has been said (in 3.15): "serenity regarding that, immediately becomes absolute unity." Here now he says: in someone, who has reached knowledge born of discrimination, this unity remains, following the end of the outward-directed vision. How is that? When the sattva is pure as puruṣa, there is an absolute unity.

When the illusions of rajas and tamas have been shaken off, the brain software (buddhi-sattva) with its seeds (saṁskāras) roasted, its thinking processes and the malware in it stopped, upholds nothing but the thought of separateness from puruṣa. The brain software melts into the dignity of the thought of this separateness and then reaches a purity similar to that of puruṣa.

Although that, which consists of the three guṇas, has an opposite nature to puruṣa, and puruṣa has an opposite nature to that, which consists of the three guṇas, it is said anyway, that the brain software (buddhi-sattva), which becomes transformed into the thought of separateness from puruṣa, reaches a similar purity. In this state, absolute unity is achieved, no matter whether he has reached the divine powers, or not, no matter whether he processes the knowledge, born from discrimination, or not. That is, because in both cases, the basis of the absolute unity is present, which is nothing but the ending of ignorance.

Then, when the seeds of illusions are roasted, there is no longer any dependence on any further knowledge. He, who sees this correctly (saṁyagdarśin), realizes that everything consists of the three guṇas and that he has to escape from this thought, because it also consists of the three guṇas. And thus, he is no longer attached to all knowledge, as in the honey state. Yogic knowledge and power are described as side products, which have come about by the purity of the brain software and have been achieved in the way of striving towards the right view (saṁyag-darśana). However, the highest truth is this: By knowledge, the failure of sight ends, and when that ends, no more of the previously described illusions are present, like the "I"-ness because their range is ignorance. Without any illusions, karma bears no fruits, as has been stated in the sūtras 2.12 and 2.13: "The cause of all the objects in the store of karma is illusion" and "due to an existing root [illusion] *that store of karma ripens..."*

Therefore, this work has a correct vision as its only goal, and the glory of the knowledge is not its goal. In this state, the guṇas have ended their participation, and no longer appear in front of the puruṣa as the seen. That is the absolute unity of puruṣa when puruṣa is there alone in its true nature as pure light. "So it is" means, this part has ended.

With this, the third part of the yoga sūtras of Patañjali with the title "extraordinary abilities" ends, with the commentary of the holy Vyāsa and the commentary of the holy ruler Śaṁkara, who is a Paramahaṁsa Parivrājaka Ācārya and student of the holy ruler Govindapāda, whose feet are to be worshipped.

4

Kaivalya Pāda

Liberation

Transformation of Brain Software

Summary

In the previous three chapters, the evolution to higher versions of the brain software has been explained. Chapter four now puts this development into a cosmic context. By starting from the various kinds of living beings in the universe, the predominance of software over the hardware will be explained. The cosmic individual creates, with its consciousness (software), suitable hardware (body), and then manifests in this hardware in the form of brain software. The modern computer technology also develops in this direction with various approaches, like for example "Field Programmable Gate Arrays (FPGA)," or "Memory Driven Computing (MDC)." The software creates its required hardware in real-time.

We are very well aware that many scientists assume that initially there must be brain hardware, such, that on this hardware, the software can run, which they then call "consciousness." However, we are also aware, that in doing so, they start from an old computer paradigm: Hardware before software. This paradigm is generally no longer valid because these days software can create its hardware and modify it at any time. In this way, the hardware-software duality became obsolete. We assume, that, regarding this, the human brain works far more intelligently.

With the gradually increasing removal of malware, the brain software, on the one hand, activates the infinitely fast quantum computer in the brain; on the other hand, it is also able to run on the universe-computer ever more independently of the human brain. These abilities have been explained in Chapter three along with some of the *siddhi* techniques.

In chapter 4, now some more possibilities of the universe-computer will be illustrated, like for example, the networking of several brain software objects. It will be explained, how the memory administration of those networks is organized, and how, why, how long, the law of *karma* is applicable; how the brain software can cognize and influence not only one brain and one body but rather the whole physical reality in the cosmos.

At the end of the chapter the highest perfection will be described, where perfect, pure consciousness is freed from all its veils and impurities, independent of brain hardware and brain software, with perfect sight, and access to infinite knowledge, can know and achieve anything.

4.1

Siddhis (extraordinary abilities) arise from samādhi directly, [or] from birth, [or] by herbs, [or] mantras, [or] the urge for liberation.

जन्मौषधिमन्त्रतपःसमाधिजाः सिद्धयः

janma-oṣadhi-mantra-tapaḥ-samādhi-jāḥ siddhayaḥ

janma (n. comp.: birth) oṣadhi (f. comp.: plant, drug, herb) mantra (m. comp.: sound for meditation) tapas (n. nom. s.: urge for liberation) samādhi (m. comp.: restful alertness) ja (mf(ā)n. ,m.Nom. p.: caused by, birth) siddhi (f. nom. p.: siddhi, extraordinary ability)

Samādhi exclusively brings the *siddhi* result with it. For those without permanent *samādhi,* there are four methods, for the temporary achievement of *siddhis.*

Siddhis originate

- *By birth in another body, such as in heaven or a similar region.*
- *By consuming herbs, like soma, or the āmalaka plant.*
- *By repeating mantras, the abilities, to levitate, and to become as small as an atom, and the other (seven) are achieved.*
- *By tapas, the abilities are achieved, to take on any form and to go anywhere by willpower.*
- *By samādhi, siddhis are achieved as has already been described in chapter 3.*

4.2

From an excess of prakṛti [comes] the transformation into a related form of existence [rebirth].

जात्यन्तरपरिणामः प्रकृत्यापूरात्

jāti-antara-pariṇāmaḥ prakṛti-āpūrāt

jāti (f. comp.: birth, form of existence, fixed by birth) antara (mf(ā)n. comp.: inner, near, related) pariṇāma (m. nom. s.: change, transformation) prakṛti (f. comp.: power of creating the material world, nature; eight prakṛtis) āpūra (m. abl. s.: flooding, flood, overflow, excess)

The subtlest *prakṛti* in 1.45 has been equated with *pradhāna*, the ground state of *sattva*, *rajas*, and *tamas*.

The excited, non-balanced *prakṛti*, on the other hand, has an excess of *sattva*, *rajas*, or *tamas*. This non-balanced *prakṛti* in 2.22 has been described as "individualized" *pradhāna*, which opens a parallel universe, which is no longer there for the users of brain software versions 7 and 8.

In addition to *pradhāna*, there is an excess, and by that the *pradhāna* becomes individualized. Unfulfilled desires, for example, create this excess of *prakṛti*, which then leads to rebirth.

4.3

The undirected-ness of the prakṛtis [gets] a direction, like a farmer uses a dam [for irrigation] but consequently opens it up.

निमित्तमप्रयोजकं प्रकृतीनां वरणभेदस्तु ततः क्षेत्रिकवत्

nimittam aprayojakam prakṛtīnām varaṇa-bhedaḥ tu tataḥ kṣetrikavat

nimitta (n. nom. acc. s.: cause, the defining, motivation) aprayojaka (mf(ikā)n., n. Nom. Akk. s..: not causing, not effecting, without goal) prakṛti (f. gen. p.: power of creating the material world, nature; eight prakṛtis) varaṇa (m. comp.: rampart, mound) bheda (m. nom. s.: breaking, splitting) tu (ind.: and, but) tataḥ (ind.: from this, consequently, for this reason) kṣetrika (m. comp.: farmer, owner of the field) vat (affix: like, similar)

> Virtue is *dharma*, vice is *adharma*.

A dam contains water, to water the fields. The farmer opens and closes the dam depending on the need.

Water always flows to the lowest point, until the water levels become equal. By using a dam, this natural water flow is interrupted. A farmer, however, can open the dam at certain places, to water specific fields. Thus he gives a direction to the water. Then, at the opened places, the water flows, until the difference of heights is leveled.

It is similar with the three *guṇas*, who always strive towards the direction of *pradhāna*, their balanced state.

The imbalance of the excess of prakṛti initially does not cause anything. Then it receives a direction, for example by dharma, to balance these excesses in the direction of pradhāna, enabled by another birth.

When dharma prevails, an excess of sattva builds up (the dam fills up with water). When adharma prevails, an excess of tamas builds up (the dam fills up with mud.)

Prakṛti creates the corresponding forms of body, organs of sense and action, according to the stimulating cause of dharma or adharma.

4.4

Brain software [objects] are created exclusively from a [limited] "I"-consciousness (asmitā).

निर्माणचित्तान्यस्मितामात्रात्

nirmāṇa-cittāni asmitā-mātrāt

nirmāṇa (n. comp.: form, creating, making) citta (n. nom. acc. p.: brain software) asmitā (f. nom. s.: i-consciousness, identity) mātra (mf(ā)n., n. abl. s.: only, alone)

Every computer requires an operating system. This operating system can start, control, and end all apps (programs). The operating system treats those apps like objects. One app can simultaneously become started and run several times. Even the operating system can be the app of a superior operating system.

It is similar to the brain software. It can be the object of a superior, limited "I"-consciousness. Exactly like in today's computer technology this can also generate several brain software objects.

Every brain software object (citta) with a corresponding body and sense organs, becomes generated by one, limited "I"-consciousness. When the yogi with a limited "I"-consciousness generates several bodies with their sensory organs, then each of those bodies, become attributed to a separate brain software.

A *yogi*, therefore, is not a body, but a powerful "I"-consciousness, which can create different bodies, each with separate copies of the corresponding brain software. The *yogi*, on this level, is already liberated (brain software version 8), has no more ego, and has his individuality uploaded to the universe-computer. In this state, he has become a part of the universe-computer. He fulfills the tasks of the all-knowing and almighty in his individual way. If for the fulfillment of those tasks, several bodies are required, this *yogi* can create them.

4.5

The differences in the appearance of many [cittas] are caused by one [generating, controlling] citta.

प्रवृत्तिभेदे प्रयोजकं चित्तमेकमनेकेषाम्

pravṛtti-bhede prayojakam cittam ekam anekeṣām

pravṛtti (f. comp.: appearing, tendency, action, behavior) bheda (m. loc. s.: difference) prayojaka (n. nom. acc. s.: causing) citta (n. nom. acc. s.: brain software) eka (n. nom. acc. s.: one) aneka (n. m. gen. p.: many, much, not one)

A *yogi* can generate and control with his controlling brain software several software instances of individualized brain software.

The *yogi* really is only software and not the hardware of his body. The hardware adapts to the software. Here, it does not matter, whether the controlling software runs on a human brain or the universe-computer.

Laws of Karma

4.6

Of those [five methods of accomplishing siddhis], [only] the method dhyāna creates no store [of karma].

तत्र ध्यानजमनाशयम्

tatra dhyāna-jam an-āśayam

tatra (ind.: therein, there, in that case) dhyāna (n. comp.: Meditation) ja (mf(ā)n., m. acc. s.: created by, born of) an (ind.: not, negation) āśaya (m. acc. s.: place, deposit, seat of feelings and thoughts)

A brain software can install *siddhi* apps in five ways:

By birth, herbs, mantras, tapas, or samādhi. All, except mantras and samādhi, create a store of positive karma (merits, virtues) or negative karma (guilts, vices), or both.

Saṁskāras are like grains of sand in a gearbox; *karma* is like a heap of sand. The store of *karma* represents an imbalance of the *guṇas*, which leads to rebirth.

Siddhis arising from meditation (dhyāna), and only those, do not deposit anything in the store of karma. The yogi is free of illusions and karma. Therefore, there is no connection to good or bad, because the illusions have been removed by this yogi. Thus it was said: the store of karma has its roots in illusions (2.12). The yogi has no store of karma because no more illusions are there. However, in all other cases, there is a store of karma, because they have not removed the illusions.

4.7

The action of a yogi [brain software version 7+] is neither white nor black. For others, it is threefold [white, black, mixed].

कर्माशुक्लाकृष्णं योगिनस्त्रिविधमितरेषाम्

karma-aśukla-akṛṣṇam yoginaḥ trividham itareṣām

karman (n. comp.: action) aśukla (mf(ā)n. comp.: not white) akṛṣṇa (n. nom. acc. s.: not black) yogin (m. gen. abl. s.: yogi) trividham (mfn., n. nom. acc. s.: of threefold kind, threefold) itara (nm. gen. p.: of others)

A *yogi* (brain software versions 7 and 8) creates no facts (*karma*), which are white (virtuous) or black (vicious). However, he does act by the transformations in unity (3.12).

The others are creating facts (karma) that are white (purely mental, positive actions), black (bad) or grey (mixed).

This *sūtra* refers to the creation of new *karma*, the next (4.8) to the reaping of the results of previous *karma*.

4.8

Resulting from those [three kinds of karma] only those groups of thinking patterns (vāsanās), matching the situation, manifest.

ततस्तद्विपाकानुगुणानामेवाभिव्यक्तिर्वासनानाम्

tataḥ-tat-vipāka-anuguṇānām eva abhivyaktiḥ vāsanānām

tataḥ (ind.: from that, resulting from that) tad (n. comp.: that) vipāka (m. comp.: result, fruit, ripening) anuguṇa (mf(ā)n., m. gen. p.: of same nature, matching) eva (ind.: really, so, only, truly) abhivyakti (f. nom. s.: manifestation, distinction) vāsanā (f. gen. p.: thinking pattern)

Indeed, a saṁskāra is of a twofold nature, consisting of memories and the causing illusions. It has the name vāsanā when it occurs in its activation process in the form of virtue or vice (Śaṁkara's commentary on 3.18).

Before installing brain software version 7, a thinking pattern (*vāsanā*) causes a corresponding action (*karma*), as soon as a similar situation appears again (4.8).

Example: Someone has mostly positive (white) *karma*, consisting of more white than black *vāsanās*. As a result, he is born in a heavenly environment. However, the few black *vāsanās* are not deleted. They remain, and they do not ripen because the heavenly environment does not fit with the black *vāsanās*.

Liberation (kaivalya) has been praised, and now the illusions and karmas and vāsanās, which are the causes of the obstacles for that (liberation), must be illustrated. However, the functionality of the illusions, their antagonists, and their deletion have already been accurately described. The next sūtras, therefore, explain exactly, the functionality, the states, the antagonists and the deletion of karma and vāsanās. Only if, all of these end, liberation (kaivalya) is reached, not otherwise. Because there are three kinds of results, black, white and mixed, the result of karma that is ripened to become effective, originates only from those vāsanās that fit the result [the environment, the situation]. *These vāsanās, therefore, have a corresponding nature and a similar form to the result.*

With karmas, which are ripening to a divine, animal or human birth, the result is similar to the kind of karma that has caused it. The result arises only from those vāsanās originating from the karma ripening. It is similar to a boy, who sees a person, who looks like his mother and runs after her.

Thinking pattern (vāsanā) modifies a pure thought (pratyaya)

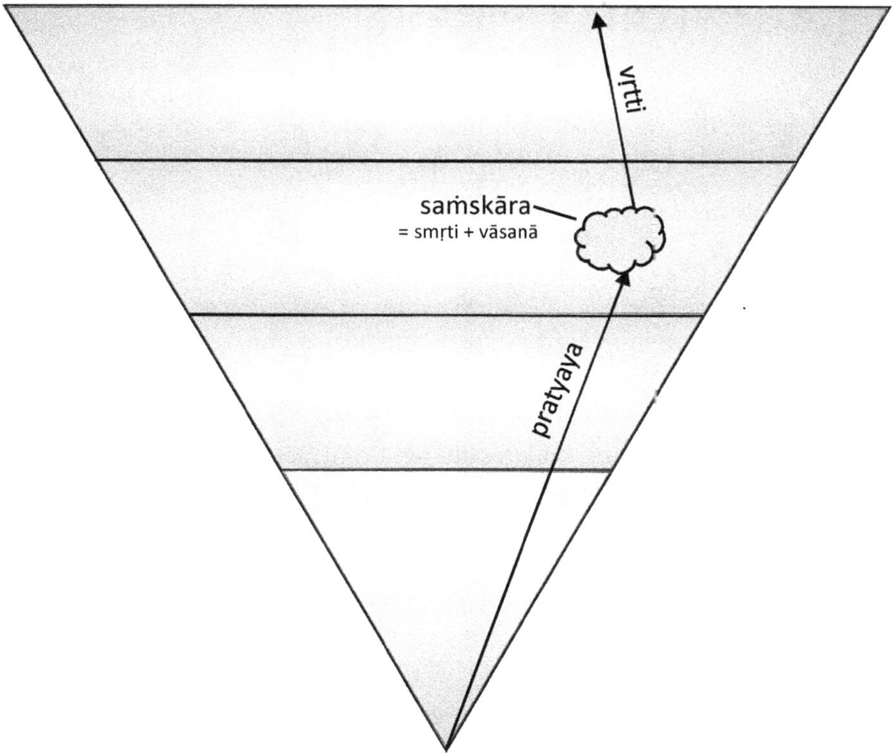

4.9

[The pairs of] memories (smṛtis) and impressions (saṁskāras) may be interrupted by birth, place or time. However, they follow a sequence in a [certain] format.

जातिदेशकालव्यवहितानामप्यानन्तर्यं स्मृतिसंस्कारयोरेकरूपत्वात्

jāti-deśa-kāla-vyavahitānām api ānantaryam smṛti-saṃskārayoḥ eka-rūpatvāt

jāti (f. Komp.: Geburt) deśa (m. Komp.: Ort, Platz) kāla (m. Komp.: Zeit, Zeitpunkt) vyavahita (m. Gen. p.: getrennt, unterbrochen, versteckt, entfernt) api (auch, sogar, selbst wenn) ānantarya (n. Nom. Akk. s.: unmittelbare Folge, Aufeinanderfolge,) smṛti (f. Komp.: Erinnerung, Gedächtnis) saṃskāra (m. Gen. Lok. d.: Eindruck) eka (eins) rūpa-tvāt (n. Abl. s.: Natur, Art, Form, Gestalt, Körper, Erscheinung)

Saṁskāras are organized by similarities of experiences, not by incarnation, place, or time. An event deposits memories and hidden impressions (*saṁskāras*). To understand the uninterrupted sequence of the *saṁskāra* ripening, one should study the *daśa* systems in *jyotiṣ*.

For the users up to and including brain software version 7, new *saṁskāras* are added to the existing *saṁskāras*, according to the *daśa* phases, making the *saṁskāras* more influential.

Saṁskāras in computer science correspond to the malware objects, and their sequence corresponds to a sequential method for the lists, containing these objects.

The impressions, in connection with illusions, lead to suffering. *Saṁskāras* are merged into groups according to the similarity of their events, whereas the *saṁskāras* may originate from various lives, times, places and causes. Thus, the tendency of that person for similar activities in the future is increased. For example, desires for a role as a leader, are stored up, and result in a future life, once more, in striving for a leading position.

4.10

And the lack of a beginning of those [vāsanās] [we conclude, is from the] eternal desire to live.

तासामनादित्वं चाशिषो नित्यत्वात्

tāsām-anāditvam ca āśiṣaḥ nityatvāt

tad (f. gen. p.: that) anāditva (n. nom. acc. s.: state without beginning) ca (ind.: and, also) āśis (f. abl. gen. s.: desire to live) nityatva (n. abl. s.: without end, eternity)

"Hope springs eternal" – the desire to live is a class (*kleśa*) of thinking patterns (*vāsanā*). Every newborn being immediately has a desire to survive. They all fear death, although, most of them, in their new life, have never had a near-death experience. Therefore, the fear of death must come from experiences of death at the end of previous lives.

The brain software has stored *vāsanās* without a beginning and is driven by those that fit in with the current situation.

Karmic Causes

The karmic causes are of different strengths.

The outer causes require means, like body and actions, like for example, adoration and greeting. The inner (mental) causes are those that begin with trust, followed by strength, memory, samādhi and intuitive prajñā knowledge (1.20). Inner causes are stronger than outer causes and, become ever stronger in the sequence from trust to intuitive knowledge. Saṁyama on friendliness and the other siddhis are inner causes, independent of body and actions, etc., and lead to the highest dharma.

4.11

In the absence of the collected causes, results, container [brain software] and supports [things], those [vāsanās] disappear.

हेतुफलाश्रयालम्बनैः संगृहीतत्वादेषामभावे तदभावः

hetu-phala-āśraya-ālambanaiḥ saṁgṛhītatvāt eṣām abhāve tat-abhāvaḥ

hetu (m. comp.: cause, reason, condition, intention) phala (n. comp.: effect, result, fruit) āśraya (m. comp.: container, receiving, refuge) ālambana (n. Ins. s.: support, dpending on, reason, cause) saṁgṛhīta-tvāt (mfn., m. abl. s.: seized, taken, collected-ness) idam (m. n. gen. p.: this) abhāva (m. loc. s.: absence [time or place related]) tad (n. comp.: that) abhāva (m. nom. s.: destruction, disappearance)

In 4.9, this collected experience structure has been described as the basis of the *saṁskāras*, if a thing or a situation appears, then the related *saṁskāra* objects become activated, for example, fear of heights on a bridge. The experience structure disappears, as soon as its causes have been removed.

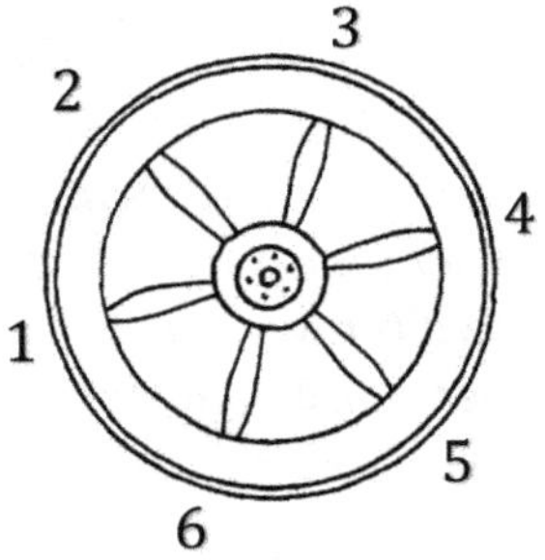

The six-spoked wheel of existence (*saṁsāra*) has the following spokes:

(1) virtue → (2) pleasure → (3) longing → (4) vice → (5) pain → (6) hate →effort.

The effort can alternatively go in both directions:

→ (1) virtue

→ (4) vice

By fleeing from the hate, someone comes back to virtue, and the wheel keeps turning.

The outer rim of this wooden wheel is ignorance (*avidyā*). As soon as the ignorance is destroyed, the whole wheel flies apart. Then the wheel of *karma* no longer turns.

As long as the brain software still has the task, of making experiences, it is in ignorance, and functions as a container for *saṁskāras*. As soon as it has recognized *puruṣa*, this task is finished.

4.12

Past and future are [subtle] forms of the present, which lead, according to their path, to various tasks.

अतीतानागतं स्वरूपतोऽस्त्यध्वभेदाद्धर्माणाम्

atīta-ānāgatam svarūpataḥ asti adhva-bhedāt dharmāṇām

atīta (n. comp.: past) ānāgata (n. nom. acc. s.: future) svarūpatas/ḥ (ind.: in own form, shape, similar, according to its nature) asti (ind.: existent, present, belongs to) adhvan (m. comp.: time, travel, way, path, place) bheda (m. abl. s.: difference) dharma (n. gen. p.: task, virtue, righteousness, character, quality, peculiarity)

Dharmin is the carrier of qualities, for example, clay. *Dharma* is the item with qualities, for example, the pot; (explained in detail in 3.13) The *dharmin* contains potentially all possible forms of expression. However, only in the *dharma*, one of these forms of expression is chosen.

> In computer science, *dharmin* corresponds to a class. *Dharma* corresponds to an object of this class.

The disappeared *saṁskāra* objects with their memories are described as past. However, they have not completely disappeared, but rather stay in a subtle form in the present. Therefore memories of previous lives are possible, even with an advanced brain software, when all the *saṁskāras* are switched off. Anything that comes into existence in the present must have waited for that, in its subtle future form. Anything that goes from the present into the past becomes transformed into its subtle past form.

Nothing can be created or destroyed. It merely becomes transformed. With brain software versions 1 to 3, there is a habit, of perceiving only the present with the sensory organs and only manifest things, although all things carry in them in a subtle form their past and future.

Similar to *sūtra* 3.52, here again, there is a hint to special relativity theory. Depending on the state of motion of the perceiver, the same thing can be viewed, as happening in the future or the past.

Items in their essence are knowledge

The pot, in its essence, is nothing but the knowledge of the potter, applied to the clay (*dharmin*). The purpose of the pot, to contain liquids, is its *dharma*. The origins of the pot are in the brain software and hands of the potter and the turn table. In the present time, products are the manifestations of a patent, an idea, etc. For brain software versions 7 and 8 an item or a thing is only knowledge.

4.13

Those [three distinct time phases] have the qualities [of being] manifest or subtle.

ते व्यक्तसूक्ष्माः गुणात्मानः

te vyakta-sūkṣmāḥ guṇātmānaḥ

tad (f. n. Nom. d.: jene, m. Nom. p.: jene) vyakta (mfn. comp.: manifest, perceivable) sūkṣma (mf(ā)n., m. nom. p.: fine, unmanifest) guṇātman (m. Nom. p.: having qualities)

Devī: I am time, I am *guṇa*, I am *ātman*.

Devī, the female personification of all natural laws, connects the changeable with the unchangeable. *Devī* holds both sides of the gap, *ātman,* and *pradhāna*.

Devī is present, past and future; *Devī* is the "material," from which time is made. The present is not subtle; it is perceived by many perceivers, and therefore its items are manifest. Past and future are subtly contained in the present.

Power of the Brain Software

4.14

From the transformation in unity (ekatva) [results] the reality of the manifest (vastu).

परिणामैकत्वाद्वस्तुतत्त्वम्

pariṇāma-ekatvāt vastu-tattvam

pariṇāma (m. comp.: change, transformation) ekatvāt (n. abl. s.: uniformity, uniqueness, alone, unity, unification) vastu (n. comp.: object, thing, manifestation) tattva (n. nom. acc. s.: principle, reality, essence)

That is the perception of the triad of future, present, and past in eternal oneness, in *brahman*-consciousness.

Ekatva is the final state of *ekāgratā* (3.12). *Brahman*-consciousness (*ekatva*) comes with the cosmic expansion of unity consciousness (*ekāgratā*). The manifest exists only in the present, whereas future and past are unmanifest.

The present is the common focal point, the here and now, assumed by multiple beings, including humans.

In 3.12, *ekāgratā* has been defined as one-pointed thinking. A similar thought is the thought of unity with all, for example: "I am you," "I am that," "I am the universe," "Everywhere I perceive my SELF."

Here now, the reality of the manifest universe is derived from that. Action in *brahman*-consciousness is attention that changes everything in the universe or leaves it as it is. This action generates no *karma* and always stays in unity.

> Action in *brahman*-consciousness is not impelled by *karma*.

In physics, the unitary transformation is completely reversible as no information is lost. In the language of the *yoga sūtras,* this means, no *karma* is generated.

4.15

Given the sameness of the manifest, any difference between two cittas gives rise to alternative paths.

वस्तुसाम्ये चित्तभेदात्तयोर्विभक्तः पन्थाः

vastu-sāmye citta-bhedāt tayoḥ vibhaktaḥ panthāḥ

vastu (n. comp.: object, substance, manifestation) sāmya (n. loc. s., nom. acc. d.: equality, sameness) citta (n. comp.: brain software) bheda (m. abl. s.: difference, different) tad (n. gen. d.: of those two) vibhakta (m. nom. s.: different, separate) pathin (m. nom. s.: way, path, world line, traveler)

Examples: From the viewpoint of virtue (dharma), mostly happiness results, according to the nature of sattva. Parents see a person as their son, generating happiness. From the viewpoint of vice (adharma), mostly suffering results, according to the nature of rajas. A competitor sees the same person as an enemy, which creates suffering. From the viewpoint of ignorance (avidyā), mostly illusion results, according to the nature of tamas. A tiger sees the same person as food, which could profoundly change the path of the person.

At each moment, the brain software chooses one of several future paths. In physics, these paths are called "word lines."

4.16

A manifest [thing] also is not the product of a single brain software, [because] what could it be without the attention [of that brain software]?

न चैकचित्ततन्त्रं वस्तु तदप्रमाणकं तदा किं स्यात्

na ca eka-citta-tantram vastu tat-apramāṇakam tadā kim syāt

na (ind.: not) ca (ind.: and, also) eka (mfn., comp.: one) citta (n. comp.: brain software) tantra (n. nom. acc. s.: main point, characteristic quality, product [created as]) vastu (n. nom. acc. s.: object, thing, manifestation) tad (n. comp.: that) apramāṇakam (apramāṇa–kam n. nom. acc. s.: non- attention, meaninglessness, without weight; kam = who, which, what) tadā (ind.: then, after) kim (ind.: n. nom. acc. s.: what) syāt (ind.: it could be)

If the Moon was merely the mental product of one observer, it would disappear when the observer looked away. In the process of liberation, the things only disappear for the liberated, but not for the others (2.22).

In physics: The perception of a thing by many observers defines the borderline between quantum physics (few particles) and classical physics (many particles).

If unified field theories were supplemented with the information network of the universe-computer, as we have suggested in 1.23 and the following *sūtras*, all these considerations would be immediately plausible. It is the cosmic software which generates, maintains, and destroys the elementary particles in the form of software objects of their respective elementary particle classes. [22]

As long as a brain software has not yet perfect access to the cosmic software that means before brain software version 8 it has no essential influence. Only the *yogi*, whose software runs on the universe-computer, whose software, therefore, is no longer an "individual brain software," functioning separately from the rest of the universe, has these possibilities. He could, at any time, create an apple in his empty hand from the vacuum (3.44).

4.17

According to the coloring of the brain software by that [manifest thing], the manifest [thing] is known or unknown.

तदुपरागापेक्षित्वाच्चित्तस्य वस्तु ज्ञाताज्ञातम्

tat-uparāga-apekṣitvāt-cittasya vastu jñāta-ajñātam

---

[22] The concept of information at the foundation of all of physics is not new. The famous John Wheeler talked about "it from bit". Today, several physicists work on theories explaining, how there could be some sort of digital calculation at a more fundamental level than quantum physics, for example Max Tegmark, MIT; James Gates, University of Maryland; Seth Lloyd, MIT.

tad (n. comp.: that) uparāga (m. comp.: colouring, darkening, eclipse) apekṣin-tva (n. abl. s.: dependency, in relation to, expectation, requirement) citta (n. gen. s.: brain software) vastu (n. nom. acc. s.: object, thing, manifestation) jñāta (mfn.: comp.: known) ajñāta (n. nom. acc. s.: unknown)

Knowledge arises, for example, by perception. In the process of perception, the item is recognized by the brain software changing its state, adapting to the item. As items are sometimes known and sometimes not, the brain software is a tool, whose state can change.

4.18

The thinking processes (vṛttis) are always known to their Lord [puruṣa] due to the non-variability of puruṣa.

सदा ज्ञाताश्चित्तवृत्तयस्तत्प्रभोः पुरुषस्यापरिणामित्वात्

sadā jñātāḥ citta-vṛttayaḥ tat-prabhoḥ puruṣasya-apariṇāmitvāt

sadā (ind.: comp.: always) jñāta (mfn., mf. nom. p.: known) citta (n. comp.: brain software) vṛtti (f. nom. p.: thought process) tad (n. comp.: that) prabhu (m. abl. gen. s.: Lord, master, ruler) puruṣa (m. gen. s.: silent SELF) apariṇāmin-tvāt (m. n. abl. s.: non-variability, unchanging)

The non-variability of *puruṣa* includes eternally knowing all the processes in the brain software (*citta*). *Puruṣa* always sees the brain software because *puruṣa* does not change. *Puruṣa* is the user of the brain software. *Puruṣa* is also the user of the cosmic software. For *puruṣa,* both the cosmic software and the brain software of all living beings in all universes are something, which he observes. This will be explained in more detail in the following *sūtra*.

4.19

That [brain software] does not radiate on its own [because] it is something observed.

न तत्स्वाभासं दृश्यत्वात्

na tat sva-ābhāsam dṛśyatvāt

na (ind.: not) tat (n. nom. acc. s.: that) sva (mf(ā)n.: own) ābhāsa (m. acc. s.: radiating, brilliance, light, appearance) dṛśyatva (n. abl. s.: visibility, sight)

Puruṣa always observes *citta*. Therefore *citta* is the observed. That means the brain software is something, observed by *puruṣa*. This observation has nothing to do with the senses, but rather is the eternal relationship between *puruṣa* and the observed *citta*. *Citta* is nothing without *puruṣa*.

4.20

And one simultaneous meeting [of puruṣa and citta] confirms both [as separate entities].

एकसमये चोभयानवधारणम्

eka-samaye ca ubhaya-avadhāraṇam

eka (mfn. comp.: one) samaya (m. loc. s.: time, meeting, connection) ca (ind.: and, also) ubhaya (mf(ī)n.: both, of both kinds) avadhāraṇa (n. nom. acc. s.: observation, confirmation, assuring, approval, affirmation)

Cognition, in principle, can only refer to one thing at one time. It can either refer to the brain software, or to *puruṣa*, the user; not simultaneously to both. It always requires a little bit of time, to direct the attention to something else. That applies before upgrading to brain software version 5. By using the activated quantum computer starting from version 5, however, everything becomes possible.

4.21

The brain software is observed internally by its main component, and a continued [observation] by [another] main component [would lead to] a confusion of memory.

चित्तान्तरदृश्ये बुद्धिबुद्धेरतिप्रसङ्गः स्मृतिसंकरश्च

citta-antara-dṛśye buddhi-buddheḥ atiprasaṅgaḥ smṛti-saṁkaraḥ ca

citta (n. comp.: brain software) antara (n. comp.: inner, neighbouring, near, gap) dṛśya (m. loc. s., n. nom. acc. d., loc. s.: visible, the perceivable, sight, perceived) buddhi (f. comp.: intellect) buddhi (f. abl. gen. s.: process of perceiving, main component of the brain software) atiprasaṅga (m. nom. s.: "infinite loop", diffuseness, confusion) smṛti (f. comp.: memory, remembrance) saṁkara (m. nom. s.: mixing) ca (ind.: and, also)

The main component of the brain software (*buddhi*) is contained in the brain software (*citta*) and internally observes the brain software. If each time another *buddhi* were required to observe the previous *buddhi*, this would require an infinite number of *buddhis*.

In computer science: In software, non-terminated loops (observation processes) lead to "stack overflow" (confusion of memory).

Evolution of Intellect

4.22

Due to pure consciousness being in unrestricted lockstep with the content of that [brain software perceived by its main component] the main component falsely assumes [this pure consciousness] to be its own.

चितेरप्रतिसंक्रमायास्तदाकारापत्तौ स्वबुद्धिसंवेदनम्

citeḥ aprati-saṅkramāyāḥ tat-ākāra-āpattau sva-buddhi-saṁVedanam

cit = citi (f. abl. gen. s.: [pure] consciousness; s. Mylius) aprati (mfn. comp.: irresistible, without resistance) saṃkrama (m. -> f.: genus adjusted to cit; m. abl. gen. s.: sequence, transition, proceeding) tat (n. comp.: that) ākāra (m. comp.: form, gestalt, outer appearance) āpatti (f. loc. s.: transformation in, mistake, fault, offence) sva (mf(ā)n.: own) buddhi (f. comp.: main component of brain software, intellect) saṃVedana (n. nom. acc. s.: feeling, perceiving)

That is the experience process of the brain software before the upgrade to version 5. The *buddhi* (main component) of those previous brain software versions sees it as follows: Pure consciousness is continually with me. Therefore it must belong to me, and therefore I call it my consciousness.

The actual process, however, is the following: Pure consciousness (*puruṣa*) continually notices the *buddhi* with all its contents.

The intellectual mistake is, that *buddhi* has merely borrowed consciousness from *puruṣa*, but believes this to be its own and that it does not need to return it. The *buddhi* identifies with *puruṣa*, although in reality, it is totally different from *puruṣa*.

This false identification is also called the „fault of the intellect".

Therefore it has been said: Neither in the netherworld, nor in the deep mountain crevices, nor in darkness, nor in the depths of the oceans is the secret cave, where the eternal brahman hides; however, it is in the mental process, if it is not discerned.

It has been said: By the mere similarity to the process of brain software (buddhi-vṛtti), the "knowledge"-process is only observed in the brain software (buddhi) and not outside it. Neither in the netherworld, nor in crevices, nor in darkness nor ocean depths, nor in any such thing, is the secret cave, in which the eternal brahman is hidden. This secret cave is not the netherworld or any other cosmic region.

What, then is the secret cave where it is hidden? It is the mental process. That is the secret cave of the brain software (buddhi), the mental process, that [falsely] *is called the SELF (ātman), that is called brahman, as long as it is not distinguished, as long as it is not cut out, as long as it is not distinguished from the process in the brain software. Thus are teachings of those, who see the difference.*

4.23

Brain software, influenced by the perceiver [puruṣa] and the perceived, has all goals.

द्रष्टृदृश्योपरक्तं चित्तं सर्वार्थम्

draṣṭṛ-dṛśya-uparaktam cittam sarva-artham

draṣṭṛ (m. comp.: perceiver, observer, seer) dṛśya (m. comp.. sight, n. comp.: seen, perceived, cognised) uparakta (mfn., m. acc. s., n. nom. acc. s.: colored, coloring) citta (n. nom. acc. s.: brain software) sarva (mf(ā)n. comp.: all) artha (m. acc. s.: meaning, aim, purpose, goal)

All goals mean both experience and liberation. Here, the state of cosmic consciousness (brain software version 5) is described. *Puruṣa* is conscious of the brain software of all living beings: He is the "witness of all thinking beings." *Puruṣa* is influenced, neither by brain software nor by the perceived object. *Citta's* nearness to *puruṣa* is experienced by *citta's* attention to the higher SELF. Expressed in our modern language: The brain software is close to its user when it directs its attention to its user. That means, the communication interface adapts to its user, not vice versa.

In the *prajñā* knowledge of the user of brain software versions 7 and 8, in addition to the knowledge impulses (what were previously outer items), always the cognition of *puruṣa* is present as well. Clear distinction (not mixing) of the knower (*puruṣa*), the process of knowing and the known, leads to absolute unity (*kaivalya*).

4.24

Although that [brain software] is tainted by countless vāsanās, it has another purpose caused by its relationship [of being the servant of puruṣa].

तदसंख्येयवासनाभिश्चित्रमपि परार्थं संहत्यकारित्वात्

tat-asaṅkhyeya-vāsanābhiḥ citram api para-artham saṁhatya-kāritvāt

tad (n. comp.: that) asaṅkhyeya (mfn. comp.: countless) vāsanā (f. Ins. p.: thinking pattern) citra (n. nom. acc. s.: tainted, spoilt, impurity) api (ind.: also, even, although) para (mf(ā)n.: other) artha (m. acc. s.: meaning, goal, purpose) saṃhatya (ind.: connected, joined with, combined, together with) kāritva (m. n. abl. s.: cause, origination, causing)

Citta is not an end in itself but serves *puruṣa*.

Brain software is not an end in itself, but serves the user.

4.25

For those who know the difference [between buddhi and puruṣa], contemplation of SELF-realization ends.

विशेषदर्शिन आत्मभावभावनाविनिवृत्तिः

viśeṣa-darśinaḥ ātmabhāva-bhāvanā-vinivṛttiḥ

viśeṣa (m. comp.: difference, peculiarity) darśin (mfn., m. gen. abl. s, nom. p.: seeing, knowing, cognizing, observing ; aḥ ā => a ā) ātmabhāva (m. comp.: ātman as a goal, SELF-Realisation) bhāvanā (f. nom. s.: contemplation, feeling of devotion, deliberation) nivṛtti (f. nom. s.: ending, halting, vanish)

Users of brain software versions 7 and 8 have reached the goal, know the difference and hence do not think about the goal any more.

4.26

Then, the brain software with deeply discriminating cognition tends towards unity.

तदा विवेकनिम्नं कैवल्यप्राग्भारं चित्तम्

tadā viveka-nimnam kaivalya-prāgbhāram cittam

tadā (ind.: then) viveka (m. comp.: correctly-discriminating-cognition) nimna (mf(ā)n., n. nom. acc. s.: depth, thoroughness) kaivalya (n. comp.: unity consciousness, liberation) prāgbhāra (m. acc. s.: tendency, inclination) citta (n. nom. acc. s.: brain software)

The brain software distinguishes between its main component, *buddhi* and its user, *puruṣa*. By this distinction (3.35), it tends towards unity. Why? That is because, by this distinction, the changing (*buddhi*) is recognized as an expression of the unchanging (*puruṣa*). Then, only the unity of *puruṣa* = *ātman* remains.

Starting from cosmic consciousness, a deeper and more fundamental distinction between *buddhi* and *puruṣa* leads to unity consciousness.

4.27

At the time of interruption of that [deep discrimination], intermediate thoughts [arise] from saṁskāras.

तच्छिद्रेषु प्रत्ययान्तराणि संस्कारेभ्यः

tat-chidreṣu pratyaya-antarāṇi saṁskārebhyaḥ

tad (n. comp.: that) chidra (mf(ā)n., n. loc. p.: by time and place: hole, gap) pratyaya (m. comp.: thought) antara (mf(ā)n., n. nom. acc. p.: inner, bordering, near) saṃskāra (m. dat. abl. p., impression)

When unity consciousness is there only as a temporary state, in the intermediate periods, when the *yogi* is not practicing discrimination, thoughts arise from *saṁskāras*.

As long as unity consciousness is not stabilized, distracting *saṁskāras* can again take the *yogi* out of this one-pointed transformation.

4.28

The ending of these [thoughts from saṁskāras] [happens] as explained for the illusions [kleśas].

हानमेषां क्लेशवदुक्तम्

hānam eṣāṃ kleśavat uktam

hāna (mfn., n. nom. acc. s.: ending, abandon) idam (mn. gen. p.: of these) kleśa-vat (m. comp.: like [vat] illusions) ukta (mfn., m. acc. s., n. nom. acc. s.: explained, described)

Unity consciousness results from the ending of ignorance (*avidyā* 2.24, 2.25). In *sūtra* 2.26, we have described the method of uninterrupted, correctly-discriminating cognition (*viveka khyāti*). Then we determined in 2.28 that in the eight areas of *yoga* a purification must happen before *viveka khyāti* is fully realized.

Thus, it became clear, that *viveka khyāti* is an advancing process, and here, in *sūtras* 4.27 and 4.28, now is the instruction for the *yogi*, what to do, when his unity consciousness occasionally becomes disturbed by thoughts from *saṁskāras*. He should go about it, in the same way as with the battle against the illusions, and immediately again apply *viveka khyāti*. See also the summary of the *yoga* methods in 2.33 and one more in 4.29.

Perfection

4.29

One who does not even expect anything from his meditation, by applying correctly-discriminating cognition [reaches] a samādhi with the name "rain cloud of dharma."

प्रसंख्यानेऽप्यकुसीदस्य सर्वथा विवेकख्यातेर्धर्ममेघः समाधिः

prasaṅkhyāne api akusīdasya sarvathā viveka-khyāteḥ dharma-meghaḥ samādhiḥ

prasaṁkhyāna (n. loc. s., n. nom. acc. d.: meditation, pondering) api (ind.: also, even, although, not even) akusīda (mfn., mn. gen. s.: no interest, desirelessness, not expecting) sarvathā (ind.: in every respect, anything) viveka (m. comp.: distinction, discrimination) khyāti (f. abl. gen. s.: knowledge, clarity, cognition) dharma (n. comp.: virtue) megha (m. nom. s.: mass, rain cloud) samādhi (m. nom. s.: restful alertness)

From communication with perfect beings, we have heard that the term "rain cloud of *dharma*" must refer to "refined cosmic consciousness," brain software version 6.

Filled with myriad little drops of *samādhi* with a wonderful taste – Heaven on Earth!

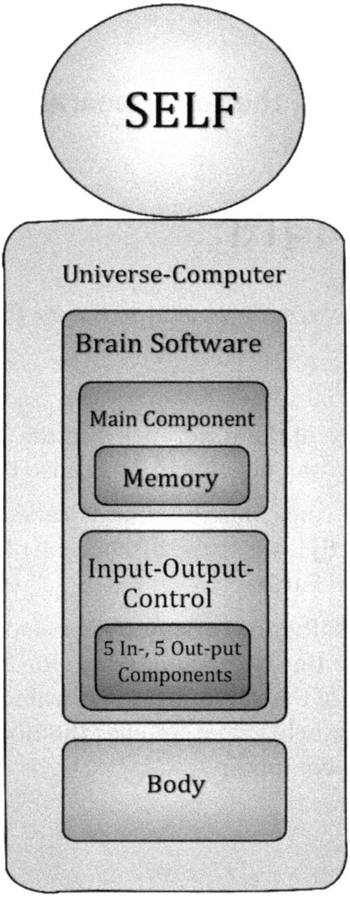

Brain software version 6

4.30

From that [follows] the disappearance of the illusions (kleśas) and the karma.

ततः क्लेशकर्मनिवृत्तिः

tataḥ kleśa-karma-nivṛttiḥ

tataḥ (ind.: from that) kleśa (m. comp.: illusion) karman (n. comp. s:) nivṛtti (f. nom. s.: disappearance)

From the knowledge of the difference and the "rain cloud of *dharma*," illusions, the roots of *karma*, disappear. Thus, also the *karma* disappears.

The higher state of consciousness that is called cosmic consciousness (brain software version 5) leads to the dissolution of all illusions and *karma*, while the *yogi* is alive on Earth.

We call that brain software version 6. See also the illustration on the previous page. Compare this to the illustration for version 5 (see the introduction, before the test of the version of your brain software, page 38). The SELF has expanded so much, that it touches the nonself, which it now recognizes as the universe-computer.

4.31

Then, freed from all veils and impurities, in the infinity of knowledge only a tiny bit of ignorance remains.

तदा सर्वावरणमलापेतस्य ज्ञानस्यानन्त्याज्ज्ञेयम् अल्पम्

tadā sarva-āvaraṇa-mala-apetasya jñānasya ānantyāt jñeyam alpam

tadā (then) sarva (mf(ā)n.: all, total) āvaraṇa (mfn., n. comp.: covering, envelope, veil) mala (n. comp.: dirt, impurity) apeta (mfn., mn. gen. s.: free of) jñāna (n. gen. s.: unenlightened knowledge) ānantya (mfn., n. abl. s.: endlessness, eternity) jñeya (mfn.: to be known, to be learnt, to be understand) alpa (mf(ā)n., m. acc. s., n. nom. acc. s.: small, little, unimportant)

"Only a tiny bit of ignorance" means *leśa avidyā*. It is not something to maintain, but something to be removed by infinite knowledge. The individual in unity consciousness lives with a body and is yet free.

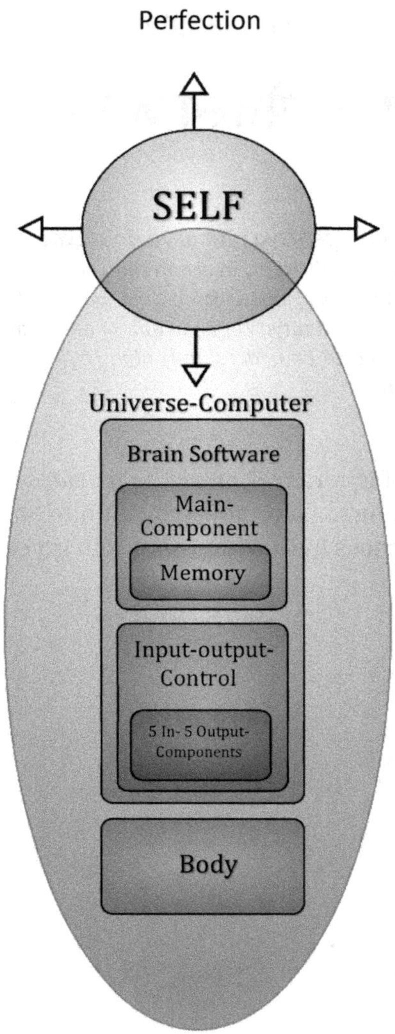

Brain software version 7

Guṇas and Kaivalya

4.32

With that [knowledge of the difference and the rain cloud of dharma], the guṇas have achieved their goals, and their continuous transformation has ended.

ततः कृतार्थानां परिणामक्रमसमाप्तिर्गुणानाम्

tataḥ kṛtārthānām pariṇāma-krama-samāptiḥ guṇānām

tataḥ (ind.: through that, by that, as a consequence) kṛtārtha (mf(ā), n. gen. p.: goal accomplished, intentions accomplished, successful) pariṇāma (m. comp.: change, transformation) krama (m. comp.: sequence, flow) samāpti (f. nom. s.: ending, fulfillment) guṇa (m. gen. p.: Tendenz)

The goals of the *guṇas* are experiences and liberation. With that accomplished, they cannot continue, even for a moment. The list of transformations in 3.11, 3.12, 3.13 and 4.29, now comes to its grand finale. The unity of consciousness reaches the status of absolute unity consciousness, which is also called *brahman*-consciousness, described by us as brain software version 8. Basically, it is not even brain software, but rather cosmic software, which additionally is connected to a brain, living on Earth. The difference between brain software and cosmic software has disappeared. The *yogi* now is a cosmic individual. All fullness of power and all knowledge from the universe-computer is available to him.

4.33

The transformation of sequentially following moments has ended and [then] their flow is recognized.

क्षणप्रतियोगी परिणामापरान्तनिर्ग्राह्यः क्रमः

kṣaṇa-pratiyogī pariṇāma-aparānta-nirgrāhyaḥ kramaḥ

kṣaṇa (m. comp.: moment) pratiyogin (mfn., m. nom. s.: correlative, being related, connected; any object dependent upon another and not existing without it) pariṇāma (m. comp.: transformation, change) aparānta (m. comp.: extreme end) nirgrāhya (m. nom. s.: perceivable, to be traced or found out) krama (m. nom. s.: sequence, process, flow)

Guṇas as *dharmin* (as clay) remain, but as *dharma* (pot) they disappear and then change no more. The world comes to an end for the liberated, not for the others.

The flow of world events has ended and is replaced by a far more interesting game of knowledge impulses. All *karma* has ended, perfect freedom is gained.

The world comes to an end for the user of brain software version 8, however, not for the users before version 8.

From the viewpoint of physics, one can understand it in this way:

The methods of quantum physics derived from the Schrödinger equation describe the whole world as a transformation of moments, which can be as short as 5.39106×10^{-44} seconds, to be exact. That is the period of the shortest vacuum fluctuations.

With the achievement of the highest state of consciousness, the physical world ends. That corresponds to the time-independent Schrödinger equation, where only unitary transformations of eigenvalues occur. Unitary transformation of eigenvalues means: the resulting state coincides with the beginning state and has stable energy values.

4.34

The guṇas, having returned to their original state, serve no [further] purpose for puruṣa, and unity consciousness has settled in its own nature. That is the power of consciousness – and so it is.

पुरुषार्थशून्यानां गुणानां प्रतिप्रसवः कैवल्यं स्वरूपप्रतिष्ठा वा चितिशक्तिरिति

puruṣa-artha-śūnyānām guṇānāṁ pratiprasavaḥ kaivalyaṁ svarūpa-pratiṣṭhā vā citi-śaktiḥ iti

puruṣārtha (m. comp.: purpose of puruṣa) śūnya (mf(ā)n., n. gen. p.: non-existence, emptiness) guṇa (m. gen. p.: tendency) pratiprasava (m. nom. s.: returning to the original state) kaivalya (n. nom. acc. s.: absolute unity consciousness, liberation) svarūpa (n. comp.: own nature) pratiṣṭhā (f. nom. s.: basis, standing still, based on) vā (ind.: or) citi (f. abl. gen. s.: [only] consciousness) śakti (f. nom. power, force, energy) iti (so it is)

Brahman-consciousness is there when the brain software runs exclusively on the universe-computer, and the quantum computer of the brain (*buddhi-sattva*) has become insignificant.

The individuality is still there. However, without the ego, it has expanded into cosmic realms. The cosmic individual has reached its absolute status. In the *brahma-sūtras, Śaṁkara* comments how far this freedom of the cosmic individual goes. The *yogi* in *brahman*-consciousness has total freedom, to choose his bodily existence in three different varieties.

He can:

- ⇨ Exist with one body.
- ⇨ Exist without any body.

⇨ Exist with arbitrarily many bodies, while staying the one, individual *yogi*, who controls all those bodies according to sūtra 4.4 and 4.5.

There never was a time when I was not,
nor you, nor these rulers of men. Nor
will there ever be a time when all of
us shall cease to be.

Bhagavad Gīta (2.12)

May the force be with you!

With the "so it is" the instruction ends.

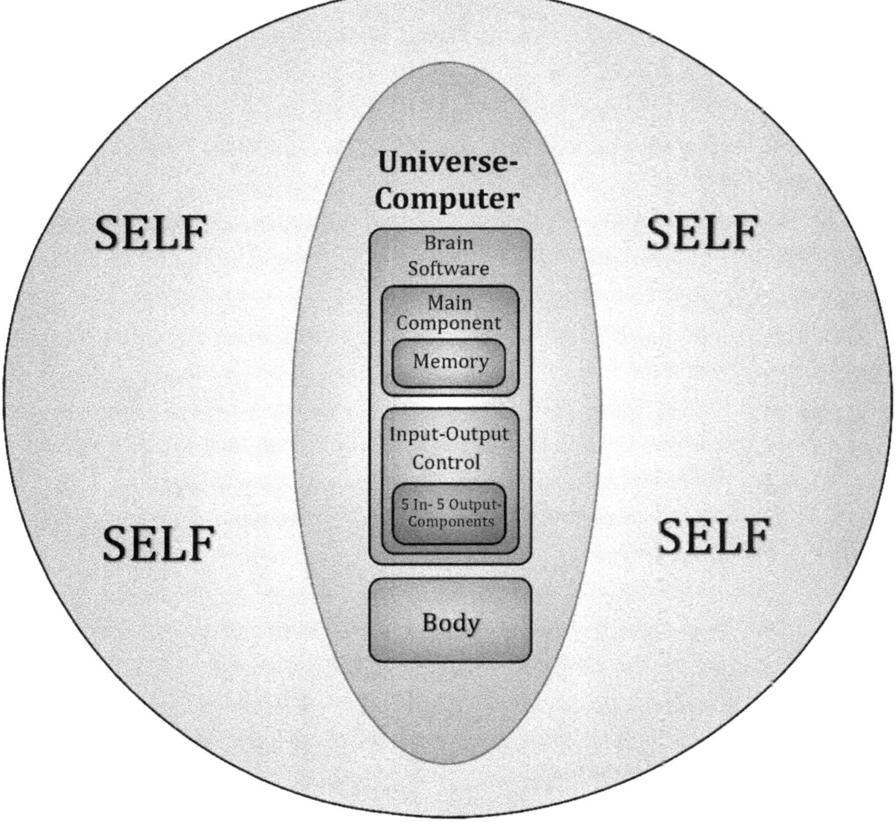

Brain software version 8

Eulogy

Whose expressive word is auṁ, from whom all action is made fruitful,

Who, himself without illusions or fruition of karma, brings about everything as the fruit of actions,

Lord of lords, controller of preservation and coming into being and cessation of all creations, may he have regard to our good deeds and annul our bad.

He has given life to the three worlds.

A fraction of his unimaginable power became in this world The Fish and other Avatāras reckoned to be ten;

Tormented by the continuous chain of the three sufferings arising from the illusions, we go for refuge to Him who has Śeṣa, the cosmic serpent, as his couch.

Salutations to Patañjali, Lord of the yogis, Lord of serpents (being an incarnation of Śeṣa) by the power of the gem in his hoods lights everywhere on Earth, in the sky, and in space,

Who by yoga has removed impurities of the mind, by his grammar those of speech, and by his (classic on) medicine those of the physical body – to that highest of sages, Patañjali, be this bow with my folded hands.

The Sage Patañjali is supreme, by whom all the seekers of ends attain their highest good; the joy which he brings removes the three burning afflictions, by the rain cloud of dharma (samādhi);

Who to remove the heat of the dharmas of illusory action of those traversing the path of worldly existence appeared as the water-bearer of the yoga which leads to the rain cloud of dharma – to that Ṛṣi Patañjali I bow down.

I bow down to him on whose continence is a full Moon, the teacher, the Lord, who is not decorated with wealth and who is without the necklace of serpents, the incomparable Śaṁkara whose feet are to be worshipped.

With this, the fourth part, on "Liberation," of the sub-commentary on the commentary to the yoga sūtras of Patañjali, by the holy Lord Śaṁkara, who is a Paramahaṁsa Parivrājaka Ācārya and student of holy Lord Govindapāda whose feet are to be worshipped, is complete.

Appendix

A - Yoga Sūtras at a Glance

Chapter 1 – Levels of Silence

1.1 Now begins the instruction in *yoga*.

1.2 Yoga [is] the calming of thought processes (*vṛttis*) in the brain software (*citta*).

1.3 Then the perceiver is grounded in his own nature.

1.4. Otherwise [not in the *yoga* state], [*ātman* appears to] conform to the thinking process (*vṛtti*).

1.5 The thinking processes (*vṛttis*) are fivefold [and] pain-inducing or non-pain-inducing.

1.6 [The five kinds of thinking processes (*vṛttis*) are] *pramāṇa* (correct knowledge), *viparyaya* (misunderstanding), *vikalpa* (imagination), *nidrā* (deep sleep), *smṛti* (memory).

1.7 Correct knowledge (*pramāṇa*) is [defined as] direct perception (*pratyakṣa*), inference (*anumāna*) [or] knowledge from an authority (*āgama*).

1.8 Misunderstanding is the illusory knowledge that does not conform to facts.

1.9 Imagination (*vikalpa*) is something following on from verbal knowledge, [but] not based on any existent thing.

1.10 Deep sleep is the mental process based on the thought of nonexistence.

1.11 Memory is the not losing of an item of experience.

1.12 By practice and serenity, the calming of those [*vṛttis*] is accomplished.

1.13 In that, staying with those two [practice and serenity], there is practicing with zeal.

1.14 If [the *yogi*] practices for a long time without interruption carefully and diligently, [he] becomes firmly grounded.

1.15 Intentionally not longing for seen or heard things is known as serenity (*vairāgya*).

1.16 Beyond that [serenity], from the cognition of *puruṣa* [there is] an absence of desires for the *guṇas*.

1.17 *Saṁprajñāta* [*samādhi*] is a state of unboundedness accompanied by [four] sequentially [subtler] levels of thinking: speech comprehension (*vitarka*), subtle thinking (*vicāra*), bliss (*ānanda*), limited "I"-consciousness (*asmitā*).

1.18 If one has practiced the thought of stopping before, a residue of *saṁskāras* remains – that is the other [*samādhi*].

1.19 [*Asaṁprajñāta samādhi*] arises from birth in the *videhas* (the unembodied) and in the *prakṛtilayas* (nature beings).

1.20 For others before [*asaṁprajñāta samādhi*] comes trust, strength, memory, [*saṁprajñāta*] *samādhi* and intuitive knowledge (*prajñā*).

1.21 [For those] with intense striving for [*samādhi*], [it is] near.

1.22 Resulting from a mild, medium, or intensive [striving] there is also a difference [regarding the closeness to *asaṁprajñāta samādhi*].

1.23 Or by attention to *Īśvara* [*samādhi* is achieved].

1.24 Untouched by illusions, actions, results, and stores of *karma* [but] distinct from *puruṣa* is *Īśvara*.

1.25 In him [*Īśvara*] [is] the seed of unsurpassed all-knowingness.

1.26 He [*Īśvara*] is even the teacher of the previous [teachers], unlimited by time.

1.27 His [*Īśvara's*] sound characteristic is *praṇava*.

1.28 The repetition of that [seed] realizes that goal [of supreme all-knowingness].

1.29 From that [practice comes] the mastery of inner consciousness and also the disappearance of [any] obstacles.

1.30 Illness, stubbornness, doubt, negligence, laziness, greed, confusion, failure to attain stages of development and instability in maintaining a state, cause mental distractions; these are the obstacles.

1.31 Pain, discomfort, body tremors, irregular breathing out and breathing in [sighing, gasping, panting] appear with a mental distraction.

1.32 The practice [is to be applied on] one principle [at a time], to prevent those [mental distractions].

1.33 Applying the feelings of friendliness, compassion, happiness, and indifference respectively to the happy, the suffering, the virtuous and the vicious calms the software in the brain [and heart].

1.34 Also [calming] by exhaling or retention of the breath.

1.35 Also by researching an item of attention [and] staying [with it] continuously, a fascination arises calming the input-output component (*manas*) of the brain software.

1.36 Also, the suffering is ended by bright inner light.

1.37 Also [by focusing on] a brain software user who is free from longing for sense objects.

1.38 Also [calming by] realizing the knowledge of dreaming and deep sleep.

1.39 Also by *dhyāna* on any proper, revered item.

1.40 Mastery of [*dhyāna*] [ranges from] the smallest to the biggest [items].

1.41 Attention (*samāpatti*) [means]: Just as a clear crystal takes on the color [of its environment], [brain software] with calmed thinking that rests on the perceiver, the perception process, or the perceived, takes on their qualities.

1.42 There [in *samāpatti*] mixed with [mental] speech, knowledge of its meaning, and imagination [*vikalpa*] [is] *savitarka* [gross] *samāpatti.*

1.43 Purified from memory, in its own form, as if empty, the complete goal appears. It defines *nirvitarka* [*samāpatti*].

1.44 Similarly, *savicāra* [*samāpatti*] and *nirvicāra* [*samāpatti*] are defined, [when applied to] the subtle perceived.

1.45 The measure of subtlety ends in the non-perceivable *prakṛti.*

1.46 Those [four] truly [are called] *samādhi* with seeds.

1.47 Skill [in] *nirvicāra* lets the highest SELF (*ātman*) clearly shine.

1.48 The intuitive knowledge within this [*nirvicāra samādhi*] contains truth.

1.49 Intuitive knowledge (*prajñā*) is different from [generally valid] authority, or inference [because *prajñā*] refers to specific facts.

1.50 The impression created through that [*nirvicāra* practice] stops other impressions.

1.51 With the halting even of those [impressions from *nirvicāra*] all [impressions] are calmed, which defines *nirbīja* [seedless] *samādhi.*

Chapter 2 – Removal of Ignorance

2.1 The urge for liberation, self-study of the *Veda* and attention to *Īśvara* are defined as the *yoga* of action.

2.2 The goal [of the *yoga* of action] is to achieve *samādhi* and to reduce the illusions (*kleśas*).

2.3 The illusions are ignorance, [limited] "I"-consciousness, longing, hate and the survival instinct.

2.4 Ignorance is the fertile ground of the other [four *kleśas*]; [all five are either] asleep, weak, interrupted or active.

2.5 Ignorance is seeing the impermanent as if eternal, the impure as if pure, suffering as if happiness, the non-SELF as if the SELF.

2.6 [Limited] "I"-consciousness [means mixing] the power of the seer [the unchanging SELF] and the power of the process of seeing [the intellectual activity] as if they were one SELF [one identity].

2.7 Pleasure leads to longing.

2.8 Suffering leads to hate.

2.9 The survival instinct is inherent, even in the wise [one].

2.10 Those weakened [illusions] must be dissolved at their cause.

2.11 *Dhyāna* removes the thinking processes of those [illusions].

2.12 The cause [of all objects] in the store of *karma* is illusion and [it] will be lived in the visible [present] or an invisible [future] life.

2.13 Due to an existing root [*kleśa*], that [store of *karma*] ripens as births, lives, and experiences.

2.14 The fruits of those [births, lives, and experiences] are pleasure and pain caused by merit and guilt.

2.15 Change, fear, *saṁskāras*, suffering, arising from the action patterns due to the battle of the [three] *guṇas* are to the discriminating (*vivekin*) nothing but suffering.

2.16 Future suffering [is to be] avoided.

2.17 The connection between the perceiver and the perceived is the cause [of the suffering and is] to be avoided.

2.18 [With the] striving [of the three *guṇas*] towards clarity, action, and steadiness, the perceived consists of the elements (*mahābhūtas*) and the senses for experience and liberation.

2.19 The states of the *guṇas* [are] special, general, structured (*liṇga*), measurable (*mātra*) and unstructured (*pradhāna*).

2.20 Although the perceiving power of the perceiver [*draṣṭṛ* = *puruṣa*] is pure, he notices thoughts.

2.21 The purpose of that [noticing of thoughts] actually is the perceivable SELF.

2.22 For him [the *yogi*], who has reached the goal, it [the goal] has finished, but not so for others [the unskilled] because of their commonality [of collective consciousness].

2.23 Due to the connection of the possession [thinking processes] with the owner [SELF], they are perceived [only] in the form of the possession.

2.24 The cause of that [connection] is ignorance.

2.25 By the disappearance of that [ignorance], the connection disappears. That ends in the unity of consciousness (*kaivalya*).

2.26 The method for liberation is uninterrupted correctly-discriminating cognition (*viveka khyāti*).

2.27 The seven stages of that [correctly-discriminating cognition] lead to the highest level of intuitive knowledge.

2.28 By the practice of the areas of *yoga*, with the reduction of impurity, knowledge radiates until correctly-discriminating cognition [is established in each corresponding area].

2.29 The eight areas of *yoga* are self-control (*yama*), rules of living (*niyama*), body postures (*āsana*), breathing techniques (*prāṇāyāma*), withdrawing the senses from the objects (*pratyāhāra*), focusing the brain software (*dhāraṇā*), meditation (*dhyāna*) and absolute silence (*samādhi*).

2.30 Nonviolence, truth, non-stealing, sexual and sensual abstinence, non-greediness [define] self-control.

2.31 The great rule of behavior [with relation to 2.30] means that they, [the self-controls,] are valid over the whole Earth and are unlimited by birth, place, time and convention.

2.32 The rules of living are attention to bodily purity, contentment, urge for liberation, self-study of the *Vedas*, and devotion to *Īśvara*.

2.33 Dubious [thinking] is removed by pondering over its opposite.

2.34 Dubious [thoughts] of violence etc. – whether to be carried out, incited, or allowed – having arisen from greed anger, or insanity, to a mild, medium, or intensive extent, result in unending suffering and ignorance. Therefore think of their opposite.

2.35 In the vicinity of someone established in total nonviolence [all] enmity disappears.

2.36 [When] established in truthfulness, actions have corresponding results.

2.37 [When] established in non-stealing, all wealth flows to him.

2.38 Established in sexual and sensual abstinence, he gains vitality.

2.39 Steadiness in non-greediness leads to the cognition of the circumstances of birth.

2.40 From bodily purification [there arises] a disinterest in the limbs of the body [the imperfection of the body] and in touching others.

2.41 [From that arise] the abilities of clarity, purity, contentment, purposefulness, mastery of the senses, and SELF-cognition.

2.42 Contentment creates the highest joy.

2.43 From the urge for liberation (*tapas*), impurity disappears [and] perfection of body and senses [arises].

2.44 From the self-study of the *Vedas* and Vedic literature [arises] a connection with the personally revered *devatā* (personification of infinity).

2.45 By attention to *Īśvara* perfection of *samādhi* [results].

2.46 *Āsana* is a stable and pleasant body posture.

2.47 [That body posture] results from relaxation of effort and attention (*samāpatti*) on infinity (*anantya*).

2.48 Due to those [*āsana*], opposites do not violate.

2.49 While remaining in that [in an *āsana* position], *prāṇāyāma* is the interruption of the motion of breathing out and breathing in.

2.50 The cessation [of air coming from] outside [after fully breathing in], cessation [of air coming from] inside [after fully breathing out], and holding the breath [intermediately] are measured as long and fine, depending on the place, time and number.

2.51 Regarding the outer and the inner phase, there is a fourth [*prāṇāyāma*].

2.52 Then [as a result of *prāṇāyāma*] the covering of the light disappears.

2.53 And [as a result of *prāṇāyāma* follows] the ability, to focus (*dhāraṇā*) the input-output component of the brain software (*manas*).

2.54 Withdrawing from its objects of perception the brain software (*citta*) takes on its own [unexcited] state, and the sense organs and organs of action imitate this. That is *pratyāhāra*.

2.55 By this [*pratyāhāra*], perfect mastery over the senses [is attained].

Chapter 3 – Extraordinary Abilities

3.1 Binding of [the total] brain software in one place is *dhāraṇā*.

3.2 There [bound to the place], the expansions of one same thought are defined as *dhyāna*.

3.3 In that way, just the total goal [of 3.1 and 3.2] appears in its own form, as if empty. That is *samādhi*.

3.4 The three [*dhāraṇā, dhyāna, samādhi*] in one place are *saṁyama*.

3.5 By mastering that [triad] the brilliance of wisdom (*prajñā*) radiates.

3.6 That [*saṁyama*] is applied in stages.

3.7 The three inner areas [*dhāraṇā, dhyāna, samādhi,* are more important] than the previous ones.

3.8 Those [three] areas [are] even less important than the seedless (*nirbīja samādhi*).

3.9 The calming transformation is that which occurs when the distracting *saṁskāras* are calmed while [simultaneously] *saṁskāras* of calming appear. Then the brain software is calmed for a moment.

3.10 In that [calming transformation], from the *saṁskāra* [of calming, follows] a quiet flowing [of the brain software].

3.11 [Then follows] the *samādhi* transformation, in which the scattered state of the brain software disappears, and its one-pointed focus grows.

3.12 Then follows the one-pointed transformation [which means that] repeatedly a new thought arises in the brain software similar [to the thought] previously vanished.

3.13 By this [one-pointed transformation], the transformations of tasks, time qualities, and states of elements and sense and organs of action are explained.

3.14 The material (*dharmin*) adapts to the finished, active and indeterminable tasks (*dharma*).

3.15 The difference in the [three natural] sequences [of evolution] is the reason for the difference in the transformations.

3.16 By *saṁyama* on the three transformations [of the task, time phase, and state, there arises] knowledge about past and future.

3.17 From the mutual projections of sound sequences, meanings and thoughts [there arises] confusion. By *saṁyama* on the difference of those [three] comes the knowledge of the utterances of all beings.

3.18 By intuitive perception of an impression (*saṁskāra*) [one gains] knowledge of previous lives.

3.19 [By intuitive perception, *saṁyama* on] the thought of another, [one gains] knowledge of [the other's] brain software.

3.20 But not about the state of consciousness, that is connected to that thought, because it is not a fitting item for this *saṁyama*.

3.21 By *saṁyama* on the contour of the body, the possibility of being seen by beings is suppressed. Disconnected from the light of the eyes [of the observer, the body of the *yogi*] becomes invisible.

3.22 [*Karma* becomes] either carried out or not carried out. By *saṁyama* on that *karma* or on omens [there arises] foreknowledge of one's death.

3.23 By *saṁyama* on friendliness, etc., these powers [increase].

3.24 By *saṁyama* on the strengths, [for example] of an elephant, etc., [bodily] strengths [arise accordingly].

3.25 By attention [by *saṁyama*] on the inner light of anything, [there arises] knowledge about the subtle, hidden and remote.

3.26 By *saṁyama* on the Sun, knowledge about the cosmic regions [arises].

3.27 [By *saṁyama*] on the Moon [there arises] knowledge of the arrangement of the stars.

3.28 [By *saṁyama*] on the Pole Star [arises] knowledge about the movement of those [arrangements of stars and planets].

3.29 [By *saṁyama*] on the navel wheel (*nābhi cakra*) [arises] knowledge of the structures of the body.

3.30 [By *saṁyama*] on the throat pit, hunger and thirst disappear.

3.31 [By *saṁyama*] on the tortoise energy channel [arises] steadiness.

3.32 [By *saṁyama*] on the brightness in the top of the head [arises] vision of the perfect beings.

3.33 Or from intuition [the cognition] of everything.

3.34 [By *saṁyama*] on the heart one cognizes the brain software.

3.35 Experience is a thought that does not distinguish between [*buddhi-*] *sattva* and *puruṣa*, although they are absolutely distinct. By *saṁyama* on that [*buddhi-sattva*] which is there for the purpose of the highest, and on that which is there for its own purpose [*puruṣa*], arises knowledge of *puruṣa*.

3.36 [*Saṁyama*] there, [on the knowledge of *puruṣa*] increases intuition, [then] hearing, feeling, seeing, tasting and knowledge of events.

3.37 Those [intuition, etc. of *sūtra* 3.36, while] overshadowing [*nirvicāra*] in *samādhi* [appear as] perfections in the excited [brain software].

3.38 By [*saṁyama* on] the loosening of the cause of bondage, and knowing the playground [of another body and its environment], the brain software can remotely control other bodies.

3.39 By mastering [*saṁyama*] the upward moving live stream [*udāna*] [the *yogi* walks] untouched on water, swamps, thorns, etc., and when dying, takes the upward path.

3.40 By mastering [*saṁyama*] of the middle live stream, in the belly [*samāna*] there comes about a blazing light.

3.41 By *saṁyama* on the intimate connection between space (*ākāśa*) and hearing [arises] divine hearing.

3.42 By *saṁyama* on the intimate connection between the body (*kāya*) and space (*ākāśa*), and attention (*samāpatti*) on the lightness of cotton fiber, space goes.

3.43 The "great bodiless" is a mental process (*vṛtti*) outside of the body and not [merely] imagined. From this, the covering of the light diminishes.

3.44 By *saṁyama* on their physical form, their essential nature, their subtle form, their inheritance and their purposefulness, the [five] elements are controlled.

3.45 From that [mastery of the elements, eight abilities] arise [for example] becoming small, etc., and the perfection of the body, its tasks, and its protection.

3.46 A perfect body has a beautiful form, [insurmountable] strength and the hardness of a diamond.

3.47 By *saṁyama* on the [process of] perception [of the senses], their essential nature, their limited "I"-consciousness, their inheritance and their purposefulness, the senses are controlled.

3.48 From that [mastery of the senses] and by mastering [*saṁyama* on] *pradhāna*, arise [the abilities to travel] with the speed of thought, to exist without bodily organs, and to control nature.

3.49 By the complete cognition that *buddhi-sattva* and *puruṣa* are distinct, [the *yogi*] has power over all that exists and omniscience.

3.50 When, from serenity towards even those [omnipotence and omniscience] the seeds of impurities are destroyed, liberation (*kaivalya*) [remains].

3.51 [In the case of] invitations by the rulers of heavenly realms, one should neither get involved with them nor show pride [smiling] because, from that, unwanted results would again follow.

3.52 By *saṁyama* on the now and its two sequences of time phases comes knowledge born from discrimination.

3.53 From that [knowledge of *sūtra* 3.52] comes the discrimination between two things that are apparently the same, unidentifiable by class, quality or place.

3.54 And also in that way knowledge is born from the discrimination between all that is intuitively perceived in the starry skies and the totality of all at all times.

3.55 When *buddhi-sattva* is as pure as *puruṣa* then the absolute unity (*brahman*-consciousness, *kaivalya*) is there. So it is.

Chapter 4 – Liberation

4.1 *Siddhis* (extraordinary abilities) arise from *samādhi* directly, [or] from birth, [or] by herbs, [or] *mantras*, [or] the urge for liberation.

4.2 From an excess of *prakṛti* [comes] the transformation into a related form of existence [rebirth].

4.3 The undirected-ness of the *prakṛtis* [gets] a direction, like a farmer uses a dam [for irrigation] but consequently opens it up.

4.4 Brain software [objects] are created exclusively from a [limited] "I"-consciousness (*asmitā*).

4.5 The differences in the appearance of many [*cittas*] are caused by one [generating, controlling] *citta*.

4.6 Of those [five methods of accomplishing *siddhis*], [only] the method *dhyāna* creates no store [of *karma*].

4.7 The action of a *yogi* [brain software version 7+] is neither white nor black. For others, it is threefold [white, black, mixed].

4.8 Resulting from those [three kinds of *karma*] only those groups of thinking patterns (*vāsanās*), matching the situation, manifest.

4.9 [The pairs of] memories (*smṛtis*) and impressions (*saṁskāras*) may be interrupted by birth, place or time. However, they follow a sequence in a [certain] format.

4.10 And the lack of a beginning of those [*vāsanās*] [we conclude, is from the] eternal desire to live.

4.11 In the absence of the collected causes, results, container [brain software] and supports [things], those [*vāsanās*] disappear.

4.12 Past and future are [subtle] forms of the present, which lead, according to their path, to various tasks.

4.13 Those [three distinct time phases] have the qualities [of being] manifest or subtle.

4.14 From the transformation in unity (*ekatva*) [results] the reality of the manifest (*vastu*).

4.15 Given the sameness of the manifest, any difference between two *cittas* gives rise to alternative paths.

4.16 A manifest [thing] also is not the product of a single brain software, [because] what could it be without the attention [of that brain software]?

4.17 According to the coloring of the brain software by that [manifest thing], the manifest [thing] is known or unknown.

4.18 The thinking processes (*vṛttis*) are always known to their Lord [*puruṣa*] due to the non-variability of *puruṣa*.

4.19 That [brain software] does not radiate on its own [because] it is something observed.

4.20 And one simultaneous meeting [of *puruṣa* and *citta*] confirms both [as separate entities].

4.21 The brain software is observed internally by its main component, and a continued [observation] by [another] main component [would lead to] a confusion of memory.

4.22 Due to pure consciousness being in unrestricted lockstep with the content of that [brain software perceived by its main component] the main component falsely assumes [this pure consciousness] to be its own.

4.23 Brain software, influenced by the perceiver [*puruṣa*] and the perceived, has all goals.

4.24 Although that [brain software] is tainted by countless *vāsanās*, it has another purpose caused by its relationship [of being the servant of *puruṣa*].

4.25 For those who know the difference [between *buddhi* and *puruṣa*], contemplation of SELF-realization ends.

4.26 Then, the brain software with deeply discriminating cognition tends towards unity.

4.27 At the time of interruption of that [deep discrimination], intermediate thoughts [arise] from *saṁskāras*.

4.28 The ending of these [thoughts from *saṁskāras*] [happens] as explained for the illusions [*kleśas*].

4.29 One who does not even expect anything from his meditation, by applying correctly-discriminating cognition [reaches] a *samādhi* with the name "rain cloud of *dharma*."

4.30 From that [follows] the disappearance of the illusions (*kleśas*) and the *karma*.

4.31 Then, freed from all veils and impurities, in the infinity of knowledge only a tiny bit of ignorance remains.

4.32 With that [knowledge of the difference and the rain cloud of *dharma*], the *guṇas* have achieved their goals, and their continuous transformation has ended.

4.33 The transformation of sequentially following moments has ended and [then] their flow is recognized.

4.34 The *guṇas*, having returned to their original state, serve no [further] purpose for *puruṣa*, and unity consciousness has settled in its own nature. That is the power of consciousness – and so it is.

B - Glossary

abhiniveśa, m.	Survival instinct
adharma, m.	Guilt, sin, injustice, vice, vicious thinking pattern
āgama, m.	Knowledge of an authority
agni, m.	Fire, god of fire, digestive fire, energy
aham	I, individual self
ākāśa, m.n.	Space
ākāśa-Chronik	Information store in space
ānanda, m.	Absolute bliss
ananta, n.	Unboundedness
anantya, n.	Infinity, eternity
antarīkṣa, n.	World of stars, region between heaven and Earth
anumāna, n.	Inference
apāna, m.	Down going breath flow
asamprajñāta samādhi, m.	*Samādhi* without thinking processes, without excitation, idle mode of the brain software, transcendental consciousness (brain software version 4), absolute silence without attention to anything
āsana, n.	Body posture, sitting posture without effort with attention to infinity
asmitā, f.	Ego, limited "I"-consciousness; they ego thinks: "I do this," "I see," "I feel," "I remember," "I decide," etc.
asura, m.	Demon, natural law of fermionic behavior
ātman, m.	SELF (user of the brain software), universal SELF
auṁ	Characteristic sound of the best ruler, subtlest pattern of the cosmic software
avasthā, f.	State, situation
avatāra, m.	An incarnation of the cosmic software that shows with a body, nervous system and brain software

B - Glossary

āvatya, m.	Name of a Vedic seer
avīci, m.	Hell; an area of space, where predominantly thermionic natural laws prevail
avidyā, f.	Ignorance (class of malware)
āyus, n.	Life-force, long life
bāhya-vṛtti, f.	Outward directed mental process
bhakti, f.	Devotion
bhāvita, Adj.	Alive; a thing maintained because it is continuously called to life
bhoga, m.	Experience, pleasure
bhūta, n.	Being; demon, disease; a fermionic tendency in the body
bīja, n.	Seed, seed grain
brahmā, m.	World creator; the method of the cosmic software that leads to the creation of a universe
brahmacarya, n.	Celibacy, abstinence
brahman, m.	All comprehensive, all comprehensive totality
brahman-Bewusstsein	Brain software version 8, the consciousness of infinitely expanded unity
buddhi, f.	Intellect, main component of the brain software
buddhi-sattva, n.	Most abstract and most influential level of the brain software
buddhi-indriya, n.	Sensory and knowledge organs
chandas, n.	The perceived, meter (of a verse)
cit, f.	Pure consciousness, perceiver, knower, pure intelligence
cit-ātman, m.	Consciousness quality of the SELF
citi-śakti, f.	Power of pure consciousness
citta, n.	Brain software
darśana, n.	Sight, appearance, vision

Devanāgarī	Script of *saṁskṛt*
deva, m.	Highest personified expression of natural law, software component of the universe-computer
devatā, f.	Divine being, the process of perception
Devī, f.	Divine mother, she is *ātman* and *pradhāna*, SELF and finest level of nature
dhāraṇā, f.	Focusing the thoughts to one place
dharma, m.	Virtue, righteousness, duty, justice, virtuous thinking pattern, task, special form of the basic material (*dharmin*)
dharmin, m.	Material at the basis of *dharma*
dhruva, m.	Pole Star
dhyāna, n.	Meditation, extending the attention in one place or item
doṣa, m.	Defect, disorder, fault
dveṣa, m.	Hate
Durgā, f.	The "invincible," a form of *Devī*
ekatva, n.	*Brahman*-consciousness, unlimited unity
ekāgratā, f.	One-pointed thinking, undivided attention, unity consciousness
ekatāna, m. *ekatāna-ta, m.*	The continued direction of attention to one place; extending the flow of similar thoughts; *ekatānata* during the *dhyāna* means holding the attention to one place or one item, without allowing any distracting thoughts – but without effort. *-ta* = -ness
ekendriya, Adj.	Third stage of serenity: the desire, no longer to experience with the senses, but rather with the brain software
FPGA Chip	Field Programmable Gate Array Chip
gagana, n.	Heaven: the range of the universe between 10^{-19} m to 10^{-35} m

B - Glossary

gandha, m.	Smell
gaṇeśa, m.	*Deva* with the elephants head, remover of obstacles, ruler over natural laws and heavenly bodies, one of the main methods of the software of the universe-computer
go, f.	Cow
graha, m.	Movable heavenly bodies
guṇa, m.	Natural tendency, the three *guṇas* are *sattva, rajas, tamas*
indriya, n.	Sense or action organ
indriyas, n.	The five sense and organs of action: Hearing, touch, sight, taste, smell, and speech organ, hands, feet, reproductive organs, excretion organs
Īśvara, m.	The best ruler, source of the highest and best knowledge, the one cosmic intelligence, *īś* = ruler, *vara* = the best, the universe-computer
jambū, f.n.	Rose Apple (-tree)
japa, m.	Repeating, murmuring
jāti, f.	Birth, specific family, family member
jīvan-mukti, m.	Liberated while living
jñāna, n.	Comprehensive knowledge, all levels of knowledge
jyotiṣa, n.	Vedic astrology
kaivalya, n.	Unity, absolute freedom, final liberation
karman, n.	Activity, action, result of action, destiny
karmāśaya, m.	*Karma*-store
karmendriyas, n.	The five organs of action: speech organ, hands, feet, reproductive organs, excretion organs
kāya, m.	Body
khyāti, f.	Cognition, sight, vision
viṣaya, m.	Store, field, content, area

kleśa, m.	Illusion; the five *kleśas* are ignorance, ego, longing, hate, and survival instinct
kriya yoga, m.	Striving for liberation, self-study of the Vedas, attention on *Īśvara*
kumāra, m.	Boy, son, prince, child
līlā, f.	Cosmic game, game, sports
liṅga, n.	Sign, mark, characteristic, structure
liṅga mātra = mahat	Mathematical rules of natural laws, cosmic intellect
mahābhūta, n.	The five gross elements space, air, fire/light, water, earth; they correspond to the aggregate states spatial, gaseous, plasmatic, fluid, solid
mahat, n.	The great principle
manas, n.	Perception-action-processing, input-output control, controls sensory and organs of action
mandākinī, f.	River Ganges, River in heaven, heavenly Ganges
mātrā, f.	Measure, unit, measure unit, time unit
nāman, n.	Name, personal Name
nidrā, f.	Deep sleep
nirbīja, Adj.	Seedless; *samādhi* without excitation
nirodha, m.	Calming, stopping, obstructing, subduing
nirvicāra, Adj.	Nothing to reflect, nothing to ponder
nirvicāra samādhi, m.	Intuitive knowledge, state of pure knowledge, beyond the subtle
nirvitarka, Adj.	Without consideration, without (gross) thoughts
nirvitarka samādhi	Without speech comprehension
niyama, m.	Living rule, instruction, guideline rule
nyāya, m.	Philosophy of *Gautama*, science of Logic, means of gaining correct knowledge
Pāṇḍava, m.	Son of *Pandu*; there were five *Pāṇḍavas*
pāda, m.	Chapter, stage

pāpa, n.	Vice, sin, evil, misdeed, crime, calamity
paramātman, m.	The highest SELF
parameṣṭhin, Adj.	Main, highest
parameśvara, m.	The highest being, the highest law, the universe-computer
pariṇāma, m.	Transformation, metamorphosis, evolution, sequence
Patañjali	Author of the *yoga sūtras*
Pradhāna	*Guṇas* in their ground state in *savicāra*, subtlest state of nature
prajāpati, m.	Creator and ruler of the local Galaxy cluster chain; one of the software methods of the universe-computer
prajñā, f.	Intuitive knowledge, wisdom, SELF-referral, intuitive knowledge
prakṛti, f.	Nature; primordial matter, at the basis of the universe; it is without forms, unlimited, and is eternal
prakṛtilayas, m.	Nature beings, absorbed in nature
pramāṇa, n.	Learned knowledge, book and experiential knowledge, knowledge from authorities
prāṇa. m.	Life energy, upload going breath flow, exhaling, breath in general
praṇava, m.f.	Ancient and mighty, sound characteristics, for example, *auṁ*
prāṇāyāma, m.	Breathing practices, interruption of breathing in and breathing out
prārabdha, Adj.	Begun, undertaken
prārabdha karma	Impressions of previous actions that have again been activated
pratibhā, f.	Perfect intuition, creativity, radiant
pratisaṁvedin, Adj.	The silent observer of the intellect (*buddhi*)
pratyāhāra, m.	Withdrawal of the senses from items, control of the senses

pratyakṣa, n.	Direct perception, observation
pratyaya, m.	Thought
puṇya, n.	Merit, good deed
pūraka, m.	Breathing in, filling the lungs
purāṇa, n.	Ancient, Vedic Scriptures with instructional stories and legends
puruṣa, m.	Silence SELF, user, and observer of the brain software, eternal silence of pure consciousness, uninvolved observer
rāga, m.	Passion, longing, redness, melody
rajas, n.	One of the three *guṇas*, the tendency towards movement and activity
rasa, m.	Taste
recaka, m.	Breathing out, emptying the lungs
ṛṣi, m.	Seer, perceiver
rūpa, n.	Form, appearance
śabda, m.	Speech, voice
sādhana, n.	The six milestones of the *yoga*-practice: trust, strength, memory, *saṁprajñāta samādhi*, intuitive knowledge (*prajñā*) and *asaṁprajñāta samādhi*
śakti, f.	Power, energy, ability, strength
śakti vāda	The power of words
samādhi, m.	Ground state of absolute silence – can be together with thoughts, state of total balance, a state "as if empty" – without thoughts, idle mode of the brain software
samāna, m.	Balancing, homogeneous, movement of the digestion processes, one of the five *prāṇas*
samāpatti, f.	Attention, coming together
saṁhitā, f.	Unification, connection; totality of *ṛṣi* (perceiver), *devatā* (perception process) und *chandas* (perceived)

B - Glossary

Śaṁkara	Indian master and philosopher, founder of *Advaita*, around 800 A.D.
saṁskāra, m.	Stored mental impression, influences processes of thinking and action, as correspondence in the nervous system
saṁskṛta, n.	The language *saṁskṛt*
samyagdarśana, n.	Correct perception, insight
samyagdarśin, m.	The one with correct sight
saṁyama, m.	*Dhāraṇā, dhyāna, samādhi* applied to one place or item
saṁyoga, m.	A connection between the perceiver and the perceived
sandhi, m.	Sound adaption of the ending and beginning letters between words or syllables
śarīra, n.	Body of a person
sarva, Adj.	Every, each, all
sat, Adj.	Eternal, true, unchanging
sattva, n.	One of the three *guṇas:* the tendency towards clarity and cognition
satya, n.	Truth, truthfulness
savicāra, Adj.	With subtle thoughts, subtle perceived
savicāra samādhi, m.	State of silence, accompanied with subtle thoughts
savitarka, Adj.	With logical thinking or argumentation, with speech understanding
savitarka samādhi, m.	State of silence accompanied by logical thinking, internal speaking
siddhi, f.	Extraordinary ability, success
siddha, m.	Expert, master of extraordinary abilities
smṛti, f.	Remembrance, memory
soma, m.	Soma Plant, Moon, nectar, software method of the universe-computer that appears as virtual fluctuations of space-time
sparśa, m.	Sense of touch

sukha, n.	Joy, delight, pleasure
sūkta, n.	Vedic hymn
śūnya, Adj.	Empty, absent, zero, follow, transparent, unfathomable
suṣupta, n.	Deep sleep
sūtra, n.	Threat, formula, proposition, instruction, rule
svapna, m.	Dreaming state
śvāsa, m.	Heavy breathing, sighing, fizzling, growling
tamas, n.	One of the three *guṇas:* the tendency towards stability and persistence
tāna, m.	Extended, held tone, monotonous sound when reciting, extension
tanmātra, n.	Subtle element, for example, electromagnetic field; *tanmātras* correspond to the five physical fields not perceivable by the sensory organs (sound, touch, form, taste, smell)
tapa, m.	Heat, warmth
tapas, n.	Striving for liberation
tāraka, n.	Star, meteor
udāna, m.	One of the five *prāṇas*: upward going live stream; beginning from the feet flowing to the top of the head
upakrama, m.	Approach of the *yoga*-practices; there are three kinds: lazy, medium, intensive
upaśama, m.	Resting of the brain software, silence, ending
upāya, m.	Remedy, relief, healing method
ūrdhvareta, Adj.	Celibacy, chastity, holding back the semen
vāda, m.	Sound, words, speech, statement
vairāgya, n.	Serenity, equanimity
varga, m.	Category, class, section, group
vāsanā, f,	Thinking pattern; ripens in the form of virtue or vice
vaśīkāra, Adj.	Mastery of serenity

vāyu, m.	Wind, air, movement, momentum, god of the wind
vibhūti, f.	Extraordinary ability
vicāra, m.	Subtle thinking beyond speech; in abstract forms, colors, and sounds
videha, Adj.	Bodiless
vidyā, f.	Knowledge, science, philosophy
vikalpa, m.	Imagination (thinking processes), based on words
viparyaya, m.	Misunderstanding, fault
virāma, m.	Ending, end, halting
virāma-pratyaya	Thought of halting
viveka, m.	Correct discrimination
viveka khyāti	Correctly-discriminating cognition
vivekin, Adj.	Correctly discriminating, wise
vṛtti, f.	Thinking process; the five thinking processes are *pramāṇa* (correct knowledge), *viparyaya* (misunderstanding), *vikalpa* (imagination), *nidrā* (deep sleep), *smṛti* (memory)
Vyāsa, m.	Vedic master; commentator of the *yoga sūtras*; was living around 3000 BC
vyatikrānta, n.	A stage of serenity: Thought of having achieved the non-longing in some things, and not in others
yajña, m.	Ceremony, offering, ritual
yama, m.	Moral rule, self-control
yoga, m.	Perfection of the brain software, unification, connection
yoga-state	Calming of suffering-inducing thinking processes

C - Simulation of Malware in the Brain

The following code in the language MATLAB simulates the illusion classes, their inheritance, the generation of *saṁskāras*, the objects (instances) of the classes, activation of the objects, researching the data of *saṁskāras*, and, finally, the deletion of the class ignorance.

```
%-----------------------------------------------------------------------
% filename: ignorance.m

classdef ignorance
  %% the basic klesha class
  properties
    state;
    intensity;
    place;
    time;
    situation;
    livingBeing;
  end
  methods
    % constructor
    function obj = ignorance (st,inten,plac,tim,sit,life)
      obj.state = st;
      obj.intensity = inten;
      obj.place = plac;
      obj.time = tim;
      obj.situation = sit;
      obj.livingBeing = life;
    end
    function correctKnowledge (obj)
      % correct thought
      fprintf('Thought of correct knowledge of class %s \n',class(obj));
    end
    function misunderstanding (obj)
      % misunderstanding thought
      fprintf('Thought of misunderstanding of class %s \n',class(obj));
    end
    function imagination (obj)
      % imagining thought
      fprintf('Thought of imagination of class %s \n',class(obj));
    end
    function deepSleep (obj)
      % deep sleep thought of non-existence
      fprintf('Thought of deep sleep of class %s \n',class(obj));
    end
    function memory (obj)
```

```
      % remembering thought
      fprintf('Thought of remembering of class %s \n',class(obj));
    end
  end
end

%---------------------------------------------------------------------
% filename: ego.m

classdef ego < ignorance
  %% a klesha class inherited from the class ignorance
  methods
    % constructor
    function obj = ego (st,inten,plac,tim,sit,life)
      obj@ignorance (st,inten,plac,tim,sit,life)
    end
  end
end

%---------------------------------------------------------------------
% filename: longing.m

classdef longing < ignorance
  %% a klesha class inherited from the class ignorance
  methods
    % constructor
    function obj = longing (st,inten,plac,tim,sit,life)
      obj@ignorance (st,inten,plac,tim,sit,life)
    end
  end
end

%---------------------------------------------------------------------
% filename: hate.m

classdef hate < ignorance
  %% a klesha class inherited from the class ignorance
  methods
    % constructor
    function obj = hate (st,inten,plac,tim,sit,life)
      obj@ignorance (st,inten,plac,tim,sit,life)
    end
  end
end

%---------------------------------------------------------------------
% filename: survivalInstinct.m

classdef survivalInstinct < ignorance
  %% a klesha class inherited from the class ignorance
  methods
    % constructor
    function obj = survivalInstinct (st,inten,plac,tim,sit,life)
      obj@ignorance (st,inten,plac,tim,sit,life)
    end
```

```
  end
end

%-----------------------------------------------------------------------------
% filename: samskaraCreation.m

%% Generation of Samskara Object
% Works with an existing class ignorance (YS 2.12)
% Example of generating a samskara object of class longing
% Millions of samskaras can exist with living beings
try
  EatingIcecream = longing  ('active',...
                             0.85,...
                             'at home with mother',...
                             '4 years 3 months old',...
                             'first icecream tasted very good',...
                             'human')
  % can be continued for any amount of samskaras
  % happens continuously in life as long as klesha classes exist
catch
  % catch error message if class ignorance is deleted
  % nothing to do because class ignorance does not exist
  % no samskare objects are generated
end
%% Generates following output:

% Before applying deleteIgnorance:
% EatingIcecream =
%   longing with properties:
%
%           state: 'active'
%        intnsity: 0.850000000000000
%           place: 'at home with mother'
%            time: '4 years 3 months old'
%       situation: 'first icecream tasted very good'
%     livingBeing: 'human'

% After applying deleteIgnorance:
% >> no output <<

%-----------------------------------------------------------------------------
% filename: activateSamskaraThinkingPattern.m

%% Activation of two thinking patterns
% functions only with existing class ignorance (YS 2.13)
try
  % the command 'try' helps to catch faults,
  % corresponding to an attitude of serenity (vairagya).
  EatingIcecream.misunderstanding
  EatingIcecream.memory
catch
  % catch the error message with a non-existent class ignorance
  % nothing to do because class ignorance does not exist
end
%% generates the following output:
```

```
% Before applying deleteIgnorance:
% Thought of misunderstanding of class longing
% Thought of remembering of class longing

% After applying deleteIgnorance:
% >> no output <<

%-----------------------------------------------------------------------
% filename: samskaraResearchPreviousLives.m

%% Research of the data in previous samsakaras
% Functions as long as samskara EatingIcecream exists. (YS 3.18)
% Independent of whether or not the klesha class ignorance is deleted.
% By erasing the klesha class the data remain,
% but the methods are lost.
EatingIcecream.intensity
EatingIcecream.place
EatingIcecream.time
EatingIcecream.situation
EatingIcecream.livingBeing

%% generates the following output:
% samskaraResearchPreviousLives
% ans = 0.850000000000000
% ans = at home with mother
% ans = 4 years 3 months old
% ans = first icecream tasted very good
% ans = human

%-----------------------------------------------------------------------
% filename: deleteIgnorance.m

%% Deleting ignorance by deleting the class definition
% (YS 4.11, 4.30)
try
  % the command 'try' helps to catch faults,
  % corresponding to an attitude of serenity (vairagya).
  delete ignorance.m
catch
  % catch the error message with non-existing class ignorance.
  % Nothing to do because class ignorance does not exist.
  % ignorance has been erased already.
End

%-----------------------------------------------------------------------
Practical hint:
Store each section in a separate file.
Before testing the code on MATLAB, make a copy of the file ignorance.m,
because this file will be really erased and thus it can be restored again.
```

www.ingramcontent.com/pod-product-compliance
Lightning Source LLC
Chambersburg PA
CBHW060304030426
42336CB00011B/931
* 9 7 8 0 9 9 5 5 9 6 1 1 5 *